THIRD EDITION

Master the Boards USMLE® Step 3

Other USMLE Titles by Conrad Fischer

Books

Master the Boards USMLE® Step 2 CK

Master the Wards:
Survive IM Clerkship & Ace the Shelf

Master the Boards Internal Medicine

Master the Boards USMLE® Medical Ethics

Flashcards

USMLE® Step 1 Pharmacology Flashcards

USMLE® Diagnostic Test Flashcards:
The 200 Questions You Need to Know for the Exam for Steps 2 & 3

USMLE® Examination Flashcards:
The 200 "Most Likely Diagnosis" Questions You Will See on the Exam for Steps 2 & 3

USMLE® Physical Findings Flashcards:
The 200 Questions You're Most Likely to See on the Exam

Online

Dr. Conrad Fischer's Comprehensive Cases

USMLE® Step 3 Qbank

Other Kaplan USMLE Titles

medEssentials for the USMLE® Step 1

USMLE® Step 1 Qbook

USMLE® Step 2 CK Qbook

USMLE® Step 2 CS: Core Cases

Dr. Pestana's Surgery Notes: Top 180 Vignettes for the Surgical Wards

USMLE® Steps 2 and 3 in Your Pocket

USMLE® Step 3 Qbook

THIRD EDITION

Master the Boards USMLE® Step 3

Conrad Fischer, MD

and Sonia Reichert, MD

Obstetrics, Gynecology, and Pediatrics sections edited by Elizabeth August
Surgery and Psychiatry sections edited by Niket Sonpal
All images courtesy of Conrad Fischer, MD

Published by Kaplan Publishing, a division of Kaplan, Inc.
395 Hudson Street
New York, NY 10014

Printed in the United States of America

10 9 8 7 6 5 4 3 2

ISBN-13: 978-1-61865-375-8

Dedication

To the Reader,

This book represents the consolidation of 25 years in the classroom teaching Step 3. You can be fully confident that you have, in one volume **EVERYTHING** you need to do well on Step 3.

To Edmund Bourke, MD,

My "Fearless Leader," teacher, and protector these many years. Dr. Bourke represents the best compilation of a "Gentleman Scholar," lifelong student, and teacher. A wise counselor and loyal friend. I dedicate this book to a "man for all seasons" whose kindness spills over onto all who are in contact with him. "Oh, for a muse of fire!"

Conrad Fischer, MD

To Mum,

I dedicate this book to you, a woman who has always exemplified dedication, determination, strength, and above all, a bright spirit that has been the guiding light for many people. You taught me to have a vision, dream big, and to always reach for the farthest and brightest star. You have shown me that dreams have no limits and boundaries. I will be eternally grateful for your love and support.

Sonia Reichert, MD

To my mom and dad,

Without whose support and sacrifice I would not be where I am today.

Niket Sonpal, MD

For Test Changes or Late-Breaking Developments

kaptest.com/publishing

The material in this book is up-to-date at the time of publication. However, the Federation of State Medical Boards (FSMB) and the National Board of Medical Examiners (NBME) may have instituted changes in the test after this book was published. Be sure to carefully read the materials you receive when you register for the test. If there are any important late-breaking developments—or any changes or corrections to the Kaplan test preparation materials in this book—we will post that information online at *kaptest.com/publishing.*

Table of Contents

Acknowledgments

The author wishes to recognize the excellent support of Dr. Vladimir Gottlieb, MD, Vice Chair of Medicine at Brookdale, and the administrative and emotional support of Ms. Juliette Akal.

Section Editors

Cardiology: Hal Chadow, MD, Chief of Cardiology, Brookdale University Medical Center; Andrei Bandarchuk, MD

Endocrinology: Debabrata Sen, MD; Chris Paras, MD

Pulmonary: Sabu Varghese, MD

Ethics: Michael Farca

Rheumatology: Debabrata Sen, MD; Lawrence Bernstein, MD

Hematology: Vladimir Gotlieb, MD; Hamza Minhas, MD

Infectious Diseases: Farshad Bagheri, MD; Richard Cofsky, MD

Gastroenterology: Anjula Gandhi, MD

Neurology: Arthur Kay, MD

Nephrology: Debabrata Sen, MD

Oncology: Vladimir Gotlieb, MD: Hamza Minhas, MD

Preventive Medicine: Neeraj Abrol, MD; Herman Lebovitch, MD

Surgery: Sunil Abrol, MD; Richard Fogler, MD

Pediatrics: Sherry Sakowitz, MD

Psychiatry: Sanila Rehmatullah, MD

Emergency Medicine: Jonathan Rose, MD

Contributors

Mark Nolan Hill, MD; Adil Farooqui, MD

About the Authors

Conrad Fischer, MD, is director of the residency program at Brookdale University Hospital and Medical Center in New York City. Dr. Fischer is associate professor of physiology, pharmacology, and medicine at Touro College of Osteopathic Medicine in New York City.

Sonia E. Reichert, MD, is former director of curriculum for Kaplan Medical and is currently a practicing hematologist and oncologist in northern California. She is the director of clinical research for the greater Sacramento region at Dignity Health and the Dignity Health Research Institute. Dr. Reichert is a regular participant at National Board conferences and has years of experience in the creation of educational materials for physicians.

Niket Sonpal, MD, is former chief resident at Lenox Hill Hospital–North Shore–LIJ Health System (2013–2014) and assistant clinical professor of medicine at both Touro College of Osteopathic Medicine and St. Georges University School of Medicine. He is a fellow in gastroenterology and co-author of the best-selling review books *Master the Boards: USMLE® Step 2 CK* and *Master the Boards: Internal Medicine.* Dr. Sonpal teaches American Board of Internal Medicine Review.

Elizabeth August, MD, is chief medical officer of Bergen County for Riverside Medical and Pediatric Group and former chief resident at Hoboken University Medical Center–NY Medical College (2012–2013). She is co-author of the best-selling review book *Master the Boards: USMLE Step 2 CK.*

Introduction

About the Step 3 Exam

The USMLE Step 3 is the last in a series of 3 USMLE examinations that all physicians applying for a license to practice medicine in the United States are required to pass. After successfully completing the 3 steps of the USMLE, a physician is eligible to practice medicine in an independent, unsupervised setting (some period of U.S. postgraduate training is also required).

This test is not merely a more advanced and detailed version of the Step 2 CK or CS exams. Understanding this concept is key to this challenging exam. Step 3 tests whether a physician not only can assimilate data and diagnose clinical conditions but also has acquired the ability to make clinical decisions about patient management in a way that ensures appropriate management in an unsupervised setting. In addition, Step 3 will test your understanding of basic science correlations.

How can the Step 3 test all first-year interns if they are working in such varied subspecialty settings? The same concepts that medicine house-officers learn about managing a diabetic with heart failure can be equally applied to the postsurgical patient with heart failure.

How Is Step 3 Different?

Unlike the Step 2 exams, which emphasize diagnosis of medical conditions, Step 3 evaluates your ability to evaluate the severity of a patient's condition and discern the most appropriate clinical management based on the presenting scenario. This assessment of your *clinical judgment* distinguishes Step 3 from Step 2. In Step 3, you are required to think beyond the diagnosis (which is often implicit in the question itself) and make decisions in management. The cases presented will include options that may all appear appropriate; however, for the presented situation, there is only ever one correct answer. Your interpretation of laboratory data, imaging, and elements of the presenting history and physical examination will assist you in selecting the correct management.

Clinical Encounter Frames

Multiple-choice and case-simulation questions are presented in one of three *clinical encounter frames:* initial care, continuing care, and urgent care. The encounter frame determines the amount of history, as well as clinical and laboratory test results, that are available to you. More importantly, the encounter frame influences how you'll proceed with management. For example, a longstanding patient with a history of repeated hospitalizations for asthma who presents with shortness of breath would be approached differently than if she were presenting for the first time to a clinic complaining of periodic dyspnea or if she presented to the emergency department with an acute asthma attack. The majority of test items (50 to 60 percent) in Step 3 involve the management of continuing-care patients. In the continuing-care setting, you are tested on your ability to recognize new problems in an existing condition, assess severity, establish prognosis, monitor therapy, and perform long-term management.

Clinical Settings

There are 3 clinical settings in Step 3: office/health center, inpatient facility, and the emergency department. As with the encounter frame, knowing the clinical setting influences your management decisions. As will be discussed in the "Examination Structure" section, test questions will be arranged in blocks based on one of the three clinical settings.

Physician Tasks

For any given clinical encounter frame in a clinical setting, you'll be challenged with a finite number of skills. The 6 physician tasks that are tested on the Step 3 exam are representative of what all physicians practicing unsupervised medical management are expected to know.

Task	Tests your ability to...
Obtaining a history and performing a physical examination	• identify key facets of the history or physical exam and relate them to the presenting problem or condition. • predict the most likely additional physical finding or examination technique that would result in the finding.
Using laboratory and diagnostic studies	• select the appropriate *routine* or *initial* lab or diagnostic test either to ensure effective therapy or to establish diagnosis. • predict the most likely lab or diagnostic test result.
Formulating the most likely diagnosis	• determine the diagnosis and use it to manage the patient.
Evaluating the severity of the patient's problems	• assess the severity of a patient's condition and identify indications for consultations or further diagnostic workup. • recognize factors in history, physical exam, or lab studies that affect prognosis or determine a change in therapy.
Managing the patient	• manage a patient in the following 4 areas: 1. Health maintenance (i.e., implementing preventative measures by identifying risk factors) 2. Clinical intervention (i.e., knowing appropriate postsurgical/postprocedural management and follow-up measures) 3. Clinical therapeutics (i.e., properly utilizing pharmacotherapeutic options) 4. Legal/ethical and health care system issues, including patient autonomy, physician-patient relationships, and managed-care protocols
Applying scientific concepts	• identify processes responsible for an underlying condition and interpret results of clinical or epidemiologic experiments

Step 3 Examination Structure

The USMLE Step 3 is a 2-day computerized examination. The first day and a half tests your knowledge with a total of 480 traditional multiple-choice questions, which are arranged in blocks organized by one of the 3 clinical settings. Within a block, you may answer the items in any order, review responses, and change answers. However, after exiting a block, you can no longer review questions or change answers within that block. A link to view standard lab values, as well as access a calculator, is available at any time within the block of questions.

Day 1 includes 336 multiple-choice items divided into seven 60-minute blocks of 48 items. A total of 60 minutes is allowed for completing each block of questions, for a maximum of 7 hours of testing. A minimum of 45 minutes of break time and an optional 15-minute tutorial complete the 8-hour day. Extra break time can be gained by completing question blocks or the tutorial before the allocated time.

Day 2 includes 144 items divided into 4 blocks of 36 questions. You will have 45 minutes to complete each of these blocks. The time allotted for these blocks is 3 hours. The second day also includes 4 hours for 12 clinical case simulations (CCS), preceded by a 10-minute tutorial. CCS cases vary in length from 10 to 25 minutes in duration. As with the first day, a minimum of 45 minutes of break time is allocated for the day.

The multiple-choice questions contribute 80 percent of your score on Step 3. They are the largest component of your exam. Don't get so caught up worrying about CCS that you forget about the rest of the exam!

Traditional multiple-choice questions may either be single-item questions, multiple-item sets, or cases. As of February 2014 a new, restructured examination will also be given on 2 test days; however, examinees will be able to schedule the 2 test days on nonconsecutive days.

Day 1: Step 3 Foundations of Independent Practice (FIP). Day 1 will focus on assessment of knowledge of foundational medicine and science essential for effective health care. This test day will be entirely devoted to multiple-choice questions and will include some of the newer item formats, such as those based on scientific abstracts, pharmaceutical advertisements, and basic science correlates.

Day 2: Step 3 Advanced Clinical Medicine (ACM). Day 2 will focus on assessment of applying comprehensive knowledge of health and disease in the context of patient management. This test day will include multiple-choice questions and computer-based case simulations (CCS).

Single Items

These questions are the traditional, multiple-choice format that you encountered in Step 1 and Step 2 CK. These items include a patient vignette followed by four or five response options. Other options may be partially correct, but there is only *one best* answer.

Multiple Item Sets

A single patient-centered vignette may be associated with 2 or 3 consecutive questions that are linked to the initial patient vignette but test different points. Questions are designed to be answered independently of each other. You are required to select the one best answer for each question. As with single items, any of the options may be partially correct, but there is only *one best* answer.

Cases

A single-patient or family-centered vignette may ask 2 or 3 questions, each related to the initial opening vignette. The difference in these case sets is that additional information is added as the case unfolds. *Always* answer the questions in the order presented. You may find your response to earlier questions is altered by the additional information in subsequent questions; however, resist the urge to change your prior answers. If you do skip questions, be sure to answer earlier questions with only the information presented to that point in the case. Each question is intended to be answered independently.

Guide to the CCS

The Primum computer-based case simulations (CCS) is a testing format that allows you to provide care for a simulated patient. You decide which information to obtain and how to treat and monitor the patient's progress. The computer records each step you take in caring for the patient and scores your overall performance.

In the CCS software, you will be required to choose additional elements of the presented history, as well as select the components of the physical examination you wish to perform. You have the flexibility to order any laboratory study, procedure, request, and consultants, and you can begin medications and other therapies. Any of the thousands of possible entries that you type on the "order sheet" are processed and verified by the "clerk," and there is no limit to the number of entries into the order sheet. However, each order has a corresponding "virtual time" in which the test result may be available or procedure can be performed. Advancing the virtual time allows you to obtain results and submit the requested procedures. As virtual time passes, the patient's condition changes based on the underlying problem and the sequence and priority of your interventions. You are responsible for managing the results of tests and interventions and making subsequent management decisions based on the first sequence of tests you ordered. While you cannot go back in virtual time, you can change your orders to reflect your updated management plan. In addition, you have the option to move patients between the office, home, emergency department, intensive care unit, and hospital ward. An important aspect of correctly managing CCS patients is recognizing the most appropriate sequence of management and the most appropriate location where that patient should be treated.

The challenge of the CCS is twofold:

1. You need to manage the case itself. The management steps are case-dependent and based on acceptable standards of care. It is assumed that you will have reviewed the management of the most common presenting complaints during your year of internship and/or during your Step 3 review.
2. You will manage a patient by initiating the most appropriate course of action, such as ordering tests or transferring the patient to another setting. The computer will not cue you on what to do—*you* must decide independently what you need to do and the sequence in which it should be done.

Each case can be divided into 3 parts: the case introduction, vital signs, and initial history (first 1 to 2 minutes); the management of the case (10 to 12 minutes maximum, often less); and the conclusion of the case (last 5 minutes).

Case Introduction Screen

The first screen is called the case introduction and provides a 1- or 2-sentence description of the patient's chief complaint, the patient's location at presentation, and time of day. After reading this screen, click the **OK** button.

Vital Signs Screen

These initial vital signs are the most important indicator of whether this condition is acute-emergent or chronic-stable. Review for any abnormalities before hitting the **OK** button.

Initial History Screen

The initial history screen gives you a comprehensive description of the history of present illness, past medical history, family history, social history, and review of systems. Read this section carefully, as key diagnostic information is given here. After reading the history of present illness, you should be able to establish a short differential diagnostic list. Make note of any key features in the past medical, family, and social history and review of systems that support or refute your differential diagnosis. At the end of the initial history, click the **OK** button; this will mark the end of the prompted section of the case.

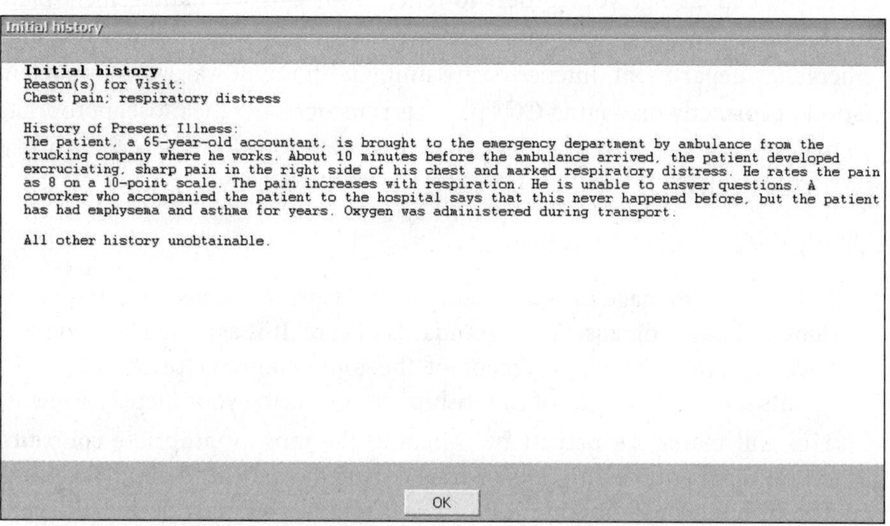
Initial history

Initial history
Reason(s) for Visit:
Chest pain; respiratory distress

History of Present Illness:
The patient, a 65-year-old accountant, is brought to the emergency department by ambulance from the trucking company where he works. About 10 minutes before the ambulance arrived, the patient developed excruciating, sharp pain in the right side of his chest and marked respiratory distress. He rates the pain as 8 on a 10-point scale. The pain increases with respiration. He is unable to answer questions. A coworker who accompanied the patient to the hospital says that this never happened before, but the patient has had emphysema and asthma for years. Oxygen was administered during transport.

All other history unobtainable.

OK

(courtesy http://www.usmle.org)

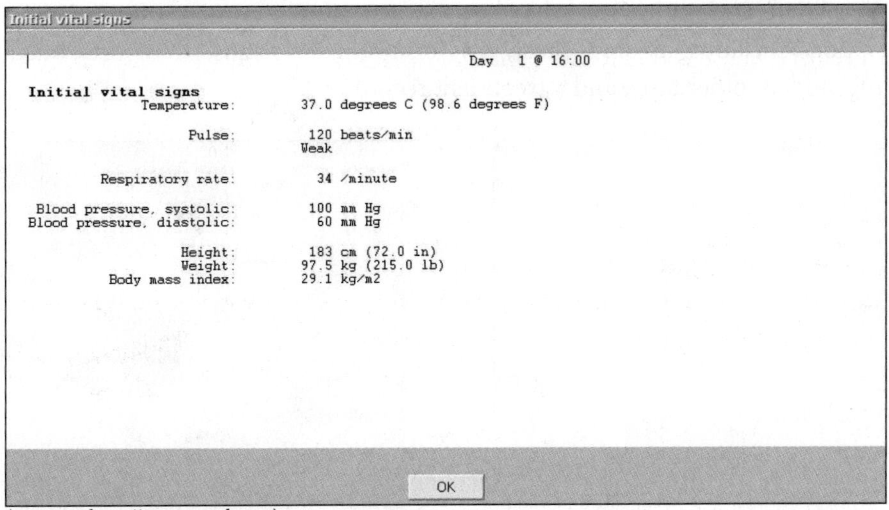
Initial vital signs

Day 1 @ 16:00

Initial vital signs

Temperature:	37.0 degrees C (98.6 degrees F)
Pulse:	120 beats/min Weak
Respiratory rate:	34 /minute
Blood pressure, systolic:	100 mm Hg
Blood pressure, diastolic:	60 mm Hg
Height:	183 cm (72.0 in)
Weight:	97.5 kg (215.0 lb)
Body mass index:	29.1 kg/m2

OK

(courtesy http://www.usmle.org)

Case Management

This section of the case is driven by your actions rather than prompts from the software. There are 4 buttons at the top of the screen, which you will use to manage the case. You will be able to access any of these buttons until the last 5 minutes, at which point you are automatically brought to the final stage.

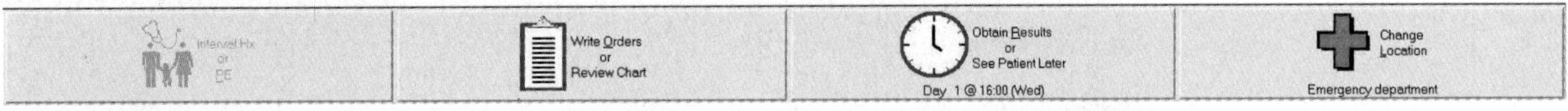

(courtesy http://www.usmle.org)

The **History/Physical** button allows you to order a follow-up history, as well as either a comprehensive or system-focused physical exam.

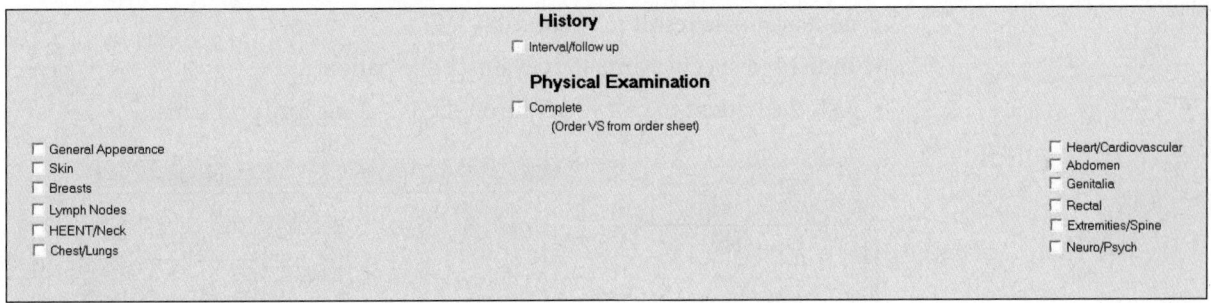

History

- [ ] Interval/follow up

Physical Examination

- [ ] Complete
  (Order VS from order sheet)

- [ ] General Appearance
- [ ] Skin
- [ ] Breasts
- [ ] Lymph Nodes
- [ ] HEENT/Neck
- [ ] Chest/Lungs
- [ ] Heart/Cardiovascular
- [ ] Abdomen
- [ ] Genitalia
- [ ] Rectal
- [ ] Extremities/Spine
- [ ] Neuro/Psych

(courtesy http://www.usmle.org)

The **Write Orders/Review Chart** button brings up a number of other chart options, including an order sheet, progress notes, vital signs, lab reports, imaging studies, other tests, and a treatment record.

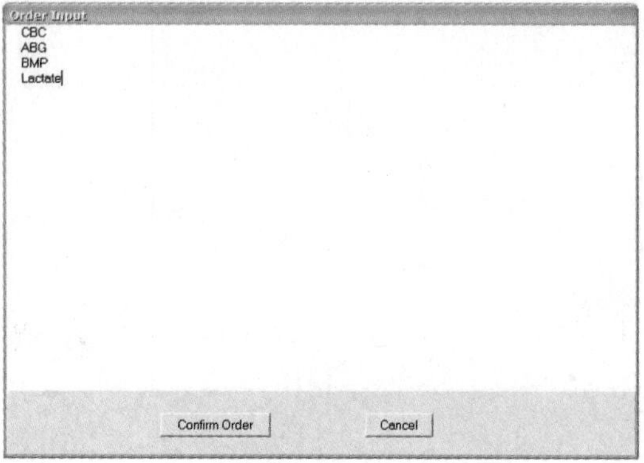

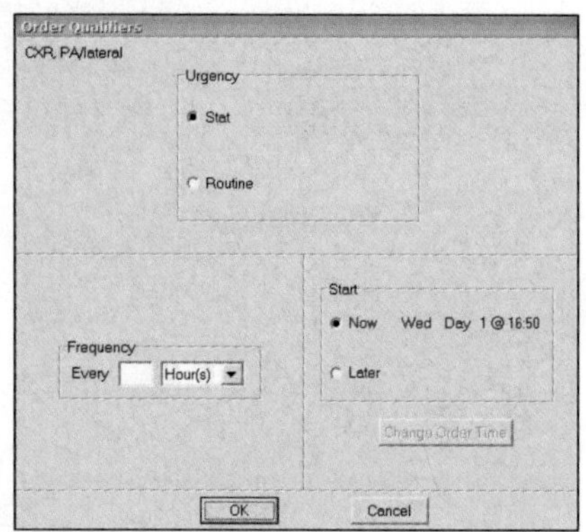

(courtesy http://www.usmle.org)

The **clock button** allows you to manipulate the **case time clock (virtual time).** This is a completely separate from the real-time clock, found at the bottom right part of the screen throughout the case. In real test time, you have up to a maximum of 10 to 25 minutes to manage the case from beginning to end. But to get results or schedule a time to reevaluate the patient, you'll need to move the **case time clock** ahead. You may move the clock ahead in any of the following ways:

- Move the clock ahead to a selected time so that you can get a specific result back.
- Move the clock automatically to when the first result comes back. Remember that you will still need to manage the case in the interim period before the next available result may come back.
- Indicate a specific time to reevaluate the patient.
- Ask the patient to call you if he or she is having any problems.

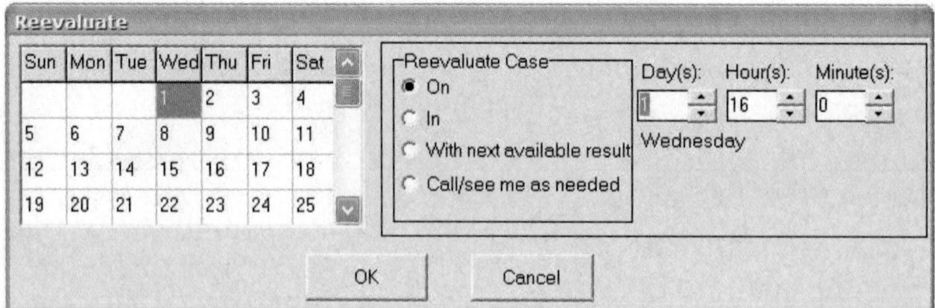

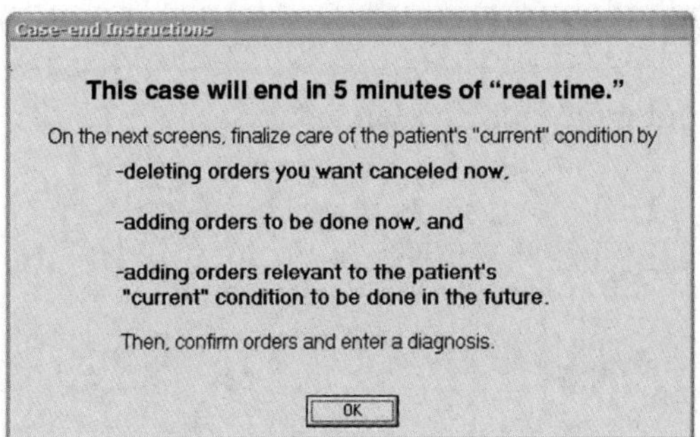

At the end of the case, you must enter your diagnosis on the screen provided. When you click **OK,** the case closes, and you move onto the next case.

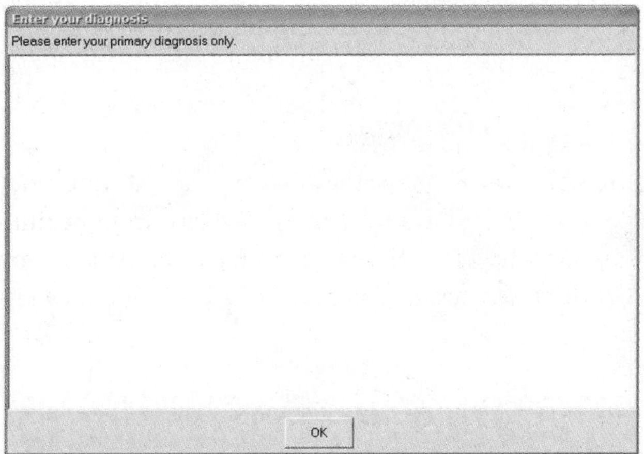

Score Reporting

The minimum passing score for Step 3 is 190. This corresponds to answering approximately 60 to 70 percent of the items correctly. The USMLE does not report performance as percentiles. There will be a 3-digit score on your score report. A graphical report of performance on the reverse side of your score sheet indicates relative strengths and weaknesses. This graphical report is not seen by anyone but you and is not provided to institutions or licensing bodies.

Registration for Step 3

For registration and more information, contact:

FSMB
Department of Examination Services
Website: *www.fsmb.org*
Telephone: (817) 868-4041
Fax: (817) 868-4098
Email: usmle@fsmb.org
or your state **medical licensing authority** (see the USMLE website at *http://usmle.org*).

Section 1
Internal Medicine

Infectious Diseases

1

Introduction to Antibiotics

Staphylococcus aureus: Bone, Heart, Skin, Joint

- **Sensitive staph (MSSA):**
  - IV: Oxacillin/nafcillin, or cefazolin (first-generation cephalosporin)
  - Oral: Dicloxacillin or cephalexin (first-generation cephalosporin)
- **Resistant staph (MRSA):**
  - Severe infection: Vancomycin, linezolid, daptomycin, ceftaroline, tigecycline, or telavancin. Linezolid causes thrombocytopenia. Daptomycin causes myopathy and a rising CPK.
  - Minor infection: Trimethoprim/sulfamethoxazole (TMP/SMX), clindamycin, doxycycline
- **Penicillin allergy:**
  - Rash: Safe to use cephalosporins
  - Anaphylaxis: Macrolides (azithromycin, clarithromycin) or clindamycin
  - Severe infection: Vancomycin, linezolid, daptomycin, telavancin
  - Minor infection: Macrolides (azithromycin, clarithromycin), clindamycin, TMP/SMX

> Telavancin is a vancomycin derivative with similar efficacy.

Basic Science Correlate

- Telavancin is a bactericidal lipopolysaccharide. Telavancin inhibits bacterial cell wall synthesis by binding to the D-Ala-D-Ala terminus of the peptidoglycan in the growing cell wall.
- Ceftaroline, like all cephalosporins, inhibits cell wall growth by binding the penicillin-binding protein.
- Linezolid inhibits protein synthesis.
- TMP-SMX is a folate antagonist.

If the organism is sensitive, oxacillin and nafcillin are superior to vancomycin.

Streptococcus

The medications above will cover *Streptococcus* as well as *Staphylococcus*. The following medications are *specific* for *Streptococcus*:

- Penicillin
- Ampicillin
- Amoxicillin

Gram-negative bacilli (rods): *Escherichia coli, Enterobacter, Citrobacter, Morganella, Pseudomonas, Serratia*

All of the following medications are essentially equal in their efficacy for gram-negative bacilli.

Cephalosporins	Penicillins	Monobactam	Quinolones	Aminoglycosides	Carbapenems
Cefepime Ceftazidime	Piperacillin Ticarcillin	Aztreonam	Ciprofloxacin Levofloxacin Moxifloxacin Gemifloxacin	Gentamicin Tobramycin Amikacin	Imipenem Meropenem Ertapenem Doripenem

Exceptions

- **Ertapenem** is the only carbapenem that does *not* cover *Pseudomonas.*
- **Piperacillin** and **ticarcillin** *also* cover streptococci and anaerobes.
- **Levofloxacin, gemifloxacin,** and **moxifloxacin** are *excellent* pneumococcal drugs.
- **Aminoglycosides** work *synergistically* with other agents to treat staph and enterococcus.
- **Carbapenems** are *excellent* antianaerobic medications. They cover streptococci and all sensitive staphylococcus (MSSA).
- **Tigecycline** covers MRSA and is broadly active against gram-negative bacilli. Tigecyline is weaker than other anti-MRSA drugs.

Gemifloxacin is a quinolone for pneumonia.

Basic Science Correlate

Mechanism of Beta-Lactam Antibiotics

The 4 beta-lactam antibiotics all inhibit the cell wall by binding the penicillin-binding protein. The 4 classes are:

- Penicillin
- Cephalosporins
- Carbapenem
- Monobactam (the only one is aztreonam)

Anaerobes

- **Gastrointestinal anaerobes (*Bacteroides*)**
  - **Metronidazole** is the *best* medication for abdominal anaerobes.
  - **Carbapenems, piperacillin,** and **ticarcillin** are equal in efficacy for abdominal anaerobes compared to metronidazole.
  - **Cefoxitin** and **cefotetan** (in the cephamycin class) are the *only* cephalosporins that cover anaerobes.
- **Respiratory anaerobes (anaerobic strep)**
  - **Clindamycin** is the *best* drug for anaerobic strep.
- **Medications with no anaerobic coverage**
  - **Aminoglycosides, aztreonam, fluoroquinolones, oxacillin/nafcillin,** and all the **cephalosporins** *except* cefoxitin and cefotetan

Adverse Effects
Daptomycin: myopathy
Linezolid: low platelets
Imipenem: seizures

CCS Tip: CCS does *not* require you to know doses, but you *are* expected to know the route of administration.

A man is admitted for endocarditis. His blood cultures grow *S. aureus,* and vancomycin is started while awaiting sensitivity testing. He develops red skin, particularly on the neck. What should you do?

Answer: Slow the rate of the infusion. Vancomycin is associated with "red man syndrome," which is red, flushed skin from histamine release. This happens from rapid infusion of vancomycin. There is no specific therapy, and you do not need to switch the medication. If the rate of infusion is slowed, the reaction will not occur. Telavancin does not cause red man syndrome.

Antiviral Agents

- **Acyclovir, valacyclovir,** and **famciclovir** (herpes simplex, varicella zoster): All 3 of these agents are equal in efficacy.
- **Valganciclovir, ganciclovir,** and **foscarnet (cytomegalovirus [CMV]):** These are essentially equal in efficacy. They also cover herpes simplex and varicella. **Valganciclovir** is the best long-term therapy for CMV retinitis. They can have the following **adverse effects:**
  - Valganciclovir and ganciclovir: Neutropenia and bone marrow suppression
  - Foscarnet: Renal toxicity
- **Simeprevir, boceprevir, sofosbuvir, ledipasvir:** All are oral agents for chronic hepatitis C. None is used as a single agent. Sofosbuvir and ledipasvir do not need to be combined with interferon.
- **Oseltamivir** and **zanamivir** (neuraminidase inhibitors): Influenza A and B
- **Ribavirin:** Hepatitis C (in combination with interferon), respiratory syncytial virus (RSV). Ribavirin causes anemia.
- **Lamivudine, interferon, adefovir, tenofovir, entecavir,** and **telbivudine:** Chronic hepatitis B

Echinocandin's unique mechanism: 1,3 glucon inhibition in fungi only.

Basic Science Correlate

Mechanisms of Oral Hepatitis C Medications

- **Sofosbuvir:** RNA polymerase inhibitor
- **Simeprevir, boceprevir,** and **telaprevir:** Protease inhibitors that prevent viral maturation by inhibiting protein synthesis

Antifungal Agents

- **Fluconazole:** *Candida* (not *Candida krusei* or *Candida glabrata*), *Cryptococcus,* oral and vaginal candidiasis as an alternative to topical mediations
- **Itraconazole:** Largely equal to fluconazole but less easy to use; rarely the best initial therapy for anything
- **Voriconazole:** Covers all *Candida;* best agent against *Aspergillus.* Adverse effect:
  - Some visual disturbance
- **Posaconazole:** Also covers mucormycosis or Mucorales
- **Echinocandins** (caspofungin, micafungin, anidulafungin):
  - *Excellent* for neutropenic fever patients.
  - Does *not* cover *Cryptococcus.*
  - Better than amphotericin for neutropenia and fever (less mortality).
  - Adverse effect—Echinocandins have *no* significant human toxicity because they affect/inhibit the 1,3 glucan synthesis step, which does not exist in humans.

Basic Science Correlate

Mechanism of Antifungal Medications

Azole antifungals inhibit conversion of lanosterol to ergosterol. Ergosterol is the major component of the cell wall of fungi. Disrupting ergosterol damages the cell membrane and increases its permeability, resulting in cell lysis and death.

- **Amphotericin:** Effective against *all Candida, Cryptococcus,* and *Aspergillus:*
  - The last 2 main indications for amphotericin are **Cryptococcus** and **mucormycosis.**
  - **Aspergillus:** Voriconazole superior to amphotericin
  - **Neutropenic fever**: Caspofungin superior to amphotericin
  - **Candida:** Fluconazole is equal to amphotericin for efficacy but has *far fewer* adverse effects.

- *Adverse effects* of amphotericin—renal **toxicity** (increased creatinine); hypokalemia; metabolic acidosis; fever, shakes, chills

Basic Science Correlate

Mechanism of Renal Toxicity of Amphotericin

Amphotericin is directly toxic to the tubules. Distal tubule toxicity results in renal tubular acidosis. Distal RTA gives excess potassium and magnesium loss and hydrogen ion retention. When renal toxicity is described, the answer is "Switch to liposomal amphotericin."

Osteomyelitis

Is the infection in the soft tissue (skin) only? Or has it spread into the bone?

Osteomyelitis in adults almost always presents in a patient with **diabetes, peripheral arterial disease, or both with an ulcer or soft tissue infection.** You can also think about osteomyelitis in patients with direct trauma and a history of orthopedic surgery, but the case with diabetes and peripheral vascular disease is more likely to show up on the exam. The "Next best step?" question fundamentally asks if you know what to do to distinguish the difference between a soft tissue infection and a contiguous spread into the bone.

Diagnostic Testing

- Best **initial test:** Plain **x-ray**
- Best **second test** (if there is clinical suspicion and x-ray is negative): **MRI**
- Most accurate test: bone biopsy and culture

You must lose more than 50 percent of the calcium content of the bone before the x-ray becomes abnormal. Although it may take up to two weeks for osteomyelitis to become severe enough to make the x-ray abnormal, the x-ray is *still* the first test. (You would not skip an EKG and go straight to a stress test; you would not skip a chest x-ray and go straight to a chest CT scan.)

Which of the following is the earliest finding of osteomyelitis on an x-ray?

a. Periosteal elevation
b. Involucrum
c. Sequestrum
d. Punched-out lesions
e. Fracture

Answer: **A.** The earliest finding of osteomyelitis on an x-ray is elevation of the periosteum. Involucrum and sequestrum are terms applied to the formation of abnormal new bone in the periosteum and chunks of bone chipped off from the infection. Punched-out lesions are seen in myeloma, not osteomyelitis. Osteomyelitis does not have an association with fracture.

On Step 3, you can get the x-ray result in 2 ways as part of a question:

1. Single best answer: The stem of the question simply states, "x-ray of the bone is normal."
2. CCS: You move the clock forward, and the x-ray result will pop up as you pass the time when it says "report available."

A 67-year-old man with diabetes and peripheral arterial disease comes in having had pain in his leg for 2 weeks. There is an ulcer with a draining sinus tract. The x-ray is normal. What is the next best step in determining a diagnosis?

a. Bone scan
b. CT scan
c. MRI
d. ESR
e. Biopsy

Answer: The MRI **(C)** is the next best test to do to determine the diagnosis of osteomyelitis if the x-ray is normal. A bone scan does not have the specificity of an MRI.

X-ray is *always* the best initial test. If the x-ray is normal, an MRI is *far* superior to a bone scan with a nuclear isotope. The bone scan is very poor at distinguishing between infection in the bone and infection of the soft tissue above it.

The sedimentation rate is the best method of following a response to therapy. Remember that osteomyelitis is *most* commonly caused by **direct contiguous spread from overlying tissue,** but hematogenous (blood) infection can also be present as a cause or result of osteomyelitis, so a blood culture (especially if the patient looks septic) is not a bad idea. However, perform the MRI first.

Which test has greater sensitivity, the MRI or the bone scan? They are **equal** in sensitivity. The MRI and bone scan both have an equal ability to exclude osteomyelitis if they are normal. The MRI, however, is *far* more specific. A swab of the ulcer for culture is extremely inaccurate. We cannot tell what is growing inside the bone for sure by growing something from the superficial ulcer. Would you allow yourself to be treated for weeks to months with intravenous antibiotics with only a 50/50 chance that you are treating the right organism?

Basic Science Correlate

Mechanism of Diagnostic Testing in Osteomyelitis

MRI is based on water content. When the bone is infected, it swells and increases water content. This happens within 48 hours of infection. Water changes the spin of hydrogen ions in tissue, and that is why MRI and bone scan become abnormal at the same time. Nuclear bone scan is based on osteoblasts depositing technetium in tissue. Osteomyelitis and cancer both destroy and form bone. Bone scans need new bone formation to light up after 48 hours. CT scans and x-rays are based on calcium loss; this takes 1–2 weeks.

How do we know how long to treat if 90 percent of patients have no fever and a normal white cell count? By following the sedimentation rate. If the sedimentation rate (ESR) is still markedly elevated after 4–6 weeks of therapy, further treatment and possible surgical debridement is necessary.

Never culture the draining sinus tract or swab an ulcer.

Treatment

Staphylococcus: This is still the *most* common cause of osteomyelitis. If the organism is sensitive, **oxacillin** or **nafcillin** intravenously for 4–6 weeks is the treatment. MRSA is treated with **vancomycin, linezolid, ceftaroline,** or **daptomycin.** You *cannot* use oral therapy for staphylococcal osteomyelitis.

- **Gram-negative bacilli** (***Salmonella*** and ***Pseudomonas*** are the ones to consider): This is the *only* form of osteomyelitis that can be successfully and reliably treated with oral antibiotics.
  - You *must* confirm it is gram-negative with a bone biopsy.
  - The organism *must* be sensitive to antibiotics.
  - There is no urgency to treating chronic osteomyelitis. You can obtain the biopsy, move the clock forward, and treat what you find on the culture.

To treat osteomyelitis appropriately, a bone biopsy/culture must be performed.

Head and Neck Infections

Otitis Externa

Presents with **itching** and **drainage** from the external auditory canal. This is a form of cellulitis of the skin of the external auditory canal. It is often difficult to visualize the tympanic membrane because of the swelling of the canal. It is also painful, especially when the tragus of the ear is manipulated.

It is associated with **swimming,** because swimming washes out the acidic environment normally found in the external auditory canal. Other causes include **foreign objects** in the ears (e.g., repeated use of cotton swabs, hearing aids, etc.).

Diagnostic Testing

No specific tests are necessary; diagnosis is based on exam. Do *not* perform a routine culture of the ear canal.

Treatment

Topical antibiotics, such as *ofloxacin, ciprofloxacin,* or *polymyxin/neomycin.* Add **topical hydrocortisone** to decrease swelling and itching. Adding **acetic acid and water solution** to reacidify the ear can help eliminate the infection.

The function of cerumen (earwax) is to make the external auditory canal acidic. Acid wax suppresses bacteria; it is like the lactobacilli in the vagina in this regard. Cerumen blocks water (hydrophobic), and a low-water environment suppresses bacteria. *Pseudomonas* likes to grow in water.

Malignant Otitis Externa

This is an *extremely* different disease from simple otitis externa. Malignant otitis externa is really **osteomyelitis of the skull** from *Pseudomonas* in a patient with diabetes. It is an extremely serious disease, because it can lead to a brain abscess and destruction of the skull. Diagnose it like osteomyelitis: MRI or bone biopsy/culture.

Diagnostic Testing

- Best **initial** test: **CT** or **MRI**
- Most **accurate** test: **Biopsy**

Treatment

Treat with **surgical debridement** and **antibiotics active against *Pseudomonas*** such as ciprofloxacin, piperacillin, cefepime, carbapenem, or aztreonam.

Basic Science Correlate

Quinolone antibiotics, such as ciprofloxacin, work by inhibiting DNA gyrase (topoisomerase). DNA gyrase unwinds DNA so it can be replicated. By preventing DNA from unwinding, you prevent DNA from copying and reproducing itself.

Otitis Media

Key features include the following:

- Redness
- Bulging
- Decreased hearing
- Loss of light reflex
- Immobility of the tympanic membrane

Although all of the findings above can be present, the *most* sensitive is the presence of **immobility of the tympanic membrane.** If the tympanic membrane is freely mobile on insufflations of the ear, then otitis media is not present. The physical exam may also describe the absence of the light reflex.

Diagnostic Testing

There is *no* radiologic test to confirm the diagnosis, which is based entirely on physical examination. Patients may complain of decreased or muffled hearing.

Treatment

- Best initial therapy: **Amoxicillin.** Usual course is 7–10 days; longer for younger patients and shorter for older patients.
- Next step: Perform the most accurate test, **tympanocentesis and aspirate of the tympanic membrane for culture.** This is rarely necessary and is only done for recurrent or persistent cases that fail therapy.

Basic Science Correlate

Otitis media is caused by swelling of the Eustachian tube. When the narrowest portion (or isthmus) becomes inflamed, it blocks the egress of secretions. Pneumococcus, nontypeable Haemophilus, and Moraxella are the most common causes. Haemophilus vaccine does not prevent the type of infections that cause sinusitis and otitis. Vaccine prevents only invasive group B Haemophilus.

CCS Tip: On CCS, advance the clock forward 3 days. If the infection is not improving, switch the amoxicillin to one of the following:

- Amoxicillin-clavulanate
- Cefdinir
- Ceftibuten
- Cefuroxime
- Cefprozil
- Cefpodoxime

Sinusitis

Look for a patient with nasal discharge, headache, facial tenderness, tooth pain, bad taste in the mouth, and decreased transillumination of the sinuses. Most cases are viral, but bacterial causes include the same group that cause otitis media: *Streptococcus pneumoniae, Haemophilus influenzae,* and *Moraxella catarrhalis.*

Diagnostic Testing

- Best initial test: **x-ray**
- Most accurate test: **Sinus aspirate for culture.** This is *more* accurate than a CT or MRI; you cannot stain or culture a radiologic test.

Treatment

- Same as for otitis media, but add inhaled steroids
- Use **amoxicillin/clavulanate** if there is
  - fever and pain;
  - persistent symptoms despite 7 days of decongestants; and
  - purulent nasal discharge.

Basic Science Correlate

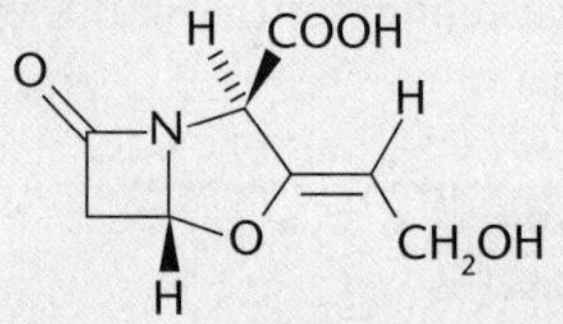

Clavulanic acid (pictured here) is a beta-lactamase inhibitor that confers a broader spectrum of antimicrobial activity to penicillin. Clavulanic acid is similar in structure to the beta-lactam ring of penicillin. The enzyme beta lactamase destroys the clavulanic acid instead of the penicillin. This is why it is a "suicide inhibitor." The other beta-lactamase inhibitors, tazobactam and sulbactam, work the same way.

Pharyngitis

The diagnosis of streptococcal pharyngitis is certain if the following are present:

- **Pain/sore throat**
- **Exudate**
- **Adenopathy**
- *No* cough/hoarseness

Diagnostic Testing

- Best initial test: **"Rapid strep test."** A positive rapid strep test is just as specific as a positive throat culture. The rapid strep test is performed instantly and can tell if the organism is of the type (group A strep) that might lead to rheumatic fever or glomerulonephritis. In adults, the sensitivity of the rapid strep test is enough. If the rapid strep test is negative in an adult, no further testing or treatment with antibiotics is necessary.
- Most accurate test: **Culture**

Treatment

- **Penicillin** or **amoxicillin**
- **Penicillin allergy:** Use azithromycin or clarithromycin; use cephalexin if allergy is just a rash

Influenza

Look for a patient with **arthralgia, myalgia, cough, headache, fever, sore throat,** and **feeling of tiredness.**

Diagnostic Testing

- **Viral rapid antigen detection** testing of a nasopharyngeal swab. This is the best next step if the diagnosis is unclear.

Treatment

Oseltamivir or **zanamivir** if the patient presents within the first 48 hours after the onset of symptoms. These are neuraminidase inhibitors that work against *both* influenza A and B. Amantadine and rimantadine will be *wrong* answers; they are only effective against influenza A.

Vaccination Against Influenza

Influenza vaccine is **acceptable** in the general population at any age. The strongest indications are:

- COPD, CHF, dialysis patients, steroid use, health care workers, everyone > 50
- Step 3 will expect you to know that there is a live attenuated vaccine administered by inhalation. The live vaccine is only efficacious in those < age 50 with none of the medical problems described above. Anyone with illness and or those > age 50 need the injected inactivated virus. Egg allergy is no longer an absolute contraindication to flu vaccine.

> An egg allergy is no longer an absolute contraindication to flu vaccine.

Skin Infections

Impetigo

This is the *most superficial* of the bacterial skin infections. It is caused by *Streptococcus pyogenes* or *Staph. aureus* infecting the epidermal layer of the skin. Because it is so superficial, there is **weeping, crusting,** and **oozing** of the skin.

Diagnostic Testing

A specific microbiologic diagnosis is rarely made or necessary. Look for "weeping, oozing, honey-colored lesions."

Treatment

- **Topical mupirocin or retapamulin** (mupirocin has greater activity against MRSA, bacitracin has less efficacy as a single agent)
- Severe disease: **Oral dicloxacillin or cephalexin**
- Community-acquired MRSA (CA-MRSA): **TMP/SMZ;** clindamycin is sometimes useful; linezolid is definitely effective.
- **Penicillin allergy: What to use?**
  - Rash: Cephalosporins are safe.
  - Anaphylaxis: Clindamycin, doxycycline, linezolid
  - Severe infection with anaphylaxis: Vancomycin, telavancin, linezolid, daptomycin

Erysipelas

The face is often the site of erysipelas.

This is a **group A (pyogenes) streptococcal infection** of the skin. The skin is **very bright red** and **hot** because of dilation of the capillaries of the dermis due to locally released inflammatory mediators. As with most bacterial skin infections, a specific microbiologic diagnosis is rarely made.

Diagnostic Testing

Blood cultures may be positive in erysipelas. Order blood cultures in CCS, but go straight to treatment on the single best multiple-choice answer.

Can erysipelas lead to rheumatic fever? No. Only pharyngeal infection can lead to rheumatic fever. Skin infections can lead to glomerulonephritis, however. Remember: Skin (erysipelas) goes to kidneys (glomerulonephritis) only. Throat (pharyngitis) goes to kidneys (glomerulonephritis) *and* heart (rheumatic fever).

Treatment

- Best initial treatment: **Oral dicloxacillin or cephalexin.** Topical antibiotics are useless.
- If the organism is *confirmed* as group A beta hemolytic streptococci, you may treat with **penicillin VK.**

Cellulitis

Look for a **warm, red, swollen, tender skin.** Likely to present in the arm or leg but can present in any skin.

Diagnostic Testing

If presented with a case of cellulitis in a leg, make sure you order a **lower extremity Doppler** to exclude a blood clot. *Both* clotting and cellulitis can cause a fever.

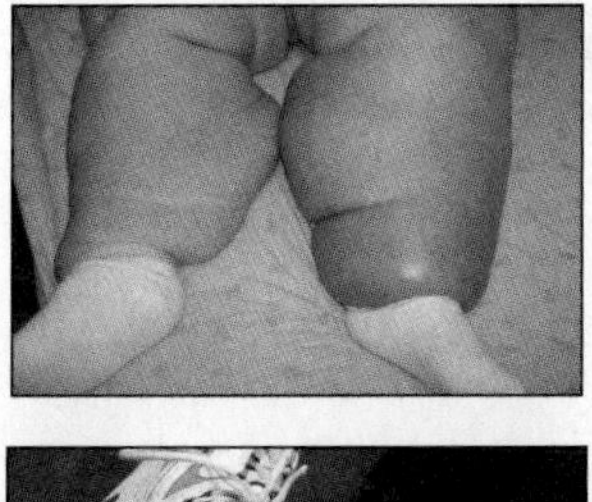

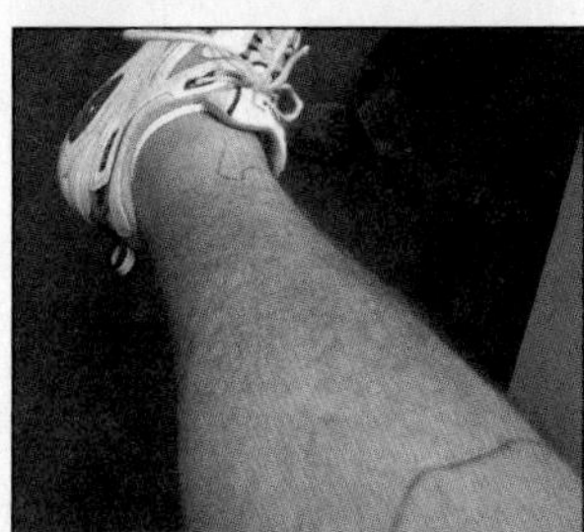

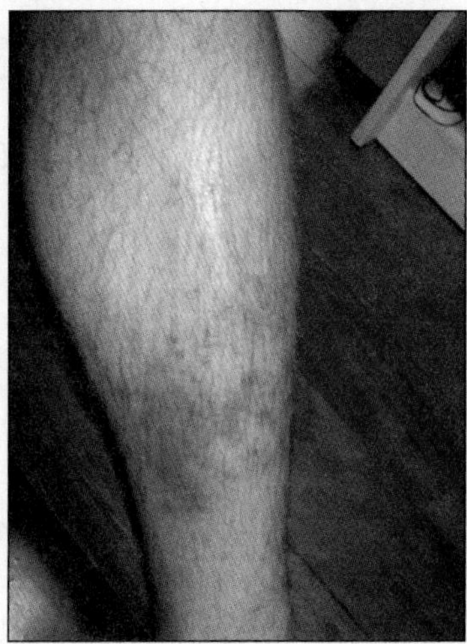

Staphylococcus aureus and *Streptococcus pyogenes* are nearly equal in the cause of cellulitis.

Retapamulin:
- topical antibiotic
- only for impetigo

Treatment

- Minor disease: **Dicloxacillin or cephalexin orally**
- Severe disease: **Oxacillin, nafcillin, or cefazolin IV**
- **Penicillin allergy:**
  - Rash: Use cephalosporins such as cefazolin or ceftaroline.
  - Anaphylaxis: Use vancomycin, linezolid, or daptomycin. For minor infections, macrolides or clindamycin can be useful.

What skin infection does Staphylococcus epidermidis *cause?* None. *S. epidermidis* is a normal commensal inhabitant of the skin. It lives there and does *not* cause skin infection.

Folliculitis < Furuncles < Carbuncles < Boils

These are **aureus-related skin infections** beginning at the hair follicle. The only difference between them is *size.* Folliculitis is the smallest and most minor. Furuncles are larger, carbuncles larger than that, and boils even larger. An "abscess" would be considered the largest.

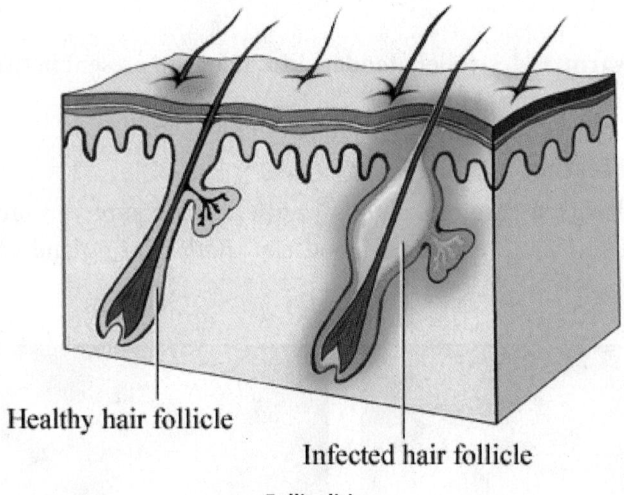

Folliculitis

Diagnostic Testing

Diagnosis of these skin infections is based on appearance.

Treatment

Antibiotic therapy is **identical to that described for cellulitis.** Larger infections, such as boils, respond to **drainage.** As with all other skin infections, the patient can develop post-streptococcal glomerulonephritis but not rheumatic fever.

Fungal Infections of Skin and Nails

Common symptoms in skin infections are severe itching of the scalp, dandruff, and bald patches where the fungus has rooted itself in the skin. In onychomycosis, nails may be thickened, yellow, cloudy, and appear fragile and broken.

Diagnostic Testing

- Best initial test: KOH preparation
  1. Scrape the skin or nail.
  2. Place the scraping on a slide with KOH and acid and heat it.
  3. The epithelial cells will dissolve and leave the fungal forms behind, visible on the slide.

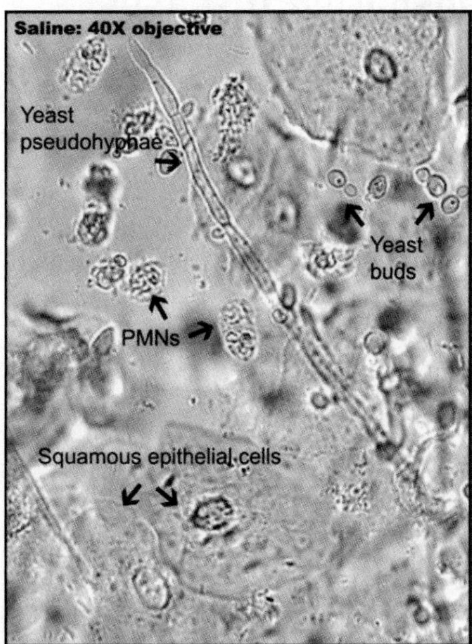

KOH Prep

Basic Science Correlate

Fungi have chitin in their outer wall. Chitin is a polymer that will not break down with KOH. Chitin is what makes up crab and lobster shells. Epithelial cells melt and fungi remain behind in a KOH prep because the chitin in the fungus is tougher than epithelial cells.

Treatment

- **Topical antifungal medication** (if no hair or nail involvement): **Clotrimazole, miconazole, ketoconazole, econazole, terconazole, nystatin,** or **ciclopirox**
- **Oral antifungal medication** for scalp (tinea capitis) or nail (onychomycosis)
  - **Terbinafine:** Causes increased liver function tests
  - **Itraconazole**
  - **Griseofulvin** (for tinea capitis): Has less efficacy than either terbinafine or itraconazole

Sexually Transmitted Diseases

Urethritis

Look for a **urethral discharge.** There can also be symptoms of dysuria, such as frequency, urgency, and burning. Discharge *without* dysuria is still considered urethritis. With dysuric symptoms but not discharge, the patient does not necessarily have urethritis; the patient could just have cystitis (i.e., a urinary tract infection).

Diagnostic Testing

- **Urethral swab** for Gram stain, WBC count, culture, and DNA probe
- **Nucleic acid amplification** tests (NAATs) are highly effective as well. NAAT can be done on urine sample in a man.

Disseminated gonorrhea gives:

- Polyarticular disease
- Petechial rash
- Tenosynovitis

Treatment

Urethritis should be treated with 2 medications. Use one drug active against **gonorrhea** and one drug active against **chlamydia,** because these are very often present in coinfection.

Gonorrhea medications	Chlamydia medications
• Ceftriaxone IM	• Azithromycin (single dose) • Doxycycline (for a week)
Pregnant patients • Ceftriaxone IM	Pregnant patients • Azithromycin

A patient develops recurrent episodes of gonorrhea. What should he be tested for?

a. Presence of a spleen
b. HIV
c. Terminal complement deficiency
d. Steroid use
e. Malabsorption

Answer: **C.** Terminal complement deficiency predisposes a patient to recurrent episodes of *Neisseria* infection. This includes any form, including genital and CNS infection.

Nucleic acid amplification test (NAAT) is a "DNA probe." NAAT is the single best test for both gonorrhea and chlamydia.

Cervicitis

Diagnostic Testing

This presents with **cervical discharge.** Swab for stain, WBC count, culture, and DNA testing in the same way as for urethritis. Self-administered blind vaginal swab for nucleic acid amplification testing (NAAT) is just as accurate as a speculum examination.

Treatment

Treat in exactly the same way as **urethritis.**

Pelvic Inflammatory Disease (PID)

Patients present with **lower abdominal pain, tenderness, fever,** and **cervical motion tenderness.** They may also have dysuria and/or vaginal discharge.

Diagnostic Testing

- There are no specific blood tests. **Leukocytosis** is a measure of severity.
- **Best initial test: Pregnancy test,** then **cervical culture** and **DNA probe (NAAT)** for chlamydia and gonorrhea.
- **Most accurate test: Laparoscopy.** This is rarely needed. Only done for recurrent or persistent infection despite therapy or for cases in which the diagnosis is not clear.

Basic Science Correlate

Leukocytosis in infection is caused by demargination of WBCs from the side of blood vessels. Half of WBCs are in circulation and half are on the walls on endothelial cells. Catecholamines (epi, norepi) and cortisol take WBCs off the margins of blood vessels and put them in circulation, meaning stress alone potentially doubles the WBC count.

A 30-year-old woman comes to the emergency department with lower abdominal pain and tenderness, fever, leukocytosis, and cervical motion tenderness. What is the next best step in the management of this patient?

a. Cervical culture
b. Pelvic sonogram
c. Urine pregnancy test
d. Laparoscopy
e. Ceftriaxone and doxycycline

Answer: **C.** The most important thing to do in a woman with lower abdominal pain or tenderness is to **exclude an ectopic pregnancy.** Perform a urine pregnancy test first and then get a cervical culture and start therapy.

Treatment

- Outpatient: **Ceftriaxone (IM)** and **doxycycline (oral)**
- Inpatient: **Cefoxitin (IV)** and **doxycycline** and maybe metronidazole. Cefotetan can be used instead of cefoxitin.
- Penicillin allergic: **Clindamycin** and **gentamicin**

NAAT can be done on voided urine for men or self-administered blind vaginal swab for women.

Basic Science Correlate

Mechanism of Infertility and Ectopic Pregnancy in PID

The tubes become scarred and narrowed. Sperm cannot travel in to fertilize the egg. Fertilized eggs get caught and implant in the wrong place—all from loss of ciliary action, fibrosis, and occlusion.

Antibiotics that are **safe in pregnancy**:

- Penicillins
- Cephalosporins
- Aztreonam
- Erythromycin
- Azithromycin

Epididymo-Orchitis

Presents with an extremely **painful and tender testicle** with a **normal position** in the scrotum. Testicular torsion is different, because it presents with an elevated testicle in an abnormal transverse position.

Treatment

- < 35 years of age: **Ceftriaxone** and **doxycycline**
- > 35 years of age: **Fluoroquinolone**

Ulcerative Genital Diseases

All forms of ulcerative genital disease can be associated with enlarged lymph nodes. Sexual history is not as important as the presence of ulcers.

Chancroid

The ulcer will be **painful** (*Haemophilus ducreyi*).

Diagnostic Testing

The best initial test is a **swab for Gram stain** (gram-negative coccobacilli) and culture (will require specialized medium: Nairobi medium or Mueller-Hinton agar).

Treatment

Single **IM shot of ceftriaxone** or single **oral dose of azithromycin.**

Lymphogranuloma venereum (LGV)

Large tender nodes are present in addition to the ulcer. The enlarged nodes, sometimes called "buboes," may develop a suppurating, draining sinus tract.

Diagnostic Testing

Diagnose with serology for *Chlamydia trachomatis.*

Treatment

Aspirate the bubo. Treat with doxycycline or azithromycin.

> **Basic Science Correlate**
>
> **Mechanism of Erythromycin Adverse Effects**
>
> Why don't we use erythromycin for chlamydia? First, its efficacy is less than that of azithromycin. Second it causes severe nausea, vomiting, and diarrhea. Erythromycin increases the release of motilin, a hormone that increases GI motility between meals. Erythromycin abnormally increases it to where there is excess GI motility. This is why it works for hypomotility disorders such as diabetic gastroparesis.

Herpes Simplex Virus Type 2 (HSV2) (Genital Herpes)

A 34-year-old man comes to the clinic with multiple vesicles on his penis. There is enlarged adenopathy in the inguinal area. What is the next step in management?

a. Tzanck prep
b. Viral culture
c. Valacyclovir
d. Valganciclovir

Answer: **C.** When there are clear vesicular lesions present, there is no need to do a specific diagnostic test for herpes. If the question describes multiple vesicles, then treatment with **acyclovir, valacyclovir,** or **famciclovir for 7–10 days** is the next best step in management. Daily suppressive therapy can be prescribed for recurrent genital herpes. If the roofs come off the vesicles and the lesion becomes an ulcer of unclear etiology, then the best initial diagnostic test is a Tzanck prep. The most accurate test for herpes is a viral culture. If there are clear vesicles, this is not necessary; go straight to treatment. Valganciclovir is therapy for cytomegalovirus (CMV). Patients with frequent recurrence should be placed on chronic suppressive therapy. Acyclovir resistant herpes is treated with foscarnet.

> Acyclovir is safe in pregnancy. Use acyclovir in pregnancy if there is evidence of active lesions at 36 weeks.

Serological testing for herpes antibody has no clinical utility.

Syphilis

The responsible pathogen is *Treponema pallidum.*

A man comes to the clinic having had a **painless, firm genital lesion** for the last several days. The inguinal adenopathy is painless.

What is the most accurate diagnostic test?

a. VDRL
b. RPR
c. FTA
d. Darkfield microscopic exam

Answer: **D.** The VDRL and RPR are only 75 percent sensitive in primary syphilis. There is a false negative rate of 25 percent. The most accurate test in primary syphilis is darkfield microscopy. Darkfield microscopy is far more sensitive than a VDRL or RPR in primary syphilis.

Primary Syphilis

- Symptoms: **Chancre, adenopathy**
- Initial diagnostic test: **Darkfield**, then **VDLR/RPR**
- Treatment: **Single IM shot of penicillin**. Use doxycycline for the penicillin-allergic. Some patients will develop a **Jarisch-Herxheimer reaction**, with fever, headache, and myalgia developing 24 hours after treatment for early stage syphilis. It is a benign, self-limited reaction caused by the release of pyrogens from dying treponemal. Treat with aspirin and continue the treatment.

FTA is more sensitive than VDRL for neurosyphilis.

Secondary Syphilis

- Symptoms: **Rash, mucous patch, alopecia areata, condylomata lata**
- Initial diagnostic test: **RPR** and **FTA**
- Treatment: **Single IM shot of penicillin.** Use doxycycline for the penicillin-allergic.

Tertiary Syphilis

- Neurological involvement: **Tabes dorsalis, Argyll-Robertson pupil, general paresis,** rarely a gumma or aortitis
- Initial diagnostic test: **RPR** and **FTA, lumbar puncture** for neurosyphilis (test CSF with VDRL and FTA). CSF VDRL is only 50 percent sensitive.
- Treatment: **IV penicillin.** Desensitize if penicillin-allergic.

If the patient is allergic to penicillin, desensitization is the answer for:

- Neurosyphilis
- Pregnant women

A man comes in with a painless ulcer and adenopathy. The edges of the ulcer are firm. The VDRL is negative. What is the next best step in management?

a. Repeat the VDRL
b. RPR
c. FTA
d. Darkfield microscopic exam
e. Order antiphospholipid antibody

Answer: D. Perform a darkfield examination. The VDRL and RPR can be negative in 25 percent of cases of primary syphilis.

Syphilis by Stage			
Stage	**Primary**	**Secondary**	**Tertiary**
Presentation	Chancre	• Rash • Alopecia • Condylomata lata • Mucous patch	• Neurosyphilis: Tabes doralis, general paresis, Argyll-Robertson pupil • Gummas • Aortitis
Test	• Darkfield (most sensitive) • RPR or VDRL • FTA	• RPR or VDRL • FTA	• RPR or VDRL • FTA • Lumbar puncture
Treatment	1. Single IM penicillin 2. Doxycycline if allergic	1. Single IM penicillin 2. Doxycycline if allergic	1. IV penicillin 2. Desensitization if allergic

Granuloma Inguinale

This is indicated by a **rare, beefy red genital lesion that ulcerates.**

Diagnostic Testing

- **Biopsy** or **"touch prep,"** ***Klebsiella granulomatis,*** **"Donovan bodies"**

Treatment

- **Doxycycline, TMP/SMX,** or **azithromycin**

> Neurosyphilis is excluded with a negative CSF FTA.

Pediculosis and Scabies	
Pediculosis	**Scabies**
• Larger • In hair-bearing areas, such as the pubic area or axilla • Visible on the surface	• Small • Burrows in web spaces • Scrape and magnify
Treat with permethrin, pyrethrins, or lindane.	Treat with permethrin, lindane, or ivermectin.

Warts

All warts (condylomata acuminata, verrucous wart, molluscum contagiosum) are diagnosed by **how they look.** They are caused by human papillomavirus (HPV). They are treated with **mechanical removal.**

- Perform surgical removal if large.
- Imiquimod is an immunostimulant that leads to sloughing off of the wart.
- Cryotherapy, laser removal, and melting with podophyllin are other options.

Basic Science Correlate

Imiquimod stimulates the release of cytokines such as interferon, TNF-alpha, and interleukin-6. It also stimulates natural killer cells to get rid of HPV infected cells and malignant cells that are not melanoma. Imiquimod is indicated for basal cell cancer, actinic keratosis, and minor squamous cell cancer, in addition to venereal warts.

Urinary Tract Infection

First line in cystitis:

- fosfomycin
- nitrofurantion

Cystitis

This often presents with **urinary frequency, urgency, burning,** and **dysuria.** Young, otherwise healthy women are the most common presenting cases.

Diagnostic Testing

- Best initial test: **Urinalysis**
- Most accurate test: **Urine culture**

Treatment

- **Uncomplicated cystitis** is treated with **TMP/SMX orally for 3 days,** if *E. coli* resistance in that area is low. If resistance is > 20 percent, then use **ciprofloxacin** or **levofloxacin.** Other options are **nitrofurantoin and fosfomycin**. Quinolones work, but we want to preserve their use for more serious infections. Fosfomycin and nitrofurantoin are considered safe in pregnancy and are class B.
- **"Complicated" cystitis** is treated with **7 days of TMP/SMX** or **ciprofloxacin.** *Complicated* means an anatomic abnormality is present, such as a stone, stricture, tumor, or obstruction.

A 25-year-old, generally healthy woman comes to the office with burning on urination. There are 50 white cells on the urinalysis. What is the next best step in management?

a. Wait for results of urine culture.
b. Obtain urine culture.
c. Treat with TMP/SMX for 3 days.
d. Treat with ciprofloxacin for 7 days.
e. Perform a renal ultrasound.

Answer: **C.** When there are clear symptoms of cystitis and white cells in the urine, it is not necessary to obtain a urine culture or to wait for results of either the culture or a sonogram. For uncomplicated cystitis, go straight to treatment for 3 days. Ultrasound is important in male patients, as it is unusual for a male patient to have a urinary tract infection in the absence of an anatomic abnormality.

Asymptomatic bacteriuria: Only pregnant women should be treated. Do *not* treat asymptomatic bacteriuria, unless the patient is pregnant.

Pyelonephritis

Patient presents with urinary frequency, urgency, burning, and dysuria in the same way as cystitis, *and* there is **flank pain** and **tenderness.** Pyelonephritis is also a more severe disease, so there is a higher fever and the patient is much more ill.

Diagnostic Testing

- Urinalysis and urine culture the same as for cystitis

Treatment

Any of the medications for gram-negative bacilli are effective. **Ciprofloxacin** is recommended for outpatient treatment. For inpatient therapy use ceftriaxone, ertapenem, quinolones, ampicillin, and gentamicin.

Radiologic Testing and Urinary Tract Infections

Neither cystitis nor pyelonephritis is diagnosed by a radiologic study (sonogram or CT). Sonography and CT scanning are used to determine the etiology of a urinary tract infection.

If there is pyelonephritis...Is there a stone? Stricture? Tumor? Obstruction? Is there an anatomic defect that has led to the infection that must be corrected so that the infection will not recur?

- Dysuria + white cells in urine + suprapubic tenderness = **cystitis**
- Dysuria + white cells in urine + flank pain + fever = **pyelonephritis**

> Urinalysis: For infections, the concern is mainly with the presence of **white cells (WBC).** Numerous squamous epithelial cells suggest an improperly collected specimen, and unless symptomatic, do not treat.
>
> **Leukocyte esterase** is derived from granulocytic white blood cells and serves as indirect evidence of the presence of bacteriuria.
>
> **Nitrites** are indicative of gram-negative bacteria. Protein is very nonspecific in a urinalysis. Protein can be from both infection and glomerular disorders. Red cells are nonspecific as well.

Perinephric Abscess

This is a rare complication of pyelonephritis. Look for a patient with pyelonephritis who **does not respond to treatment after 5–7 days.** The patient remains febrile and still shows white cells on urinalysis. Perform a sonogram or CT of the kidneys to find the collection.

Diagnostic Testing

- **Biopsy:** This is the only way to determine a precise microbiologic diagnosis to guide therapy.

Treatment

- Treat with a **quinolone** and **add staphylococcal coverage** such as oxacillin nafcillin, or vancomycin, because treatment with antibiotics for gram-negative organisms preferentially selects out for staphylococci.

Prostatitis

This is indicated by **frequency, urgency,** and **dysuria** and **perineal or sacral pain.** There is tenderness of the prostate, and it may be described as "boggy" on examination.

Diagnostic Testing

- Best initial test: Urinalysis
- Most accurate test: Urine WBCs after prostate massage

Treatment

Treat with **ciprofloxacin** or **TMP/SMX** for an extended period of time (2 weeks for acute; 6 weeks for chronic). Prostatitis is like an abscess. Use the same drugs as for cystitis and pyelonephritis but extend the length of therapy.

Infective Endocarditis

Clinically, endocarditis is diagnosed by meeting **Duke's criteria** (2 major and 5 minor criteria). The diagnosis of endocarditis is made by the presence of 2 major, 1 major *and* 3 minor, or 5 minor criteria.

Duke's Criteria for Endocarditis	
Major	**Minor**
Two positive blood cultures with • *Staphylococcus aureus* • Viridans streptococci, ***Streptococcus bovis/epidermis,*** enterococci, gram-negative rods, **Candida** HACEK organisms are generally culture-negative. • ***Haemophilus aphrophilus/parainfluenzae*** • ***Actinobacillus actinomycetemcomitans*** • ***Cardiobacterium hominis*** • ***Eikenella corrodens*** • ***Kingella kingae***	Fever (> 38.0°C)
Abnormal echocardiogram: • Intracardiac mass or valvular vegetation OR • Abscess OR • New partial dehiscence of prosthetic valve	Presence of risk factors: • IV drug use (IDU) • Presence of structural heart disease • Prosthetic heart valve • Dental procedures involving bleeding • History of endocarditis
	Vascular findings: • Janeway lesions • Septic pulmonary infarcts • Arterial emboli • Mycotic aneurysm • Conjunctival hemorrhage
	Immunological findings: • Roth spots • Osler's nodes • Glomerulonephritis
	Microbiologic findings • Positive blood culture but does not meet major criteria

Look for a patient with a risk such as the following:

- Prosthetic heart valve
- Injection drug use
- Dental procedures that cause bleeding
- Previous endocarditis
- Unrepaired or recently repaired cyanotic heart disease

Fever + Murmer = Possible endocarditis. **Do blood cultures.**

2 positive blood cultures + Positive echo = Endocarditis.

When there is **fever** and a **new murmur or change in a murmur,** the "best next step" in management is to **perform blood cultures first.** If the blood cultures are positive, then perform an **echocardiogram** to look for vegetations.

Other physical findings are rarely seen but are useful in establishing the diagnosis of endocarditis if the blood cultures are negative:

- Roth spots (retina)
- Janeway lesions (flat, painless in hands and feet)
- Osler's nodes (raised, painful, and pea shaped)
- Splinter hemorrhages (under fingernails)

Diagnostic Testing

	Transthoracic Echocardiogram (TTE)	Transesophageal Echocardiogram (TEE)
Sensitivity	60%	90–95%
Specificity	90–95%	90–95%
	If TTE is negative, then proceed to TEE.	

The most common causes of culture-negative endocarditis are no longer the HACEK group of organisms. The most common causes are Coxiella and Bartonella, which together account for 80% of cases. *Clostridium septicum* is even more frequently associated with colonic pathology than *Streptococcus bovis.*

Treatment

- The *best* empiric therapy is **vancomycin and gentamicin in combination.** This will cover the most common organisms, which are *S. aureus,* MRSA, and viridans group streptococci. You do *not* need to cover empirically for fungi or resistant gram-negative rods, since these are less common. Treatment is for 4–6 weeks.
- ***S. bovis* or *Clostridium septicum:*** Perform **colonoscopy.** Both are is associated with colonic pathology.
- **Surgery (valve replacement):** The strongest indications for surgery are **anatomic defects,** which are hard or impossible to correct with antibiotics alone, including:
  - Valve rupture
  - Abscess
  - Prosthetic valves
  - Fungal endocarditis
  - Embolic events once already started on antibiotics

Endocarditis Prophylaxis

The *only* **cardiac defects** that need prophylaxis are the following:

- Prosthetic valves
- Unrepaired cyanotic heart disease
- Previous endocarditis
- Transplant recipients who develop valve disease

The *only* **procedures** that need prophylaxis are the following:

- Dental procedures that cause bleeding: The prophylactic antibiotic to use for dental procedures is **amoxicillin.** For penicillin-allergic patients, clindamycin is the drug of choice.
- Respiratory tract surgery
- Surgery of infected skin

The following **procedures** do ***not*** need prophylaxis:

- Dental fillings
- All flexible scopes
- All OB/GYN procedures
- All urinary procedures, including cystoscopy

The following **cardiac defects** do ***not*** need prophylaxis:

- Aortic stenosis or regurgitation
- Mitral stenosis or regurgitation
- Atrial or ventricular septal defects
- Pacemakers and implantable defibrillators
- Mitral valve prolapse, even if there is a murmur
- HOCM (IHSS)

What is **the drug to give** as prophylaxis?

- Dental/oral procedures:
  - Amoxicillin
  - If rash to penicillin: Cephalexin
  - If anaphylaxis to penicillin: Azithromycin, clarithromycin, or clindamycin
- Skin procedures:
  - Cephalexin
  - If allergic to penicillin: Vancomycin

HIV/AIDS

Following are the "must know" facts about HIV:

- Adverse effects of medications
- Needle-stick injury management
- Pregnancy/perinatal HIV management

When to start therapy?

- CD4 count < 500 without exception
- Symptomatic patients with any CD4 count or viral load
- Pregnant women: All of them, any stage of pregnancy, any CD4
- Needle-stick scenario, where patient is known to be HIV-positive
- Optional at any CD4 count, even > 500

Monotherapy with AZT alone is **never** the right answer for anyone.

Start **triple highly active antiretroviral therapy (HAART),** which is one of the following:

- Tenofovir *and* emtricitabine *and* an integrase inhibitor
- Tenofovir *and* emtricitabine *and* efavirenz (single combination pill with all of these)
- Tenofovir *and* emtricitabine *and* atazanavir (or darunavir)

When a protease inhibitor such as atazanavir or darunavir is used in combination with tenofovir and emtricitabine, you should add a small amount of ritonavir to boost the level of the other protease inhibitors.

Dolutegravir, elvitegravir, and raltegravir are integrase inhibitors that are used with two nucleosides, such as tenofovir and emtricitabine. This three-drug combination is considered equivalent to the combination with efavirenz or a protease inhibitor. The precise combination is not as important as knowing the adverse effects of the medications.

Class	Nucleoside Reverse Transcriptase Inhibitors	Protease Inhibitors	Nonnucleoside Reverse Transcriptase Inhibitors	Integrase Inhibitors
Adverse effects of the class	Lactic acidosis	Hyperglycemia Hyperlipidemia	Drowsiness (efavirenz)	
Individual medications	Zidovudine: Anemia Didanosine: Pancreatitis and peripheral neuropathy Stavudine: Pancreatitis and neuropathy Lamivudine: None Abacavir: Rash Emtricitabine Tenofovir: Renal toxicity	Indinavir: Kidney stones Ritonavir Lopinavir Nelfinavir Saquinavir Darunavir Tipranavir Amprenavir Atazanavir	Efavirenz Nevirapine Etravirine Rilpivirine	Raltegravir Elvitegravir Dolutegravir

Basic Science Correlate

Raltegravir, elvitegravir, and dolutegravir are integrase inhibitors. This agent prevents the integration of the genetic material of the HIV virus from being integrated into the CD4 cell chromosome. HIV is an RNA virus. Reverse transcriptase turns it into DNA, and this viral DNA must be integrated into human DNA in order to be reproduced. This is the step blocked by the integrase inhibitor raltegravir.

Basic Science Correlate

Chemokine receptor 5 (CCR5) is the mechanism whereby the HIV virus enters the CD4 cell. CCR5 is the attachment point of the GP120 on the surface of the HIV virus whereby it finds its way into human cells. Maraviroc is an entry inhibitor: Maraviroc blocks the CCR5 receptor.

Needle-Stick Injury (Postexposure Prophylaxis)

With any significant exposure to HIV-positive blood via a needle, scalpel, or penetrating injury, the answer is the same: **HAART for a month.** Tenofovir and emtricitabine are combined with raltegravir or a protease inhibitor.

This would also be true for the **exposure of mucosal surfaces** to HIV-positive blood or after **unprotected sexual contact** with a person known to be HIV-positive.

Basic Science Correlate

Ritonavir inhibits hepatic p450 systems—the route through which protease inhibitors are metabolized. A small amount of ritonavir blocks metabolism of the other protease inhibitors, allowing higher blood levels with less frequent dosing.

Pregnancy/Perinatal

- If the patient is already on antiretroviral therapy for her own health, then simply continue the same therapy.
- Mother-to-child transmission with fully suppressive anti-retroviral therapy is < 1%. Every HIV-positive pregnant woman should be on HIV medications regardless of the stage of her pregnancy or her CD4 count. Efavirenz is avoided in pregnancy. Protease inhibitors with 2 nucleosides—such as zidovudine and lamivudine—are best. Do not wait for the second trimester of pregnancy to start therapy.

Start HIV+ pregnant women on HIV medications in the first trimester and continue.

All HIV+ pregnant women at any CD4 or viral load need treatment.

Prophylaxis

Pneumocystis jiroveci Pneumonia (PCP) (< 200 CD4 cells)

- **TMP/SMX** is the *best* prophylaxis for PCP by far.
- If TMP/SMX causes a rash, switch to **atovaquone** or **dapsone.** (Dapsone *cannot* be used if there is G6PD deficiency.)
- Aerosolized pentamidine has the *poorest* efficacy and is rarely used. There is the most amount of breakthrough.

Mycobacterium Avium-Intracellulare (MAI) (< 50 CD4 cells)

- Use **azithromycin** once a week orally.

Opportunistic Infections

PCP

This presents with **shortness of breath, dry cough, hypoxia,** and **increased LDH.**

Diagnostic Testing

- Best initial test: A **chest x-ray** will show increased interstitial markings bilaterally.
- Most accurate test: **Bronchoalveolar lavage**

Treatment

- **IV TMP/SMX**
- If there is a rash, use **IV pentamidine** or the combination of clindamycin and primaquine.
- **Atovaquone** can be used for *mild* pneumocystis.
- **Dapsone** is not intravenous and is used for prophylaxis, *not* treatment.
- If PCP is severe ($pO_2 < 70$ or A-a gradient > 35), then give **steroids.**

> Ganciclovir: low WBC
> Foscarnet: high creatinine

Toxoplasmosis

Look for headache, nausea, vomiting, and focal neurologic findings. Best initial test is a **head CT with contrast** showing "ring" or contrast-enhancing lesions.

Treat with **pyrimethamine and sulfadiazine for 2 weeks** and repeat the CT scan. If the lesions are smaller, then this is confirmative of toxoplasmosis. If the lesions are unchanged in size, then perform a brain biopsy, since this is most likely lymphoma.

Cytomegalovirus (CMV)

HIV with < **50 CD4 cells** and **blurry vision.** Perform a dilated ophthalmologic examination. CMV is diagnosed by the appearance of the lesions on examination.

Treat with **ganciclovir** or **foscarnet.**

Maintenance therapy is with **oral valganciclovir lifelong,** unless the CD4 goes up with HAART. If the CD4 rises, you can stop the CMV medications.

Cryptococcus

HIV and < **50 CD4 cells** with **fever and headache.** Neck stiffness and photophobia are not always present. Perform a **lumbar puncture,** finding an increase in the level of lymphocytes in the CSF. The best initial test is an **India ink stain,** which has about a 60 percent sensitivity. The most accurate test is a **cryptococcal antigen test,** which is over 95 percent sensitive and specific.

Echinocandins such as caspofungin do **not** cover cryptococcus.

Treat initially with **amphotericin and 5-FC,** followed by **fluconazole.** The fluconazole is continued lifelong unless the CD4 count rises. If the CD4 count rises, all opportunistic infection treatment and prophylaxis can be stopped. The only treatment that cannot be stopped is the antiretrovirals.

HIV test everyone, no matter their risk.

Progressive Multifocal Leukoencephalopathy (PML)

HIV and < **50 CD4 cells** with **focal neurologic abnormalities.** The best initial test is a **head CT** or **MRI.** The lesions do *not* show ring enhancement and there is no mass effect. PCR of CSF for JC virus is most accurate.

There is *no* specific therapy available for PML. Treat with HAART. When the CD4 count rises, PML will resolve.

Mycobacterium Avium-Intracellulare (MAI)

HIV and < **50 CD4 cells.** There is wasting with **weight loss, fever,** and **fatigue. Anemia** is frequent from invasion of the bone marrow. Increased alkaline phosphatase and GGTP with a normal bilirubin is characteristic of hepatic involvement.

Below this box is the 90th percentile area. This is lower-yield material. If you *only* need to pass the exam, you do not need to read this. If you do not have a residency yet, and your Step 3 grade will be seen to make an admission decision, you should read and learn the material below to try to get a 95 or higher.

Diagnostic testing: **Bone marrow** is more sensitive. **Liver biopsy** is the most sensitive. Blood culture is the least sensitive.

Treatment: **Clarithromycin and ethambutol.** Prophylaxis with **azithromycin. Rifabutin** is sometimes added to therapy.

Animal-Borne Diseases

Leptospirosis

This is a spirochete. There is some form of **exposure to animals** in the history. The patient has eaten food contaminated by the urine of infected animals. There is **fever, abdominal pain,** and **muscle aches** as well. Severe disease leads to altered mental status.

Diagnostic Testing and Treatment

Diagnose with serology. Treat with **ceftriaxone** or **penicillin.**

Animal exposure + Jaundice + Renal = Leptospirosis

Tularemia

Involves contact with **rabbits** in the summer. Look for a hunter or someone who has touched a small, furry animal. There is an **ulcer at the site of contact** and **enlarged lymph nodes. Conjunctivitis** is another clue.

Diagnostic Testing and Treatment

Diagnose with **serology.** Note that taking a culture is dangerous, as spores can cause severe pneumonia in lab personnel. Treat with **gentamicin** or **streptomycin**

Cysticercosis

Diagnostic Testing and Treatment

The CT scan of the head will show **thin-walled cysts,** which are most often **calcified.** This disease is often transmitted by **infected pork** that is ingested. Infection is most likely in those who have eaten pork in endemic areas such as Mexico, South America, Eastern Europe, or India.

Treat with **albendazole.**

If there are no active lesions and the patient only presents with calcifications and seizures, then all that is necessary is anti-epileptic therapy. Many people have had cysticercosis in the past. After the active infection is gone, all that remains is calcification.

Camping/hiking + Target-shaped rash = Lyme disease

Tick-Borne Diseases

Lyme

For USMLE, **camping and hiking** is a marker for the presence of **ticks.** Only 20 percent of those with Lyme disease remember the tick bite, because it is so small. The **rash** is shaped like **a target with a pale center and a red ring on the outside.** The cause is a spirochete named *Borrelia burgdorferi,* which is carried by the *Ixodes* genus (deer) tick. The question may say something about vacationing in the Northeast or Midwest. States in this region are Connecticut, Delaware, Maine, Maryland, Massachusetts, Minnesota, New Hampshire, New York, New Jersey, Pennsylvania, and Wisconsin.

The proper term is "**erythema migrans,**" but this is not a term that has a precise meaning.

A 43-year-old man presents with a target-shaped rash that has developed over the last several days. He was on a camping trip in the woods last week in Maine. What is the next best step in management?

a. Serology for IgM
b. ELISA
c. Western blot
d. Doxycycline
e. Ceftriaxone

Answer: **D.** A rash suggestive of Lyme is enough to indicate treatment. A 5-cm-wide target-shaped rash, particularly with a history of camping/hiking, is enough to indicate the need for antibiotic treatment with doxycycline. A characteristic rash is more specific than serology. Ceftriaxone is used for CNS or cardiac Lyme.

Long-term manifestations/complications of Lyme are as follows:

- Joint involvement—the most common **late** manifestation
- Cardiac—most common is **AV conduction block/defect**
- Neurologic—most common is **7th cranial nerve palsy (Bell's palsy)**

Diagnostic Testing

Manifestation of Lyme are diagnosed with serology, such as IgM, IgG ELISA, Western blot, or PCR.

Treatment

- Rash, joint, Bell's palsy: **Oral doxycycline, amoxicillin,** or **cefuroxime**
- CNS or cardiac involvement: **IV ceftriaxone**

There is *no* "chronic" Lyme disease.

Babesiosis

Babesiosis is transmitted by the same *Ixodes* (deer) tick that transmits Lyme. As a result, it is also common in the northeast. It manifests with **hemolytic anemia** and is severe in asplenic individuals.

Basic Science Correlate

Asplenic patients have more Babesia because a functional spleen removes infected cells from circulation. When Babesia infects a red cell, it further deforms the cell. The spleen detects this deformity and removes the cell before Babesia can reproduce.

Diagnostic Testing

Diagnose with a **peripheral blood smear** looking for tetrads of intraerythrocytic ring forms or do a **PCR.**

Treatment

- **Azithromycin** and **atovaquone**

Ehrlichia/Anaplasma

This, too, is transmitted by the *Ixodes* tick. There is **no rash.** Instead, there are elevated liver function tests (ALT and AST), **thrombocytopenia** (decreased platelets), and **leukopenia** (decreased white blood cells).

Diagnostic Testing

Diagnose with a **peripheral blood smear** looking for "morulae," which are inclusion bodies in the white cells, or do **PCR.**

Treatment

- **Doxycycline**

Malaria

This disease is rarely domestic. Look for a traveler recently returning from an endemic area with **hemolysis. GI complaints** are always present.

Diagnostic Testing

- **Blood smear**

The same drugs can be used for acute treatment and prophylaxis of **malaria**:

- Mefloquine
- Atovaquone/proguanil

Treatment

- **Acute disease** is treated with **mefloquine** or **atovaquone/proguanil** or **quinine/doxycycline** in very severe cases.
- **Prophylaxis** is with **mefloquine** (weekly) or **atovaquone/proguanil** (Malarone; administered daily). Daily doxycycline has been used for prophylaxis but would not be the best answer. Those being given mefloquine should be advised of neuropsychiatric side effects, sinus bradycardia, and QT prolongation.

Respiratory Diseases

Nocardia

Nocardia gives **branching, gram-positive filaments** that are weakly acid fast.

This involves **immunocompromised people** (leukemia, lymphoma, steroid use, HIV). Respiratory/pulmonary disease may disseminate to any organ, with skin and brain being the most common.

Diagnostic Testing

- Best initial test: **Chest x-ray**
- Most accurate test: **Culture**

Treatment

- **TMP/SMX**

Actinomyces

Host has a **normal immune system.** There is a history of **facial or dental trauma,** which inoculated these organisms into the cervicofacial area. *Actinomyces* is a part of normal mouth flora. Trauma, such as a tooth extraction, can put it into the facial area, thorax, and abdomen.

Diagnostic Testing

Diagnose with **Gram stain** and confirm with **anaerobic culture.** Like *Nocardia, Actinomyces* is a **branching, filamentous bacteria.**

Treatment

- **Penicillin**

Histoplasmosis

Look for **wet areas,** such as the Ohio and Mississippi River valleys. This lung disease that can present as a viral syndrome is also associated with **bat droppings from caves.** A physical exam will show **palate and oral ulcers** and **splenomegaly.**

The disseminated disease enters the bone marrow and causes **pancytopenia.** Anything tuberculosis can do, histoplasmosis can do.

Diagnostic Testing

- Best initial test: **Histoplasmosis urine antigen**
- Most accurate test: **Biopsy with culture** is most accurate for *both* histoplasmosis and tuberculosis

Treatment

- Acute pulmonary disease is transient and requires *no* therapy.
- The disseminated disease is treated with **amphotericin.**

Coccidioidomycosis

This is an acute respiratory illness that occurs in **very dry areas** like Arizona. It causes **joint pain** and **erythema nodosum.**

Treatment

- **Itraconazole**

Blastomycosis

This is an acute pulmonary disease in the **rural southeast.** Look for **broad budding yeast.**

Bone lesions are common.

- Broad budding yeast = blastomycosis

Treatment

- Antifungal agents, such as **amphotericin** or **itraconazole**

Allergy and Immunology

2

Anaphylaxis

Anaphylaxis is a hypersensitivity/allergic reaction that is potentially life threatening. The most common causes are foods (e.g., peanuts, shellfish, etc.). Other causes include:

- **Insect stings/bites**
- **Medications** (e.g., penicillin, allopurinol, sulfa-containing drugs)

Anaphylaxis presents as **hemodynamic instability** with **hypotension and tachycardia** as well as **difficulty breathing.**

Treatment

Anaphylaxis treatment has been unchanged for decades. The best initial therapy is to administer all of the following:

- **Intramuscular epinephrine in a 1:1,000 concentration**
- **Corticosteroids**
- H1-inhibiting antihistamines, such as **diphenhydramine** or **hydroxyzine**

CCS Tip: Remember that CCS does *not* require you to know doses, but you must know the route of administration and the type of the medication. Hence, you must know to give the epinephrine **intramuscularly.**

Basic Science Correlate

Epinephrine will cause vasoconstriction through alpha-1 receptor stimulation. The beta-2 receptor stimulation effect dilates bronchi. Corticosteroids need 4–6 hours to work, and they increase vasoconstriction by up-regulating alpha-1 receptors. Steroids also inhibit leukotriene release.

Angioedema

Angioedema is a **sudden swelling of the face, palate, tongue, and airway** in association with **minor trauma to the face or hands** or the **ingestion of ACE inhibitors.** The question may describe a **person hit in the face with a pillow** or **wood chips hitting the arm.** The hereditary form occurs from **deficiency of C1 esterase inhibitor.** Other symptoms include:

- Stridor
- Abdominal pain
- A lack of response to steroids

Consider placing people with angioedema in the ICU.

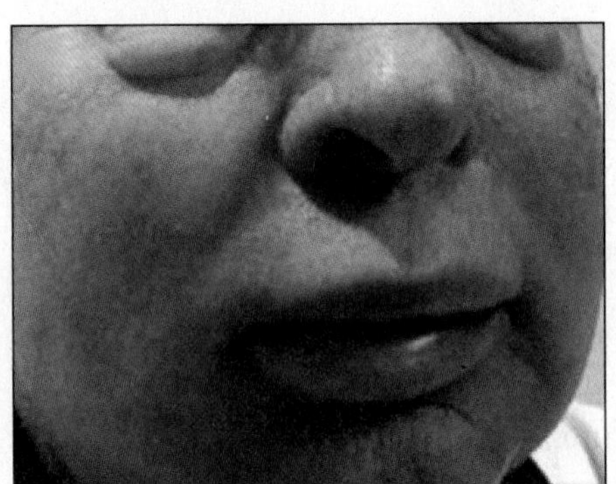

Angioedema Face

Diagnostic Testing

The diagnosis of angioedema arising from C1 esterase deficiency is based on finding **low levels of C2 and C4 in the complement pathway.** They are chronically depleted because of the deficiency of the C1 esterase inhibitor. An elevated white cell count is *not* specific.

Treatment

- **Infusion of fresh frozen plasma** (acute episodes)
- Chronic episodes: Ecallantide and icatibant are the drugs of choice for hereditary angioedema. **Androgens** are also used for chronic therapy. C1 inhibitors concentrate is also available. Androgens, for unknown reasons, raise the levels of C1 esterase inhibitor. The most frequently used androgens are **danazol** and **stanazol.**

Ecallantide, an inhibitor of kallikrein, is the best initial therapy for angioedema. Ecallantide blocks bradykinin production.

A patient comes to the emergency department with shortness of breath, facial swelling, and lip swelling 30 minutes after a bee sting. There was no response to epi-pen injection in the field. Six hours after a bolus of steroid and diphenhydramine, the patient is still short of breath and still has lip swelling.

Where should the patient be placed?

Answer: This patient should be placed in the intensive care unit. If the patient comes with anaphylaxis from any cause, the placement of the patient for CCS is based entirely on the response to therapy that occurs after treatment. In this case, the source of the allergic reaction, an insect sting, is irrelevant. What matters is that after moving the clock forward, the symptoms do not resolve. Any persistent lip, facial, or hemodynamic involvement after initial therapy should place the patient in the ICU.

A man comes in with neurosyphilis. He has a history of life-threatening anaphylaxis to penicillin. He has a history of essential tremor and is on propranolol. He has asthma and is on an inhaled beta agonist and inhaled steroids.

Which of the following is most appropriate?

a. Use ceftriaxone instead of penicillin
b. Stop propranolol prior to desensitizing him
c. Bolus with oral steroids prior to penicillin use
d. Add long acting beta agonists to treatment

Answer: **B.** Neurosyphilis is only effectively treated with penicillin. The patient must be desensitized. Prior for desensitization it is important to stop propranolol and all beta blockers. This is because epinephrine may have to be used in the event of anaphylaxis when you desensitize the patient. Bolusing with steroids in inappropriate, because anaphylaxis is treated first with epinephrine.

Allergic Rhinitis

Allergic rhinitis presents with **recurrent episodes of nasal itching, stuffiness, rhinorrhea, and paroxysms of sneezing.** There is also often **eye itching** and **dermatitis.** Allergic rhinitis may be associated with the development of asthma. Many patients present with wheezing as well.

Treatment

Avoidance

The mainstay of all therapy for those with extrinsic allergies is the **avoidance of the allergen.** It is important to close windows and stay in air-conditioned rooms to avoid pollen. In addition, an allergy to animal dander may mean avoiding a pet. Mattresses and pillows must be covered with mite and dust-proof casings.

Drug Therapy

- **Intranasal corticosteroids**
- **Antihistamines** such as loratadine, fexofenadine, and cetirizine
- **Intranasal antihistamines** (azelastine)
- **Cromolyn**
- **Ipratropium bromide**
- **Leukotriene inhibitors** (e.g., montelukast)
- **Nasal saline spray and wash**

Intranasal steroids are the single most effective treatment for allergic rhinitis.

Basic Science Correlate

Cromolyn and nedocromil work by stabilizing mast cells. They prevent degranulation of mast cells so that histamine and leukotrienes are not released. This mechanism is entirely preventive in nature: After exposure to the allergen has stimulated the mast cells, cromolyn will not work.

Immunotherapy

For extrinsic allergens that cannot be avoided, **desensitization** therapy may work. Use of beta blockers *must* be stopped before desensitization. If anaphylaxis occurs during desensitization, then epinephrine is used—*but* if the person is on a beta blocker, it will block the action of epinephrine. The need to stop beta blockers before desensitization is a favorite Step 3 question.

Primary Immunodeficiency Syndromes

Common Variable Immunodeficiency (CVID)

CVID presents in *both* men and women and may only present when the patient is an adult. Both CVID and X-linked agammaglobulinemia present with **recurrent episodes of sinopulmonary infections,** such as bronchitis, sinusitis, pneumonia, and pharyngitis. In addition, CVID causes a **spruelike abdominal disorder.** There is malabsorption, steatorrhea, and diarrhea. Lymph nodes, adenoids, and the spleen are present and may be enlarged.

Diagnostic Testing

The machinery to make immunoglobulins is intact. The nodes and both B and T cells are present, but they do not make enough antibody. Hence **total IgG levels are low.**

Treatment

CVID is treated with **infusions of intravenous immunoglobulins.**

X-Linked Agammaglobulinemia (Bruton's)

This presents in **male children with recurrent sinopulmonary infections.**

Diagnostic Testing

Lymph nodes, adenoids, and the spleen are diminished in size or absent. **B cells** are missing, as are the **immunoglobulins.**

Treatment

Like CVID, X-linked agammaglobulinemia is treated with **infusions of intravenous immunoglobulins.**

IgA Deficiency

This is the most common primary immunodeficiency. Many people are asymptomatic. Some have **recurrent sinopulmonary infections.** There is also a **spruelike malabsorption syndrome** as well as an increased incidence of **atopic conditions.** Some people present with **anaphylaxis** when receiving blood from donors who are not IgA deficient.

Treatment

Treat the infections as they arise. Intravenous immunoglobulins will not work since it has little IgA in it.

Hyper IgE Syndrome

Hyper IgE syndrome presents with **recurrent skin infections caused by *Staphylococcus.***

Treatment

Treat the infections as they arise.

A 3-year-old boy comes in with recurrent sinopulmonary infections. There are no nodes palpated in the cervical area and no tonsils seen on oral exam. The child has been treated for an infection nearly every 1–2 months since birth. There are no skin infections.

What is the most likely diagnosis?

a. Hyper IgE syndrome
b. IgA deficiency
c. X-linked agammaglobulinemia
d. Common variable immunodeficiency

Answer: **C.** X-linked agammaglobulinemia is exclusively in male children, whereas common variable immunodeficiency presents in adults. The absence of skin infection in this case goes strongly against hyper IgE syndrome. These patients are best managed with intravenous immunoglobulin infusions on a regular basis and with antibiotics for infections as episodes arise.

Cardiology

3

Ischemic Heart Disease

Coronary artery disease (CAD) is the most common cause of death, by far, in the United States, and kills 10 times more women than breast cancer.

Risk factors are useful for 2 things:

1. Helping answer diagnostic questions in equivocal cases
2. Modifying them can lower mortality

For family history to be significant as a risk factor, the family member must be young (female relatives < 65, male relatives < 55).

Emotional stress is *not* a clear risk factor. It is not possible to measure precisely.

Coronary artery disease (CAD) presents with chest pain that does *not* change with body position or respiration. CAD is *not* associated with chest wall tenderness. The single worst or most dangerous factor for CAD is diabetes. When any one of the following 3 features is present, the patient does *not* have CAD.

Risk factors include the following:

- Diabetes mellitus
- Hypertension
- Tobacco use
- Hyperlipidemia
- Peripheral arterial disease (PAD)
- Obesity
- Inactivity
- Family history

Pleuritic Pain (changes with respiration)	Positional Pain (changes with bodily position)	Tenderness (pain on palpation)
Pulmonary embolism Pneumonia Pleuritis Pericarditis Pneumothorax	Pericarditis	Costochondritis

The most common cause of chest pain that is *not* cardiac in etiology is a gastrointestinal (acid reflux) problem.

a. A patient comes to the emergency department with chest pain. The pain also occurs in the epigastric area and is associated with a sore throat, a bad metallic taste in the mouth, and a cough. What do you recommend?
b. An alcoholic patient comes to the emergency department with chest pain. There is nausea and vomiting and epigastric tenderness. What do you recommend?
c. A patient comes to the emergency department with chest pain. There is right-upper quadrant tenderness and mild fever. What do you recommend?

Answers:

a. Give a proton pump inhibitor.
b. Check amylase and lipase levels.
c. Order an abdominal sonogram for gallstones.

Besides chest pain, other **clues to ischemic disease** as the cause of chest pain are as follows:

- Dull pain
- Lasts 15–30 minutes
- Occurs on exertion
- Substernal location
- Radiates to the jaw or left arm

Physical Findings

There is nothing unique or pathognomonic about the physical findings of ischemic heart disease. Physical findings such as tenderness only tell you the patient does *not* have ischemic disease. There is no buzzword for physical examination of CAD that indicates, "Aha! This is coronary disease." However, for CCS, it is critical to know what could be abnormal so you know which pieces of the physical to choose.

Piece of Physical Exam	Findings That *Could* Be Abnormal
Cardiovascular (CV)	S3 gallop: Dilated left ventricle S4 gallop: Left ventricular hypertrophy Jugulovenous distention Holosystolic murmur of mitral regurgitation
Chest	Rales suggestive of congestive heart failure
General exam	Distressed patient, short of breath, clutching chest
Extremities	Edema

Basic Science Correlate

The mechanism of an S3 gallop is rapid ventricular filling during diastole. As soon as the mitral valve opens, blood rushes into the ventricle, causing a splash sound transmitted as an S3.

S4 gallop is the sound of atrial systole into a stiff or noncompliant left ventricle. It is heard just before S1 and occurs with any type of left ventricular hypertrophy. S4 is the bang of atrial systole.

Holosystolic Murmur

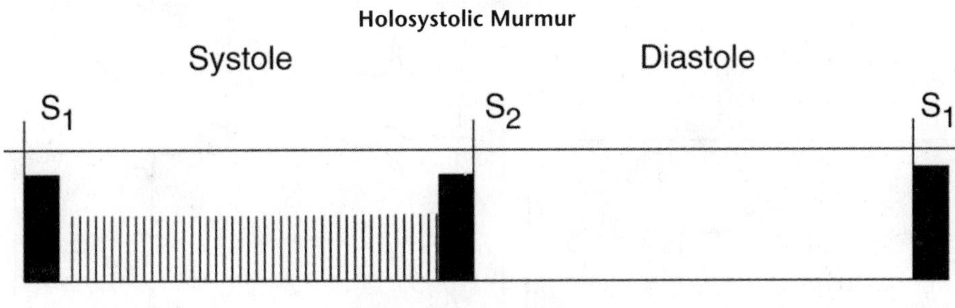

Mitral Regurgitation

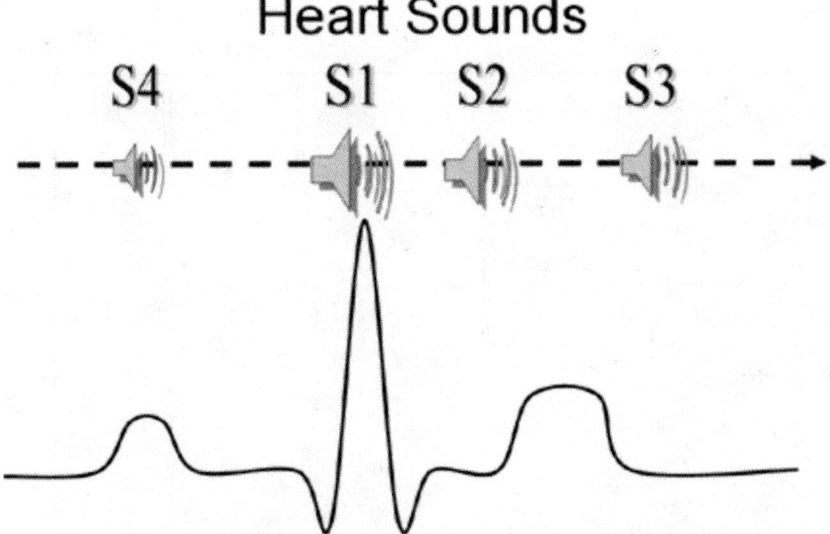

CCS Tip: Jugular veins on Step 3 CCS are in the CV exam, *not* the HEENT exam.

Diagnostic Testing

The vast majority of chest pain cases on Step 3 will hand you a clear case in terms of diagnosis and ask you what to do next in the management. An EKG is *always* the best initial diagnostic test for ischemic-type pain. If the case presented to you is **very clearly a case of ischemic pain** and the examiners ask you to **choose** between an EKG and aspirin, nitrates, oxygen, and morphine, then choose **treatment first.**

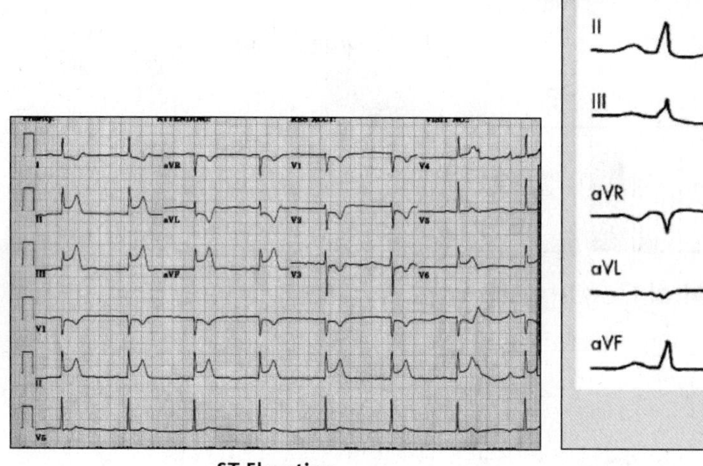

ST Elevation

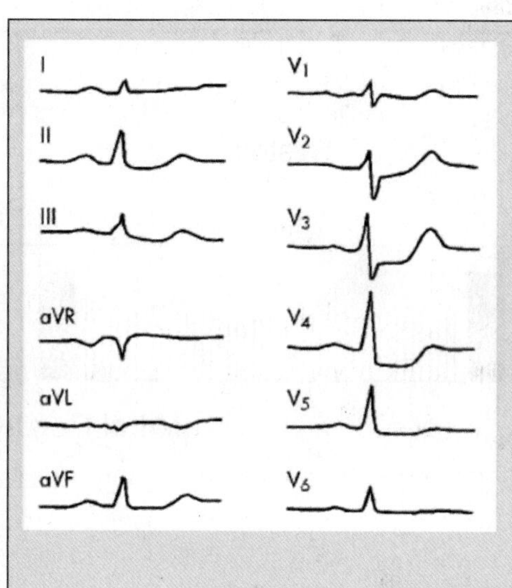

ST Depression

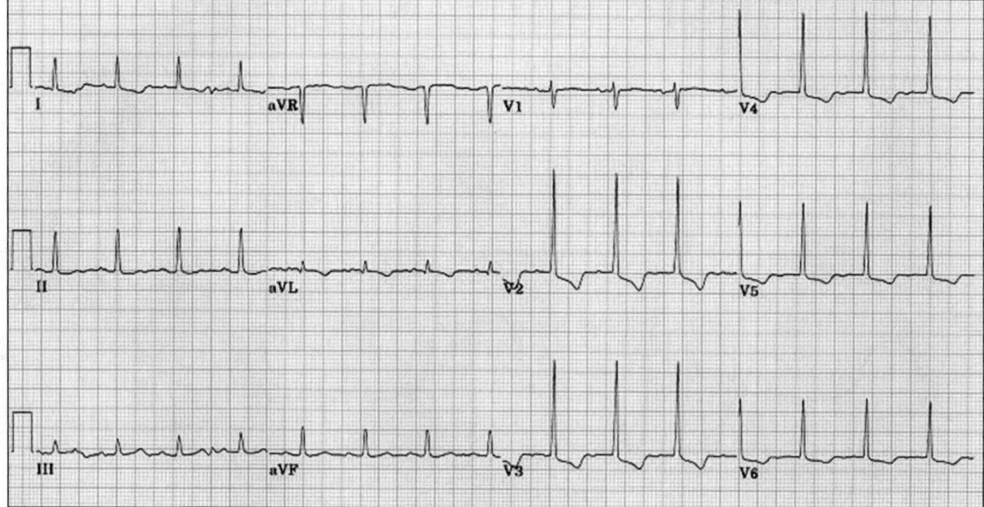

T Wave Inversion

The *wrong* "best initial tests" or steps are troponin, CK-MB, stress testing, echocardiogram, or angiography. These tests do *not* eliminate the need to **give aspirin first.** In a computerized CCS, however, answer *all* of these at the same time.

> Do not answer "consultation" for single best answer questions. However, "consultation" is okay to answer as a part of CCS management. In single best answer questions, a consultant should not be necessary when ordering an EKG, checking enzymes, and giving aspirin to a patient with acute coronary syndrome.

CCS Tip: When the question asks what the *most accurate* test is, answer CK-MB or troponin.

CK-MB and troponin levels both rise at 3–6 hours after the start of chest pain. They have nearly the same specificity. The **main difference between CK-MB and troponin** is that CK-MB only stays elevated 1–2 days while troponin stays elevated for 1–2 weeks. Therefore, CK-MB testing is the best test to detect a reinfarction a few days after the initial infarction.

CCS Tip: *Always* the wrong answer: LDH level or LDH isoenzymes.

Basic Science Correlate

Troponin C: Binds to calcium to activate actin:myosin interaction

Troponin T: Binds to tropomyosin

Troponin I: Blocks or inhibits actin:myosin interaction

Myoglobin elevates as early as 1–4 hours after the start of chest pain. Myoglobin is the answer to the question "Which of the following will rise first?" when the choices are all cardiac enzymes.

Stress testing is the answer when the case is *not* acute and the initial EKG and/or enzyme tests do *not* establish the diagnosis.

A 56-year-old man comes to the office a few days after an episode of chest pain. This was his first episode of pain, and he has no risk factors. In the emergency department, he had a normal EKG and normal CK-MB and was released the next day. Which of the following is most appropriate in his further management?

a. Repeat CK-MB
b. Statin
c. LDL level
d. Stress (exercise tolerance) testing
e. Angiography

Answer: **D.** Stress test when the case is equivocal or uncertain for the presence of CAD. Do not do an angiography unless the stress test is abnormal. Exercise tolerance, or "stress," testing detects coronary artery disease when the heart rate is raised and ST segment depression is detected. This case is asking you to know that **a stress test is a way of increasing the sensitivity of detection of CAD beyond an EKG and enzymes.**

CCS Tip: Step 3 loves the phrase "further management."

When do I answer dipyridamole or adenosine thallium stress test or dobutamine echo?	When do I answer exercise thallium testing or stress echocardiography?
Patients who cannot exercise to a target heart rate of > 85% of maximum: • COPD • Amputation • Deconditioning • Weakness/previous stroke • Lower-extremity ulcer • Dementia • Obesity	EKG is unreadable for ischemia: • Left bundle branch block • Digoxin use • Pacemaker in place • Left ventricular hypertrophy • Any baseline abnormality of the ST segment of the EKG

Sestamibi nuclear stress testing is used in obese patients and those with large breasts because of the greater ability of this radioisotope to penetrate tissue.

A 63-year-old woman is in your office for evaluation of an abnormal stress test that shows an area of reversible ischemia. She has no risk factors for CAD. What is the most accurate diagnostic test, or what is the best next step in further management?

a. Troponin level
b. Angiography
c. Coronary bypass
d. Echocardiogram
e. Nuclear ventriculogram (MUGA scan)

Answer: **B.** Angiography is the next diagnostic test to evaluate an abnormal stress test that shows "reversible" ischemia. **Reversible ischemia** is the most dangerous thing that a stress test can show. If the stress test shows "fixed" defects—that is, a defect unchanged between exercise and rest—this is a scar from a previous infarction. Fixed defects do not need angiography. **Coronary bypass** is the answer only if the angiogram has already been done. **Echocardiography** is the best initial test to evaluate valve function or ventricular wall motion. **Nuclear ventriculogram** is the most accurate method to evaluate ejection fraction.

Basic Science Correlate

Mechanism of Thallium

Nuclear isotopes are picked up by the Na/K ATPase of normal myocardium. If cardiac tissue is alive and perfused, it will pick up the nuclear isotope. To the myocardium, thallium looks like potassium.

Decreased uptake = Damage

A patient admitted 5 days ago for a myocardial infarction has a new episode of chest pain. Which of the following is the most specific method of establishing the diagnosis of a new infarction?

a. CK-MB
b. Troponin
c. Echocardiogram
d. Stress testing
e. Angiography

Answer: **A.** The CK-MB level should return to normal 2–3 days after a myocardial infarction. If a reinfarction has occurred, the level will go back up again 5 days later, while the troponin level will still be up from the original infarction. Angiography can detect obstructive, stenotic lesions but cannot detect myocardial necrosis. Stress testing should **never** be performed if the patient is having current chest pain; chest pain is a reason to stop a stress test. Echo will show decreased wall movement, but this could have been present from the previous cardiac injury.

Acute Coronary Syndrome (ACS)

The definition of **acute coronary syndrome (ACS)** is as follows:

- Causes acute chest pain
- Can be with exercise or at rest
- Can have ST segment elevation, depression, or even a normal EKG
- Not based on enzyme levels, angiography, or stress test results
- Based on a history of chest pain with features suggestive of ischemic disease

Treatment

Aspirin

The best initial therapy for all cases of ACS is **aspirin.** Aspirin can be administered orally or chewed and absorbed under the tongue. It has an **instant effect on inhibiting platelets.** Aspirin alone reduces mortality by 25 percent for acute myocardial infarction and by 50 percent for "unstable angina," which may become a non-ST segment elevation myocardial infarction (NSTEMI). **Nitrates and morphine** should also be administered in acute coronary syndromes, but they do *not* lower mortality. Oxygen has no benefit if the patient is not hypoxic.

Clopidogrel or **ticagrelor** is added to aspirin for all patients with acute myocardial infarction. **Prasugrel** is given only when angioplasty is done.

> Prasugrel, clopidogrel, or ticagrelor is added to everyone getting angioplasty and a stent. These meds inhibit ADP activation of platelets.

Basic Science Correlate

Mechanism of $P2Y_{12}$ Antagonists: Clopidogrel, Prasugrel, Ticagrelor

These agents block aggregation of platelets to each other by inhibiting ADP-induced activation of the $P2Y_{12}$ receptor. Clopidogrel and prasugrel are in the thienopyridine class.

Thrombolytics and Primary Angioplasty

Step 3 is very big on knowing which treatments will *lower mortality.* Thrombolytics and primary angioplasty both **lower mortality** in ST segment elevation myocardial infarction (STEMI) and are **dependent on time;** in other words, their benefit markedly diminishes with time.

Prasugrel is added *only* for angioplasty.

Primary angioplasty means angioplasty during an acute episode of chest pain, and **infarction** is the single best evidence for mortality benefit with angioplasty. Angioplasty is one type of "percutaneous coronary intervention" (PCI). PCI *must* be performed within 90 minutes of arrival at the emergency department for a STEMI. Angioplasty has *not* been shown to decrease mortality in stable angina more than medical therapy (aspirin, beta blockers, and statins) alone.

CCS Tip: CCS requires you to know the *route* of administration of medications.

When is the answer "urgent angioplasty" or PCI?

- The question asks "what has the single greatest efficacy?" in lowering mortality in STEMI.
- The question includes a contraindication to the use of thrombolytics.

If **PCI cannot be performed within 90 minutes** of arrival in the emergency department, the patient should receive **thrombolytics.** The question will clearly state that "the patient is at a small rural hospital" or "the nearest catheterization facility is over an hour away." The question must be clear on this point. Thrombolytics are indicated when the patient has **chest pain for < 12 hours and has ST segment elevation in 2 or more leads. A new left bundle branch block (LBBB)** is also an indication for thrombolytic therapy. Thrombolytics should be given **within 30 minutes** of a patient's arrival in the emergency department with pain.

Basic Science Correlate

Mechanism of Thrombolytics

Thrombolytics activate plasminogen into plasmin. Plasmin chops up fresh or newly formed fibrin strands into D-dimers. This is why all clots elevate levels of D-dimers. After several hours, the fibrin clot has been stabilized (made more permanent) by factor XIII. Plasmin will not cleave fibrin once stabilized by factor XIII.

Beta Blockers, ACE Inhibitors, and Angiotensin Receptor Blockers

Beta blockers lower mortality, but the timing of their administration is *not* critical. Beta blockers, such as metoprolol, should be given, but they are not as urgent to give as aspirin, thrombolytics, or primary angioplasty. **ACE inhibitors** or **angiotensin receptor blockers (ARBs)** should be given to all patients with an acute coronary syndrome, but they only lower mortality if there is **left ventricular dysfunction or systolic dysfunction.** Make sure there is a lipid profile and start the patient on HMG CoA reductase inhibitors, if indicated (i.e., if LDL is not at goal).

Basic Science Correlate

Mechanism of Beta Blockers in Myocardial Infarction

The most common cause of death in both CHF and MI is a ventricular arrhythmia brought on by ischemia. Beta blockers are both anti-arrhythmic and anti-ischemic. Slower heart rate means more time for coronary artery perfusion. Increased left ventricular filling time increases both stroke volume and cardiac output.

CCS Tip: CCS and Step 3 do *not* require you to know doses.

A 72-year-old man comes to the emergency department having had chest pain for the last hour. His initial EKG shows ST segment elevation in leads V2–V4. Aspirin has been given. Which of the following will most likely benefit this patient?

a. CK-MB
b. Stress test
c. Angioplasty
d. Metoprolol
e. Diltiazem
f. Atorvastatin
g. Digoxin
h. Amiodarone
i. Oxygen, morphine, and nitrates
j. Thrombolytics

Answer: **C.** Angioplasty will lower the risk of mortality most for this patient. If it can be obtained within 90 minutes, angioplasty is the best therapy. Metoprolol lowers mortality but is not dependent on how soon you give it, as long as the patient receives it before going home.

Statins

Statin medications, such as atorvastatin, should be given to *all* patients with an **acute coronary syndrome,** regardless of what the EKG shows or troponin or CK-MB levels.

Effects of Therapy Used in Acute Coronary Syndromes		
Always Lower Mortality	**Lower Mortality in Certain Conditions**	**Do Not Lower Mortality**
• Aspirin • Thrombolytics • Primary angioplasty • Metoprolol • Statins • Clopidogrel, prasugrel, or ticagrelor	• ACE inhibitors if ejection fraction is low • ARBs if ejection fraction is low	• Oxygen • Morphine • Nitrates • Calcium channel blockers • Lidocaine • Amiodarone

Clopidogrel or ticagrelor is used when:

- There is aspirin allergy
- The patient undergoes angioplasty and stenting
- There is acute MI

Prasugrel has greater efficacy than clopidogrel but causes more bleeding.

Prasugrel increases bleeding in:

- Age > 75
- Weight < 60 kg

- When is **prasugrel, clopidogrel,** or **ticagrelor** the answer?
  - They are the answer when a platelet antagonist is to be used for acute chest pain, there is aspirin allergy, the patient is to undergo angioplasty, or an acute infarction is occurring. Ticlopidine is associated with neutropenia.
  - Add one of them to aspirin when there is an acute MI.
- When are **calcium channel blockers** (verapamil, diltiazem) the answer?
  - The patient has an **intolerance** to beta blockers, such as severe reactive airway disease (asthma).
  - There is cocaine-induced chest pain.
  - There is coronary vasospasm/Prinzmetal's angina.
- When is a **pacemaker** the answer for acute MI?
  - Third-degree AV block
  - Mobitz II, second-degree AV block
  - Bifascicular block
  - New left bundle branch block
  - Symptomatic bradycardia
- When is **lidocaine** or **amiodarone** the answer for acute MI?
  - *Only* when there is ventricular **tachycardia** or ventricular **fibrillation.**
  - Do *not* give antiarrhythmic medications to prevent ventricular arrhythmias.

Complications of Myocardial Infarction (MI)

All the complications of myocardial infarction result in **hypotension.** Step 3 rarely asks what the diagnosis is; instead, it most often hands it to you and asks what to do in further management.

Diagnosis	Diagnostic Test	Treatment
Cardiogenic shock	Echo, Swan-Ganz (right heart) catheter	ACEI, urgent revascularization
Valve rupture	Echo	ACEI, nitroprusside, intra-aortic balloon pump as a bridge to surgery
Septal rupture	Echo, right heart catheter showing a step up in saturation from the right atrium to right ventricle	ACEI, nitroprusside, and urgent surgery
Myocardial wall rupture	Echo	Pericardiocentesis, urgent cardiac repair
Sinus bradycardia	EKG	Atropine, followed by pacemaker if there are still symptoms
Third-degree (complete) heart block	EKG, canon "a" waves	Atropine and a pacemaker even if symptoms resolve
Right ventricular infarction	EKG showing right ventricular leads	Fluid loading

Basic Science Correlate

Mechanism of Septal Rupture Systolic Murmur

Left ventricular pressure is greater than right ventricular pressure. This causes left-to-right shunt of oxygenated blood. Oxygen saturation in the right ventricle is markedly increased compared with the right atrium.

Post-MI Discharge Instructions

All patients post-MI should go home on aspirin, clopidogrel (or prasugrel), a beta blocker, a statin, and an ACE inhibitor.

A patient's wife comes to take her husband home after an MI and asks how long they should wait before they have sex. What do you tell her?

a. No waiting necessary
b. 2–6 weeks
c. After echocardiography
d. They should wait for a normal angiography.

Answer: **B.** Some waiting is necessary to have sex after an infarction. Sex minimally increases the risk of infarction. The duration and the intensity of exertion are sufficient to provoke ischemia in some cases.

Non-ST Segment Elevation Myocardial Infarction

The predominant differences in the management of non-ST segment elevation MI (NSTEMI) are as follows:

- No thrombolytic use
- Heparin is used routinely. Low molecular weight (LMW) heparin is superior to IV unfractionated heparin.
- Glycoprotein IIb/IIIa inhibitors lower mortality, particularly in those undergoing angioplasty

A 54-year-old man with a history of diabetes and hypertension comes to the emergency department with crushing, substernal chest pain that radiates to his left arm. The pain has been on and off for several hours, with this last episode being 30 minutes in duration. He has had chest pain on exertion before, but this is the first time it has developed at rest. The EKG is normal. Aspirin, oxygen, and nitrates have been given. Troponin levels are elevated. Which of the following is most likely to benefit this patient?

a. Low molecular weight heparin
b. Thrombolytics
c. Diltiazem
d. Morphine
e. CK-MB levels

Answer: **A.** Heparin is the only one of these choices that has been shown to produce lower mortality. Thrombolytics do not lower mortality, unless there is ST elevation or a new LBBB. Positive cardiac enzymes are not an indication for thrombolytics. Other answers that could be right if they were choices are **GPIIb/IIIa inhibitors,** such as eptifibatide, tirofiban, or abciximab, or the use of **angioplasty/PCI.**

> The single greatest benefits from **GPIIb/IIIa inhibitors** with ACS come in combination with angioplasty and stent placement. Abciximab does *not* benefit ST segment elevation MI.

Basic Science Correlate

Mechanism of Heparin

Heparin potentiates the effect of antithrombin. Antithrombin actually inhibits almost every step of the clotting cascade. This is why it does not work with antithrombin deficiency. Heparin only prevents new clots from forming.

Chronic Angina

Office-based cases of further management will emphasize the same issues of mortality benefit.

> **Thrombolytics** are *only* used if there is ST segment elevation or a new LBBB within 12 hours of the onset of chest pain.

Treatment

Aspirin and **metoprolol** are the 2 main routinely indicated medications because of their benefit on mortality. Nitrates should be used for those with angina pain but they do *not* lower mortality.

ACE inhibitors and ARBs should only be used in further management for stable cases if the question describes any of the following:

- Congestive failure
- Systolic dysfunction
- Low ejection fraction

> ARBs are used interchangeably with ACE inhibitors, especially if the patient has a cough with ACE inhibitors. Both ACE and ARBs cause hyperkalemia.

Coronary angiography is predominantly used to determine who is **a candidate for coronary artery bypass grafting (CABG).** You do not need to do angiography to diagnose CAD. Stress testing can show "reversible ischemia." However, you *must* do angiography to see who needs CABG.

You do *not* need to do angiography to initiate the following:

- Aspirin + metoprolol (mortality benefit)
- Nitrates (pain)
- ACE/ARB (low ejection fraction)
- Clopidogrel, prasugrel, or ticagrelor (acute MI or cannot tolerate aspirin)
- Statins
- If pain persists, add ranolazine

Which of the following is the main difference between saphenous vein grafts and internal mammary artery grafts?

a. There is less need for aspirin and metoprolol with internal mammary artery grafts.
b. Warfarin is necessary with saphenous vein grafts.
c. Internal mammary artery grafts remain open for 10 years.
d. Heparin is necessary for vein grafts.

Answer: **C.** The main difference between saphenous vein grafts and internal mammary artery grafts is that vein grafts start to become occluded after 5 years but internal mammary artery grafts are often patent at 10 years. There is no difference in the need for medications.

Indications for CABG:

- Three coronary vessels with > 70 percent stenosis
- Left main coronary artery stenosis > 50–70 percent
- 2 vessels in a diabetic
- 2 or 3 vessels with low ejection fraction

> Ranolazine:
> - Anti-angina med
> - Added if other meds do not control pain

Lipid Management

CAD + LDL > 100 =
Give statins

The single strongest indication for lipid-lowering therapy is for **a statin in a patient with an acute coronary syndrome and an LDL > 100.** The goal of therapy in those with CAD is an LDL < 100. Although the evidence is strongest for an LDL > 130, you will answer "statin therapy" for *any* case of CAD *or an equivalent* with an LDL > 100. Anyone with an acute coronary syndrome needs to be on a statin.

If a question asks for the LDL goal in a patient with **diabetes,** the answer is **LDL goal < 70.**

There are also other risk factors to consider. Make sure you also know how to **calculate risk factors** to help determine LDL goals.

Risk factors in lipid management:

- Tobacco use (cigarette smoking)
- High blood pressure (≥ 140/90 mm Hg or on blood pressure medication)
- Low HDL cholesterol (< 40)
- Family history of early coronary heart disease (female relatives < 65, male relatives < 55)
- Age (males ≥ 45, females ≥ 55)

Lipid recommendations will not change until the changes become clearer.

Many medications, such as statins, cholestyramine, gemfibrozil, ezetimibe, and niacin, lower LDL, lower triglycerides and total cholesterol, and raise HDL. Which of the following is the most important reason for using statins?

a. Fewer adverse effects
b. Lower cost
c. Greater patient acceptance
d. Greatest mortality benefit
e. Greatest effect on lowering LDL

Answer: **D.** The statins have a greater effect on lowering mortality compared with the other medications. Recent guidelines will be further clarified over time. Give statins if the 10-year risk is > 7.5%. This is very hard to put in Step 3: You cannot put a risk calculator in the question.

Coronary artery disease equivalents:

- Diabetes mellitus
- Peripheral artery disease
- Aortic disease
- Carotid disease

> Step 3 will only ask **clear** questions on lipids.

When is the goal of therapy an LDL < 70?

a. CHF
b. Diabetes
c. Coronary disease and carotid disease
d. Coronary disease and diabetes
e. Diabetes and hypertension

Answer: **D.** The goal of LDL can be < 70 for patients at the very highest risk of infarction. This includes those with acute coronary syndromes or the combination of coronary disease and a very severe risk factor, such as diabetes.

The most common adverse effect of statin medications is **liver toxicity.** As many as 1 percent of patients will stop a statin because of its effect on raising transaminases. Liver function tests should be routinely checked. Rhabdomyolysis is *not* the most common adverse effect. There is no routine indication to check CPK levels.

Sex and the Heart

A man develops erectile dysfunction after an infarction. What is the most common cause?

a. Metoprolol
b. Nitrates
c. ACE inhibitors
d. Aspirin
e. Anxiety

Answer: **E.** Anxiety is the most common cause of erectile dysfunction postinfarction. Although beta blockers may be the most common medication associated with erectile dysfunction, anxiety is still a more common cause of erectile dysfunction than beta blockers.

A man develops erectile dysfunction postinfarction. You are planning to start sildenafil. Which of the following medications must you stop?

a. Metoprolol
b. Nitrates
c. ACE inhibitors
d. Aspirin

Answer: **B.** Nitrates are contraindicated when medications such as sildenafil are to be used. When used at the same time, they can cause a dangerous level of hypotension.

Congestive Heart Failure (CHF)

The mechanism that matters for congestive failure has to do with the difference in treatment between **systolic dysfunction with a low ejection fraction and diastolic dysfunction** and a **normal ejection fraction.** There is *no* clear way to distinguish systolic from diastolic dysfunction from symptoms alone. Clues in the history are **hypertension, valvular heart disease,** and **myocardial infarction.**

S3: Splash
S4: Bang

CHF presents with shortness of breath, particularly on exertion, in a person with any of the following:

- Edema
- Rales on lung examination
- Ascites
- Jugular venous distention
- S3 gallop
- Orthopnea
- Paroxysmal nocturnal dyspnea
- Fatigue

Basic Science Correlate

Mechanism of Rales

Increased hydrostatic pressure develops in the pulmonary capillaries from left heart pressure overload. This causes transudation of liquid into the alveoli. During inhalation, the alveoli open with a "popping" sound referred to as rales.

Pulmonary Edema

A 63-year-old woman comes to the emergency department with acute, severe shortness of breath; rales on lung exam; S3 gallop; and orthopnea. Which of the following is the most important step?

a. Chest x-ray
b. Oxygen, furosemide, nitrates, and morphine
c. Echocardiogram
d. Digoxin
e. ACE inhibitors
f. Carvedilol

Answer: **B.** Oxygen, furosemide, nitrates, and morphine are the mainstay of therapy for **acute pulmonary edema.** Although they are not associated with a concrete mortality benefit, they are the standard of care for pulmonary edema, which is the worst manifestation of CHF. Removing volume from the vascular system and, therefore, the lungs is more important than any form of diagnostic testing. Pulmonary edema is a **clinical diagnosis.** Shortness of breath, rales, S3, and orthopnea are more important in establishing the diagnosis than any single test.

CCS Tip: On CCS, move the clock forward *no more than 15–30 minutes* at a time for acutely unstable ICU or emergency department patients.

Basic Science Correlate

Mechanism of Carvedilol

Carvedilol is an antagonist of both beta-1 and beta-2 receptors as well as alpha-1 receptors. This makes it anti-arrhythmic, anti-ischemic, and antihypertensive.

Diagnostic Testing

All of the following should be ordered on the first screen on the CCS portion of the exam. They should be ordered with the initial therapy (i.e., with the oxygen, furosemide, nitrates, and morphine).

Initial Tests to Be Ordered	What the Tests Show
Chest x-ray	• Pulmonary vascular congestion • Cephalization of flow • Effusion • Cardiomegaly
EKG	• Sinus tachycardia • Atrial and ventricular arrhythmia
Oximeter (consider ordering arterial blood gases [ABG])	• Hypoxia • Respiratory alkalosis
Echocardiogram	• Distinguishes systolic from diastolic dysfunction

Basic Science Correlate

Mechanism of "Cephalization" of Flow

The bases or bottom of the lungs are generally more "full" of blood because of gravity. As fluid builds up in the lungs, it fills the vessels from the bottom to the top, like a cup filling with water. This moves the fluid toward the head, a process called "cephalization."

Mechanism of Dobutamine, Imamrinone, and Milrinone

Imamrinone and milrinone are phosphodiesterase inhibitors. They increase contractility and decrease afterload as vasodilators, yielding much the same effect as dobutamine. Dopamine increases contractility, but dopamine's alpha-1 agonist activity causes vasoconstriction. This increases afterload.

Mechanism of Respiratory Alkalosis in CHF

Fluid overload causes hypoxia. Hypoxia causes hyperventilation. Hyperventilation decreases pCO_2. Decreased pCO_2 causes alkalosis. Hence, hypoxia causes respiratory alkalosis.

Cases of pulmonary edema and myocardial infarction should be placed in the intensive care unit.

Digoxin is *never* the right answer as an acute treatment for pulmonary edema. Digoxin can be used to slow the rate of atrial fibrillation.

CCS Tip: On CCS, the order in which the tests and treatments are written on the screen does not matter, as long as they are written at the same time. *Pulmonary edema* is the perfect example of a CCS in which all the tests should be ordered at the same time as the treatment.

Further Management

The vast majority of patients with pulmonary edema will respond to *preload reduction alone* to control the acute symptoms.

In a small number of patients, **acute management with a positive inotrope** will be necessary. There is no evidence that any positive inotrope or contractility inducing agent will lower mortality. They are also the answer on a CCS case of pulmonary edema when furosemide, oxygen, nitrates, and morphine are given and the patient is still short of breath after the clock is moved forward.

Positive Inotropic Agents Used Intravenously in the Intensive Care Unit	
Dobutamine (drug of choice) Inamrinone Milrinone	These are used as **further management** of acute pulmonary edema cases after the clock is moved forward 30–60 minutes and there is no response to preload reduction.

An 80-year-old woman is admitted to the intensive care unit for acute pulmonary edema. She has rales to the apices and jugulovenous distention. Her EKG shows ventricular tachycardia. Which of the following is the best therapy?

a. Synchronized cardioversion
b. Unsynchronized cardioversion
c. Lidocaine
d. Amiodarone
e. Procainamide

Answer: **A.** Synchronized cardioversion is used when **ventricular tachycardia is associated with acute pulmonary edema.** The same answer would be used if the acute pulmonary edema was associated with the onset of atrial fibrillation, flutter, or supraventricular tachycardia. Unsynchronized cardioversion is used for ventricular fibrillation or ventricular tachycardia without a pulse. Medical therapy, such as lidocaine, amiodarone, or procainamide, can be used for sustained ventricular tachycardia that is hemodynamically stable.

"Synchronized" = Timing with cardiac cycle

When is nesiritide the answer?

Answer: Nesiritide is a **synthetic version of atrial natriuretic peptide that is used for acute pulmonary edema as a part of preload reduction.** It decreases symptoms of shortness of breath and is not clearly associated with a reduction in mortality. There is no clear indication that the answer is nesiritide.

When is a BNP level the answer?

Answer: BNP or "brain natriuretic peptide" level is **a blood test that can be used to establish a diagnosis of CHF in a patient who is short of breath.** If the presentation is not clear, a BNP level can be used to help distinguish between pulmonary embolus, pneumonia, asthma, and CHF. BNP level goes up in CHF but is rather nonspecific. A normal BNP level excludes CHF.

A patient comes with pulmonary edema. A right heart catheter is placed. Which of the following readings is most likely to be found?

	Cardiac Output	Systemic Vascular Resistance	Wedge Pressure	Right Atrial Pressure
a.	Decreased	Increased	Increased	Increased
b.	Decreased	Increased	Decreased	Decreased
c.	Increased	Decreased	Decreased	Decreased
d.	Decreased	Increased	Decreased	Increased

Answer:

	Cardiac Output	Systemic Vascular Resistance	Wedge Pressure	Right Atrial Pressure
a.	Decreased	Increased	Increased	Increased

Pulmonary edema is associated with a **decrease in cardiac output because of pump failure,** which results in the **backup of blood into the left atrium and an increased wedge pressure.** There is also an **increase in right atrial pressure,** which is the same as saying jugular venous distention. Increases in sympathetic outflow will increase systemic vascular resistance in an attempt to maintain intravascular filling pressure. Choice **B** represents hypovolemic shock, such as dehydration. Choice **C** represents septic shock, which is driven by massive systemic vasodilation, such as from gram-negative sepsis. Choice **D** represents pulmonary hypertension.

Basic Science Correlate

Mechanism of Increased Wedge Pressure in CHF

Wedge pressure = Left atrial (LA) pressure

The inflated balloon blocks pressure from behind catheter, making the catheter tip pick up flow from "in front," or downstream. "Downstream" for the pulmonary capillaries means the left atrium.

LV failure = Increased LA pressure = Increased wedge pressure

Chronic Management of CHF

All patients, having been stabilized from acute pulmonary edema, should have an **echocardiogram** to establish whether there is systolic dysfunction with a low ejection fraction or diastolic dysfunction with a normal ejection fraction. Long-term management of dilated cardiomyopathy or systolic dysfunction is based on the use of **ACE inhibitors, beta blockers,** and **spironolactone.** Diuretics are also used but have not been proven to lower mortality. **Digoxin** is used to decrease symptoms and decrease the frequency of hospitalization but has *not* been shown to decrease mortality in congestive failure. **ARBs** can be used interchangeably with **ACE inhibitors.** The **beta blockers** with evidence for lowering mortality in CHF are metoprolol, carvedilol, and bisoprolol. ACE inhibitors and beta blockers are indicated for CHF patients with systolic dysfunction at any stage of disease. **Spironolactone** lowers mortality but has only been proven to do so for more advanced, symptomatic disease; any patient originally presenting with pulmonary edema should get spironolactone.

Spironolactone is anti-androgenic. Spironolactone causes gynecomastia and erectile dysfunction in men; switch to eplerenone. Eplerenone is a mineralocorticoid antagonist. Eplerenone lowers mortality in CHF without the anti-androgenic side effects of spironolactone.

Diastolic dysfunction is treated with beta blockers and diuretics. However, you have to be careful *not* to overuse diuretics. The benefit of ACE inhibitors for diastolic dysfunction is not clear. Digoxin and spironolactone definitely do *not* help diastolic dysfunction.

Further management of CHF calls for the following treatments:

Systolic Dysfunction (Low Ejection Fraction)	Diastolic Dysfunction (Normal Ejection Fraction)
• ACEI or ARB • Metoprolol or carvedilol • Spironolactone or eplerenone • Diuretics • Digoxin	• Metoprolol or carvedilol • Diuretic

The single most important fact about the "further management" of CHF is that **mortality is decreased by ACE/ ARB, beta blockers, and spironolactone.** Digoxin decreases symptoms but does *not* lower mortality.

A 69-year-old man is seen in the office for further management of congestive heart failure. He currently has no symptoms and good exercise tolerance. He has been on lisinopril, metoprolol, spironolactone, and furosemide for the last 6 months. His ejection fraction is 23 percent. Which of the following is most likely to benefit this patient?

a. Intermittent dobutamine therapy
b. Digoxin
c. Cardiac transplantation
d. Implantable cardioverter/defibrillator
e. Chlorthalidine

Answer: **D.** Implantable cardioverter/defibrillators are indicated in dilated cardiomyopathy. The most common cause of death in CHF is sudden death from arrhythmia. Those with an **ejection fraction below 35 percent that persists** are candidates for implantable defibrillator placement.

When is a biventricular pacemaker the answer for CHF?

Answer: Biventricular pacemaker is associated with a decrease in mortality in those with **severe congestive failure with an ejection fraction < 35 percent and a QRS duration > 120 msec.** This is also referred to as "cardiac resynchronization therapy."

If the patient is still short of breath and QRS is wide (> 120), then resynchronize with a biventricular pacer.

Basic Science Correlate

Mechanism of Biventricular Pacemaker

Wide QRS means ventricles not beating together. Ventricles not beating together means inefficient forward flow, like trying to hop on one leg. Biventricular pacemaker means both ventricles go back to beating at same time. Effect instant.

When is warfarin the answer for CHF?

Answer: There is no place for routine anticoagulation with warfarin, no matter how low the ejection fraction may be in CHF in the absence of a clot or chronic atrial fibrillation. Warfarin is a wrong answer for CHF.

Which of the following is an absolute contraindication to the use of beta blockers?

a. Symptomatic bradycardia
b. Peripheral artery disease
c. Asthma
d. Emphysema
e. Diabetes

Answer: **A.** Symptomatic bradycardia is an absolute contraindication for the use of beta blockers. The overwhelming majority of patients with peripheral artery disease can still use beta blockers. In a patient with a myocardial infarction, the mortality benefit of metoprolol far exceeds the risk of its use when asthma, emphysema, or peripheral artery disease is present. Two thirds of asthma patients can tolerate beta blockers.

Valvular Heart Disease

All valvular heart disease presents with **shortness of breath** as the chief complaint. Look for the phrase "**worse with exertion or exercise.**" Hypertension, myocardial infarction, ischemia, increasing age, and rheumatic fever will be in the history but, with the exception of rheumatic heart disease, are probably too nonspecific to give you the diagnosis. Young patients with valvular heart disease will have mitral valve prolapse, hypertrophic obstructive cardiomyopathy, mitral stenosis, or bicuspid aortic valves.

Following are clues to the diagnosis:

Clue to Diagnosis	Likely Diagnosis
Young female, general population	Mitral valve prolapse
Healthy young athlete	Hypertrophic obstructive cardiomyopathy (HOCM)
Immigrant, pregnant	Mitral stenosis
Turner's syndrome, coarctation of aorta	Bicuspid aortic valve
Palpitations, atypical chest pain not with exertion	Mitral valve prolapse

Physical Findings

All valvular heart disease can be expected to have murmurs and rales on lung exam. Possible findings on exam are as follows:

- Peripheral edema
- Carotid pulse findings
- Gallops

Therefore, when you suspect valvular disease, select the cardiovascular, chest, and extremities portion of the physical exam.

Murmurs

The most difficult important aspect for the exam is the part of the valvular heart disease section that concerns understanding auscultation, particularly the effects of various maneuvers on these murmurs. **Systolic murmurs** are most commonly aortic stenosis, mitral regurgitation, mitral valve prolapse, and hypertrophic obstructive cardiomyopathy (HOCM). **Diastolic murmurs** are most commonly aortic regurgitation and mitral stenosis. All **right-sided murmurs** increase in intensity with inhalation. All **left-sided murmurs** increase with exhalation.

Murmur intensity increases with...	Exhalation	Inhalation
Side of murmur	Left	Right
Associated disease	Mitral and aortic valve lesions	Both stenosis and regurgitation of tricuspid valves

Effects of Valsalva, Standing, Squatting, and Leg Raise

Maneuvers predominantly affect the volume of blood entering the heart. **Squatting and lifting the legs in the air** increase venous return to the heart. **Valsalva maneuver and standing up** suddenly decrease venous return to the heart.

Valsalva maneuver is exhaling against a closed glottis, like bearing down during a bowel movement or blowing against a thumb stuck in the mouth. This **increases intrathoracic pressure,** which decreases blood return to the heart.

When you **suddenly squat,** you are squeezing the veins of the legs, which are rather large. This essentially **squeezes blood up into the heart** like squeezing on a tube of toothpaste. For those too weak to squat suddenly, the physician can **lift up the legs.** This has the same effect as squatting, which is to drain blood into the chest from the lower extremities.

The majority of murmurs increase in intensity with squatting and leg raise. Aortic stenosis (AS), aortic regurgitation (AR), mitral stenosis (MS), mitral regurgitation (MR), and all right-sided heart lesions will become **louder** with squatting and leg raising. The only two murmurs that become **softer** with these maneuvers are mitral valve prolapse (MVP) and hypertrophic obstructive cardiomyopathy (HOCM).

The following table shows the effect of venous return on murmurs.

Valvular Lesion	Effect of Change in Venous Return	
	Increase (squat, leg raise)	Decrease (stand, Valsalva)
Aortic stenosis (AS)	Increased murmur	Decreased murmur
Aortic regurgitation (AR)	Increased murmur	Decreased murmur
Mitral stenosis (MS)	Increased murmur	Decreased murmur
Mitral regurgitation (MR)	Increased murmur	Decreased murmur
Ventricular septal defect (VSD)	Increased murmur	Decreased murmur
Hypertrophic obstructive cardiomyopathy (HOCM)	Decreased murmur	Increased murmur
Mitral valve prolapse (MVP)	Decreased murmur	Increased murmur

Effects of Handgrip and Amyl Nitrate

Handgrip is a maneuver that increases afterload by compressing the arteries of the arm by contracting the muscles of the arm. Handgrip does *not* significantly increase venous return to the heart: the veins of the arms are not as large as those of the legs, so compressing them does not make much difference in venous return to the heart. Handgrip, because it increases afterload, essentially functions as the **opposite of an ACE inhibitor,** worsening the murmurs of conditions that would get better with an ACE inhibitor. For instance, AR and MR are treated with ACE inhibitors, because afterload reduction increases the forward flow of blood into the aorta. **Handgrip will, therefore, worsen AR and MR murmurs** by pushing blood backward into the heart. Handgrip will make the murmurs of AR and MR louder and more intense. The same is true for VSD. **Handgrip worsens the murmur of VSD,** because more blood now goes from the left ventricle into the right ventricle.

Amyl nitrate is a vasodilator that decreases afterload by dilating peripheral arteries. Amyl nitrate has the **opposite effect of handgrip.** Giving amyl nitrate is like giving an ACE inhibitor or ARB. If handgrip worsens AR and MR, then amyl nitrate **improves AR and MR.**

Handgrip improves or lessens the murmurs of MVP and HOCM. The murmurs of MVP and HOCM lessen when the left ventricular chamber is larger or more full. What happens to the size of the left ventricular (LV) chamber if there is increased afterload? The LV chamber will not empty and, therefore, the LV will be larger. A larger LV chamber relieves or lessens the obstruction in HOCM.

Amyl nitrate will do the opposite. It increases ventricular emptying and, therefore, decreases the size of the LV. **Amyl nitrate worsens the murmurs of MVP and HOCM** by increasing the obstruction and the degree of prolapse of the valves in MVP.

The effect of handgrip and amyl nitrate on aortic stenosis can be hard to understand. **Handgrip softens the murmur of aortic stenosis.** This happens by preventing blood from leaving the ventricle; you can't have a murmur if blood is not moving. If afterload goes up, blood can't eject from the LV, and the AS murmur will soften. Another way of saying it is that the murmur of AS is based on the **gradient** between the LV and the aorta. If the LV pressure is greater than the aorta pressure, then the gradient or difference is high. The higher the gradient, the louder the murmur and the more severe the AS is considered. Handgrip increases pressure in the aorta; therefore, the gradient or difference between the LV and aorta decreases. Handgrip is like covering up a trombone or trumpet. You can't produce music if you put a hand over the front of a wind instrument.

Amyl nitrate has exactly the opposite effect on AS compared to handgrip. **Amyl nitrate decreases afterload and decreases the pressure in the aorta, thus increasing the gradient between LV and aorta and worsening (making louder) the murmur of AS.**

Mitral stenosis (MS) is little affected by either handgrip or amyl nitrate. These generally do not affect ventricular filling, which is the major component of MS. ACE inhibitors, likewise, have very little effect on MS.

	Effect on Murmur Volume	
Valvular Lesion	**Handgrip (Increased Afterload)**	**Amyl Nitrate (Decreased Afterload)**
Aortic stenosis (AS)	Decrease	Increase
Aortic regurgitation (AR)	Increase	Decrease
Mitral stenosis (MS)	Negligible effect	Negligible effect
Mitral regurgitation (MR)	Increase	Decrease
Ventricular septal defect (VSD)	Increase	Decrease
Hypertrophic obstructive cardiomyopathy (HOCM)	Decrease	Increase
Mitral valve prolapse (MVP)	Decrease	Increase

Location and Radiation of Murmurs

One of the main clues to the identity of a murmur is the location at which the murmur is heard.

> Step 3 USMLE has multimedia—heart sounds are played that must be identified.

- **Aortic stenosis** is heard best at the **second right intercostal space and radiates to the carotid arteries.** It is classically described as a crescendo-decrescendo murmur.
- **Pulmonic valve murmurs** are heard at the **second left intercostal space.**

USMLE multimedia will show an animation of auscultation at a particular location on the chest wall and then play the sound.

- **Aortic regurgitation and tricuspid murmurs, as well as VSD murmurs,** are heard at the lower left sternal border.
- **Mitral regurgitation** (MR) is heard at the **apex and radiates into the axilla.** The apex is at the level of the 5th intercostal space, below the left nipple.

Intensity of Murmurs

- I/VI: Only heard with special maneuvers (e.g., Valsalva, handgrip)
- II/VI and III/VI: Majority of murmurs; no objective difference between them
- IV/VI: Thrill present (a thrill is a palpable vibration you can feel from a severe valve lesion)
- V/VI : Can be heard with stethoscope partially off the chest
- VI/VI: Stethoscope not needed to hear it

Diagnostic Testing

The best initial diagnostic test for valve lesions on single best answer questions is an **echocardiogram.** The most accurate test is a **left heart catheterization.** This can also measure pressure gradients, such as in aortic stenosis, most accurately. On CCS cases, you should also add an **EKG and chest x-ray** for valvular lesion assessment.

Order **transthoracic echocardiography (TTE)** first on CCS. Then order a **transesophageal echocardiogram (TEE)** if the TTE is not fully diagnostic.

Treatment

Regurgitant lesions are best treated with **vasodilator therapy,** such as ACE inhibitors, ARBs, or nifedipine. Afterload reduction will slow the progression of regurgitant lesions. If handgrip makes it worse, then ACE inhibitors are the "most effective medical therapy." If the patient still progresses despite medical therapy, then surgical replacement of the valve should be performed.

Stenotic lesions are best treated with **anatomic repair.** Mitral stenosis should undergo balloon valvuloplasty, even if the patient is pregnant. Aortic stenosis that is severe must be surgically replaced. Aortic valve replacement is well tolerated even in the very old. Diuretics can decrease pulmonary vascular congestion with stenotic lesions, but they are not as effective or important as anatomic repair.

- Valsalva improves murmur = Diuretics indicated
- Amyl nitrate improves murmur = ACE inhibitor indicated

Valvular Lesion	Standing/Valsalva	Diuretics Indicated
Aortic stenosis (AS)	Decrease	Yes (replace best)
Aortic regurgitation (AR)	Decrease	Yes
Mitral stenosis (MS)	Decrease	Yes (balloon best)
Mitral regurgitation (MR)	Decrease	Yes
Ventricular septal defect (VSD)	Decrease	Yes
Hypertrophic obstructive cardiomyopathy (HOCM)	Increase	No
Mitral valve prolapse (MVP)	Increase	No

Valvular Lesion	Amyl Nitrate	ACE Inhibitor Indicated
Aortic stenosis (AS)	Increase	No
Aortic regurgitation (AR)	Decrease	Yes
Mitral stenosis (MS)	Negligible effect	No
Mitral regurgitation (MR)	Decrease	Yes
Ventricular septal defect (VSD)	Decrease	Yes
Hypertrophic obstructive cardiomyopathy (HOCM)	Increase	No
Mitral valve prolapse (MVP)	Increase	No

Aortic Stenosis (AS)

Aortic stenosis most commonly presents with **chest pain.** Syncope and CHF are less common presentations. The patient will be **older** and often has a history of **hypertension.** Coronary artery disease will be present in as many as 50 percent of patients.

Prognosis is as follows:

- **Coronary disease:** 3- to 5-year average survival
- **Syncope:** 2- to 3-year average survival
- **CHF:** 1.5- to 2-year average survival

On CCS, the intensity, radiation, and location of the murmur will automatically be provided with the cardiovascular examination. There is no need to ask for them separately.

Basic Science Correlate

Mechanism of Syncope/Angina in AS

In AS, a stiff valve just proximal to the entry point of coronaries blocks blood flow into the vertebral and basilar arteries and carotids. No flow to brain = Passing out. Thus, AS causes LV hypertrophy. LV hypertrophy = Increased demand.

AS = Blocked flow with increased demand = Chest pain

Physical Exam

Choose the cardiovascular (CV) exam, chest, and extremities.

Normal aortic valve gradient is zero.

AS gives a crescendo-decrescendo systolic murmur. The murmur will be heard best at the second right intercostal space and radiate to the carotid arteries. The murmur will increase in intensity with leg raising, squatting, and amyl nitrate. The murmur will decrease with Valsalva, standing, and handgrip. The case may describe delayed carotid upstroke as well.

Basic Science Correlate

Mechanism of Crescendo/Decrescendo Murmur of AS

The first part of the cardiac cycle is isovolumetric contraction. With isovolumetric contraction, no blood moves. No blood moving = No murmur. Peak flow occurs in mid-systole. Peak flow = Peak noise. Hence, AS yields a diamond-shaped crescendo-decrescendo murmur.

Diagnostic Testing

The **transthoracic echocardiogram (TTE)** is the best initial diagnostic test. A **transesophageal echocardiogram (TEE)** is more accurate. **Left heart catheterization** is the most accurate diagnostic test and allows the most accurate method of assessing the pressure gradient across the valve. Mild disease is a gradient < 30 mm Hg. Moderate disease is indicated by 30–70 mm Hg, and severe disease is indicated by a gradient > 70 mm Hg. For CCS cases, also choose an **EKG** and a **chest x-ray,** which will show **left ventricular hypertrophy.**

Treatment

Balloon dilate AS **only** if the patient is too sick to undergo surgery.

Diuretics are the best initial therapy but will not alter long-term prognosis. Further, **overdiuresis is dangerous,** and use of diuretics needs to be very judicious.

The treatment of choice is valve replacement. Bioprosthetic valves (porcine, bovine) will last 10 years on average, but do *not* require anticoagulation with warfarin. Mechanical valves do *not* have to be replaced as often, but must also be treated with warfarin to an INR of 2–3. Valve replacement is well tolerated, even in the elderly. Valve replacement by catheter is done when a patient can't tolerate surgery.

Mechanical valves can wear out after 15–20 years.

Aortic Regurgitation (AR)

Hypertension, rheumatic heart disease, endocarditis, and cystic medial necrosis cause AR. Rarer causes are Marfan's syndrome, ankylosing spondylitis, syphilis, and reactive arthritis. Reactive arthritis is an inflammatory arthritis of large joints, inflammation of the eyes (conjunctivitis and uveitis), and urethritis, previously commonly referred to as Reiter's syndrome. **Shortness of breath and fatigue are the most common presentation.**

Physical Exam

Choose the cardiovascular (CV) exam, chest, and extremities.

The murmur of AR is a **diastolic decrescendo murmur heard best at the left sternal border.** There are several unique physical findings that are rarely seen with AR. The murmur will increase in intensity with leg raising, squatting, and handgrip.

- **Quincke pulse:** Arterial or capillary pulsations in the fingernails
- **Corrigan's pulse:** High bounding pulses (also known as a "water-hammer pulse")
- **Musset's sign:** Head bobbing up and down with each pulse
- **Duroziez's sign:** Murmur heard over the femoral artery
- **Hill sign:** Blood pressure gradient much higher in the lower extremities

Diagnostic Testing

TTE is the best initial diagnostic test. **TEE** is more accurate. **Left heart catheterization** is the most accurate test. For CCS cases, also choose an EKG and a chest x-ray, which will show left ventricular hypertrophy.

Treatment

ACE inhibitors, ARBs, and nifedipine are the best initial therapy. For CCS cases, you should add a **loop diuretic,** such as furosemide. **Surgery** is the answer when the ejection fraction drops below 55 percent or the left ventricular end systolic diameter goes above 55 mm; surgery should be done in patients with these criteria even if they are asymptomatic.

Basic Science Correlate

Why Does High Pressure Dilate the Aortic Valve?

The law of LaPlace says: The wall tension, or force dilating a vessel, is proportionate to the radius of the vessel times the pressure on the inside.

Tension = Radius × Pressure

The wider a vessel is, the faster it will get pulled apart. Hence, the more the aortic ring or aorta is dilated, the faster it will get pulled apart. Likewise, the higher the interior pressure is, the faster the interior will be pulled apart. This force of being "pulled apart," or dilation, is called "wall tension" in the law of LaPlace.

ACE and ARB drugs vasodilate peripheral arterioles. Lower pressure = Lower wall tension.

Mitral Stenosis (MS)

Rheumatic fever is the most common cause of MS. Look for an **immigrant patient** because of the low rates of rheumatic fever in the United States. Also look for a **pregnant patient** because of the large increase in plasma volume with pregnancy. Special features of MS are as follows:

- **Dysphagia:** Large left atrium pressing on the esophagus
- **Hoarseness:** Pressure on recurrent laryngeal nerve
- **Atrial fibrillation** leading to stroke

> **Basic Science Correlate**
>
> **Mechanism of Increased MS Symptoms in Pregnant Women**
>
> Pregnant women have a 50 percent increase in plasma volume. More volume with the same valve diameter means more pressure, backflow, and symptoms. Pregnancy also changes the hypothalamic osmolar receptors. ADH levels stay higher in pregnancy, so the collecting duct absorbs more free water.

Physical Exam

Choose the cardiovascular (CV) exam, chest, and extremities.

The murmur of MS is a **diastolic rumble after an opening snap,** which can be described as an "extra sound" in diastole. The S1 is louder. As the mitral stenosis worsens, the opening snap moves closer to S2. The murmur will increase in intensity with leg raising, squatting, and expiration.

> **Basic Science Correlate**
>
> **Mechanism of Opening Snap Earlier in Worsening MS**
>
> The mitral valve opens when LA pressure > LV pressure. Worse MS = Higher LA pressure. Higher LA pressure pushes the mitral valve open earlier.

Diagnostic Testing

TTE is the best initial diagnostic test. **TEE** is more accurate. **Left heart catheterization** is the most accurate test. For CCS cases, also choose an **EKG and a chest x-ray,** which will show left atrial hypertrophy. On chest x-ray, there is **straightening of the left heart border and elevation of the left mainstem bronchus.** There may also be a description of a double density in the cardiac silhouette (from left atrial enlargement).

Treatment

Diuretics are the best initial therapy. They do *not* alter progression. **Balloon valvuloplasty** is the most effective therapy. Pregnant women can and should be readily treated with balloon valvuloplasty. Pregnancy is *not* a contraindication to valvuloplasty.

> **Basic Science Correlate**
>
> Balloon valvuloplasty works in MS because the stenosis results from excessive fibrosis of the valve. Rheumatic fever causes cardiac endomyocardial and valvular fibrosis. Fibrosis can be stretched by the balloon. By contrast, aortic stenosis is calcified, and calcification does not stretch or rip easily with a balloon.
>
> **MS = Balloon fibrosis**
>
> **AS = Remove/replace calcification**

Mitral Regurgitation (MR)

MR is caused by **hypertension, ischemic heart disease, and any other condition that leads to dilation of the heart.** You cannot have dilation of the heart without the mitral valve leaflets separating. **Dyspnea on exertion** is the most common complaint.

> **S3 gallop** is associated with fluid overload states, such as congestive heart failure or mitral regurgitation. An S3 can be normal in patients under the age of 30.

Physical Exam

Choose the cardiovascular (CV) exam, chest, and extremities.

The murmur of MR is **holosystolic and obscures both S1 and S2.** MR is **heard best at the apex and radiates to the axilla.** The murmur increases in intensity with leg raising, squatting, and handgrip. Standing, Valsalva, and amyl nitrate decrease the intensity. S3 gallop is often present.

Diagnostic Testing

TTE is the best initial diagnostic test for MR. **TEE** is more accurate.

Treatment

ACE inhibitors, ARBs, and nifedipine are the best initial therapy and the medications most likely to decrease the rate of progression of the disease. For CCS cases, you should add a loop diuretic, such as furosemide. **Surgery** is the answer when the left ventricular ejection fraction drops below 60 percent or the left ventricular end systolic diameter goes above 40 mm. Surgery should be done in patients with these criteria even if they are asymptomatic.

The operative criteria for regurgitant lesions in asymptomatic patients are as follows (repair is preferred to replacement):

	Aortic Regurgitation	Mitral Regurgitation
Ejection fraction	< 55%	< 60%
Left ventricular end systolic diameter	> 55 mm	> 40 mm

Ventricular Septal Defect (VSD)

Asymptomatic patients may present with only a **holosystolic murmur at the lower left sternal border.** Larger defects leads to **shortness of breath.** The murmur worsens with exhalation, squatting, and leg raise.

Diagnostic Testing

Echocardiography is the diagnostic test to use first, but **catheterization** is used to determine the degree of left-to-right shunting most precisely.

Treatment

Mild defects can be left without mechanical closure.

Atrial Septal Defect (ASD)

Small ASDs are **asymptomatic.** Larger ones may lead to **shortness of breath** or signs of right ventricular failure, such as **shortness of breath and a parasternal heave.** The most frequently tested knowledge is that **ASD is associated with fixed splitting of S2.**

> **Basic Science Correlate**
>
> **Mechanism of Fixed Splitting of S2 in ASD**
>
> S2 splitting is caused by different pressures on different sides of heart. Same pressure on both sides means no splitting.
>
> **LA/RA pressure no change in respiration = No change in splitting**

Diagnostic Testing

Diagnose with an **echocardiogram.**

Treatment

Percutaneous or catheter devices are the best therapy. **Repair** is most often indicated when the shunt ratio exceeds 1.5 to 1.

Splitting of S2

Wide, P2 Delayed	Paradoxical, A2 Delayed	Fixed
• Right bundle branch block • Pulmonic stenosis • Right ventricular hypertrophy • Pulmonary hypertension	• Left bundle branch block • Aortic stenosis • Left ventricular hypertrophy • Hypertension	ASD

Cardiomyopathy

Dilated Cardiomyopathy

Dilated cardiomyopathy presents and is managed **in the same way as the case of CHF** described above.

Diagnostic Testing

Echocardiography is the best initial test to determine the ejection fraction and look for wall motion activity. MUGA or nuclear ventriculography is the most accurate method of determining ejection fraction.

Treatment

Besides **ischemia,** the most common causes of dilated cardiomyopathy are **alcohol, adriamycin, radiation, and Chagas' disease.** The treatment for *all* forms of dilated cardiomyopathy, no matter their cause, is with **ACE inhibitors, ARBs, beta blockers, and spironolactone.** Spironolactone and eplerenone are mineralocorticoid or aldosterone antagonists. They are used to decrease the work of the heart; they are not given for their diuretic effect. Spironolactone is anti-androgenic and inhibits testosterone. Eplerenone does not inhibit androgens. Digoxin decreases symptoms but does *not* prolong survival.

Hypertrophic Cardiomyopathy

This condition presents with **shortness of breath on exertion and an S4 gallop** on examination.

> **S4 gallop** is a sign of left ventricular hypertrophy and decreased compliance or stiffness of the ventricle. S4 gallop does not automatically indicate the need for additional therapy.

Diagnostic Testing

Echocardiography shows a normal ejection fraction.

Treatment

The mainstay of therapy is with **beta blockers and diuretics.** ACE inhibitors can be used, but their benefit is not as clear. Digoxin and spironolactone do *not* benefit hypertrophic cardiomyopathy.

Restrictive Cardiomyopathy

Restrictive cardiomyopathy presents with a history of **sarcoidosis, amyloidosis, hemochromatosis, cancer, myocardial fibrosis, or glycogen storage diseases. Shortness of breath** is the main presenting complaint in all forms of cardiomyopathy. **Kussmaul's sign** is present: this is an increase in jugular venous pressure on inhalation.

Amyloid
- Low-voltage EKG
- Speckled pattern on echo

Diagnostic Testing

Cardiac catheterization shows rapid x and y descent. The **EKG** shows low voltage. **Echocardiography** is the mainstay of diagnosis. **Endomyocardial biopsy** is the single most accurate diagnostic test of the etiology.

Treatment

Diuretics and correcting the underlying cause are the best treatments.

Pericardial Disease

Pericarditis

Chest pain that is **pleuritic** (changes with respiration) and **positional** (relieved by sitting up and leaning forward) is the presentation that is most often given on Step 3. The pain will be described as **sharp and brief.** Ischemic pain is dull and sore, like being punched. The vast majority of pericarditis cases are viral. Although any infectious agent, collagen-vascular disease, or trauma can be in the history, remember that Step 3 most often hands you a clear diagnosis and asks what you want to do about it, such as testing and treatment.

Physical Exam

The only pertinent positive finding is a **friction rub,** which can have 3 components. The rub is only present in 30 percent of patients. There is *no* pulsus paradoxus, tenderness, edema, or Kussmaul's sign present. Blood pressure is *normal,* and there is *no* jugular venous distention or organomegaly.

Diagnostic Testing

The best initial test is the **EKG. ST segment elevation** is present everywhere (all leads). **PR segment depression** is pathognomonic in lead II, but is not always present.

Treatment

The best initial therapy is an **NSAID,** such as indomethacin, naproxen, aspirin, or ibuprofen combined with colchicine. Advance the clock 1–2 days and have the patient visit the office. If the pain persists, add **prednisone orally** to the treatment and advance the clock 1–2 more days. Colchicine adds efficacy to NSAIDs and prevents recurrent episodes.

Pericardial Tamponade

Tamponade presents with **shortness of breath, hypotension, and jugular venous distention.** On CCS, also examine the **lungs,** because they will be clear.

Following are the unique features of tamponade:

- **Pulsus paradoxus:** This is a decrease of blood pressure > 10 mm Hg on inhalation.
- **Electrical alternans:** This is alterations of the axis of the QRS complex on EKG, manifested as the height of the QRS complex.

Basic Science Correlate

Mechanism of Pulsus Paradoxus

Inhalation increases venous return. Increased venous return expands the right ventricle (RV). Expanded RV compresses the left ventricle (LV). Compressed LV decreases blood pressure. Tamponade compresses the whole heart.

Inhale = Big RV = Smaller LV = BP drop > 10 mm Hg

Diagnostic Testing

Echocardiography is the most accurate diagnostic test. The earliest finding of tamponade is **diastolic collapse of the right atrium and right ventricle.** Remember that it is normal to have 50 mL or less of pericardial fluid, but there should be *no* collapse of the cardiac structures.

EKG will show low voltage and electrical alternans. Electrical alternans is variation of the height of the QRS complex from the heart moving backward and forward in the chest.

Right heart catheterization will show "equalization" of all the pressures in the heart during diastole. The wedge pressure will be the same as the right atrial and pulmonary artery diastolic pressure.

Treatment

- Best initial therapy: **Pericardiocentesis**
- Most effective long-term therapy: **Pericardial window placement**
- Most dangerous therapy: Diuretics

Constrictive Pericarditis

Constrictive pericarditis presents with **shortness of breath** and the following **signs of chronic right heart failure:**

- Edema
- Jugular venous distention

- Hepatosplenomegaly
- Ascites

Following are the unique features of constrictive pericarditis:

- **Kussmaul's sign:** Increase in jugular venous pressure on inhalation
- **Pericardial knock:** Extra diastolic sound from the heart hitting a calcified, thickened pericardium

Diagnostic Testing

- **Chest x-ray:** Showing calcification
- **EKG:** Low voltage
- **CT and MRI:** Showing thickening of the pericardium

Treatment

- Best initial therapy: **Diuretic**
- Most effective therapy: **surgical removal of the pericardium** (i.e., pericardial stripping)

Aortic Disease

Dissection of the Thoracic Aorta

Dissection of the thoracic aorta presents with the following symptoms:

- Chest pain **radiating to the back between the scapula**
- Pain that can be described as **very severe and "ripping"**
- **Difference in blood pressure between right and left arms**

Diagnostic Testing

- Best initial test: **Chest x-ray showing a widened mediastinum**
- Most accurate test: **CT angiography**

Treatment

When the case describes **severe chest pain radiating to the back and hypertension,** order **beta blockers** with the first screen in addition to an **EKG and chest x-ray.** No matter what the EKG shows, move the clock forward and order either **CT angiography, TEE,** or **magnetic resonance angiography (MRA):** all 3 are equally accurate.

- CT angiography = TEE = Magnetic resonance angiography (MRA)

After starting beta blockers, order **nitroprusside** to control the blood pressure.

Aortic dissection cases should be placed in the **ICU,** and a **surgical consultation** should be ordered. **Surgical correction** is the most effective therapy.

> **Abdominal aortic aneurysm** is detected by ultrasound first. AAAs are repaired when they are > 5 cm. Smaller ones are monitored.

Abdominal Aortic Aneurysm (AAA)

Screening with an **ultrasound** should be ordered in **over-65 men who are current or former smokers.**

> **Basic Science Correlate**
>
> As an aneurysm enlarges, the rate of expansion increases: Wider aorta = Widens faster.
>
> This principle is expressed in the law of LaPlace: Wall tension = Radius × Pressure.
>
> Next step: Lower BP and repair with stent or endovascular procedure when the aneurysm goes above 5 cm.

> **Spinal stenosis** will give pain that is worse with walking downhill and less with walking uphill or while cycling or sitting. Pulses and skin exam will be normal with spinal stenosis.

Peripheral Arterial Disease (PAD)

PAD presents with **claudication** (pain in the calves on exertion). The case may also describe **"smooth, shiny skin"** with **loss of hair and sweat glands,** as well as **loss of pulses in the feet.**

Diagnostic Testing

- Best initial test: **Ankle-brachial index (ABI).** (A normal ABI should be ≥ 0.9.) Blood pressure in the legs should be equal to or greater than the pressure in the arms. If there is > **10 percent difference,** then an obstruction is present.)
- Most accurate test: **Angiography**

> Pain + Pallor + Pulseless = Arterial occlusion

Treatment

- Best initial therapy:
  - **Aspirin**
  - **Blood pressure control with ACE inhibitors**
  - **Exercise as tolerated**
  - **Cilostazol**
  - **Lipid control with statins to a target LDL < 100**
- Marginally effective therapy: **Pentoxifylline**
- Ineffective therapy: Calcium channel blocker

> **Acute arterial embolus** will be very **sudden in onset** with **loss of pulse and a cold extremity.** It is also **quite painful.** AS and atrial fibrillation are often in the history for arterial embolus.

Beta blockers are *not* contraindicated with PAD. If the patient needs them for ischemic disease, they should be used.

Basic Science Correlate

Mechanism of Calcium Blockers: Why They Don't Work in PAD

In PAD, the atherosclerotic obstruction is on the inside the vessel. Calcium blockers dilate the muscular layer, which is exterior to the atherosclerosis in the center. Dilating the outer layer does not expand the inside.

CCS Tip: On CCS, move the clock forward several weeks. PAD is *not* an emergency! If initial therapies do *not* work and the pain progresses, *or* there are signs of ischemia such as gangrene or pain at rest, then perform surgical bypass.

Rhythm Disorders

Atrial Fibrillation (A-Fib)

A-fib presents with **palpitations and an irregular pulse** in a person with a history of hypertension, ischemia, or cardiomyopathy.

Diagnostic Testing

If the initial EKG does not show the answer, a patient in the hospital should be placed on **telemetry monitoring.** Outpatients who are hemodynamically stable should undergo **Holter monitoring,** which is continuous, ambulatory cardiac rhythm monitoring for 24 hours or longer.

CCS Tip: For CCS cases, other tests to order once A-fib is found on EKG are the following:

- **Echocardiography:** Looking for clots, valve function, and left atrial size
- **Thyroid function testing:** T4 and TSH levels
- **Electrolytes:** Potassium, magnesium, and calcium levels
- **Troponin or CK-MB levels:** These may be appropriate to test in some acute-onset cases.

CHADS

C = CHF

H = Hypertension

A = Age > 75

D = Diabetes

S = Stroke or TIA

CHADS score of 0 – 1 needs aspirin. At 2 or more, use warfarin, dabigatran, rivaroxaban, or apixaban.

Treatment

Unstable patients should undergo immediate **synchronized electrical cardioversion.** Unstable patients should be cardioverted with the **first screen,** without waiting for TEE or anticoagulation with heparin or warfarin. *Instability* is defined as a systolic blood pressure < 90, congestive failure, confusion related to hemodynamic instability, or chest pain.

Stable patients should have their ventricular heart rate slowed if it is > 100–110 per minute.

Rate control medications are **beta blockers** (metoprolol, esmolol), **calcium channel blockers** (diltiazem), or **digoxin.** In the acute setting, such as the emergency department, these agents should be given intravenously.

Once the rate has been controlled, **anticoagulation with warfarin or dabigatran to a target INR of 2–3** is the next best step in all patients with an atrial arrhythmia persisting beyond 2 days. If the question does not state the duration, you are to treat it as if it were persisting for longer than 2 days.

Stroke/TIA = 2 points

Dabigatran, rivaroxiban, and apixaban are oral anticoagulants with similar efficacy to warfarin but without the need to monitor the INR.

The long-term use of **rate control medications,** such as metoprolol, diltiazem, or digoxin, **combined with anticoagulation** is equal or better than cardioversion with electricity or medications.

Routine cardioversion of atrial fibrillation is *not* indicated.

CHADS$_2$ (CHF, **h**ypertension, **age** > 75, **d**iabetes, or **s**troke/TIA) is a scoring system to indicate the need for warfarin, dabigatran, rivaroxiban, or apixaban. A score of 2 or more means warfarin, dabigatran, or rivaroxaban. A score of 0 or 1 means aspirin.

When CHADS$_2$ is at 2 or more points, control the rate and anticoagulate. Novel oral anticoagulants (NOACs) such as rivaroxaban, dabigatran, or apixaban become therapeutic in a few hours: Unlike warfarin, NOACs do not need several days to reach therapeutic levels. Even when warfarin is used for atrial fibrillation, there is no need to bolus the patient with heparin. Why? Because atrial fibrillation is a long-term disease that takes months or years to develop a risk of stroke, while full-dose heparin carries a risk of bleeding. Just start the warfarin and wait a few days. It is safe.

Heparin treatment bridging to therapeutic warfarin is a **wrong answer.**

Atrial Flutter (A-Flutter)

Atrial flutter is managed **in the same way as atrial fibrillation.** The only difference is that the **rhythm is regular** on presentation.

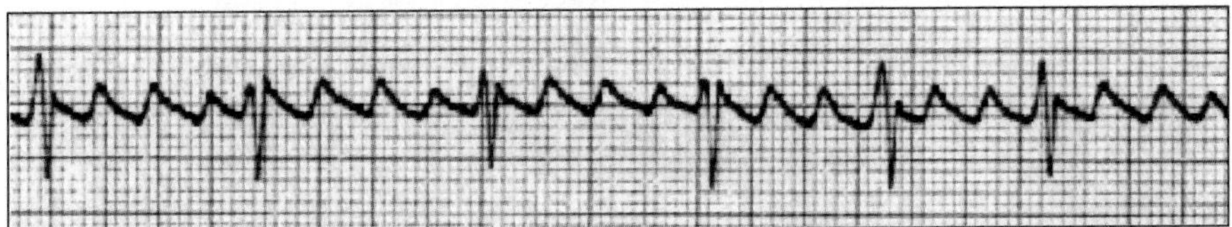

The following table shows how to choose the right rate control medication for a-fib and a-flutter.

Beta Blockers (Metoprolol)	Calcium Channel Blockers (Diltiazem)	Digoxin
• Ischemic heart disease • Migraines • Graves disease • Pheochromocytoma	• Asthma • Migraine	• Borderline hypotension

Give oxygen first for MAT.

Multifocal Atrial Tachycardia (MAT)

This condition presents like an **atrial arrhythmia in association with COPD/emphysema.** EKG will show **polymorphic P waves,** revealing different atrial foci for the QRS complexes. As the name implies, patients with MAT have **tachycardia** (heart rate > 100). MAT manifests as an **irregular chaotic rhythm** on EKG. **Do not use beta blockers.** Give oxygen first, then diltiazem.

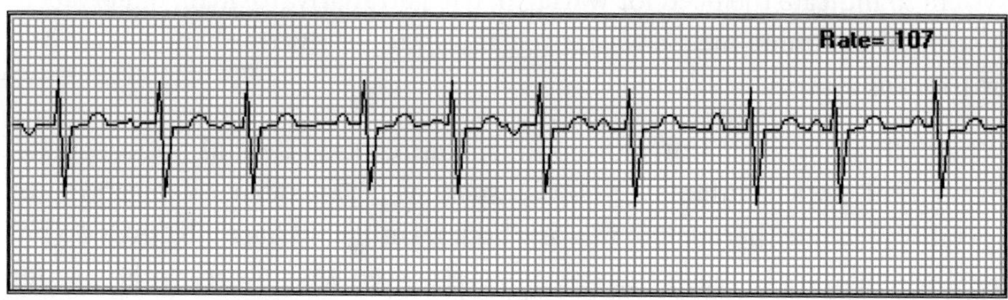

Supraventricular Tachycardia (SVT)

SVT presents with **palpitations and tachycardia** and occasionally syncope. It is *not* associated with ischemic heart disease. SVT has a **regular rhythm with a ventricular rate of 160–180.**

Diagnostic Testing

If the EKG does not show SVT, order **Holter monitor** or **telemetry** to increase the sensitivity of detection.

CCS Tip: On CCS, all cases of dysrhythmia should undergo **transthoracic echocardiography (TTE)** after the initial set of orders.

Treatment

- Best initial management for *unstable* patients: **Synchronized cardioversion**
- Best initial management for *stable* patients: **Vagal maneuvers** (carotid sinus massage, ice immersion of the face, Valsalva)
- Next best step in management if vagal maneuvers do *not* work: **Intravenous adenosine** (Note: This is the most frequently asked SVT question.)
- Best long-term management: **Radiofrequency catheter ablation**

Wolff-Parkinson-White Syndrome (WPW)

WPW presents as **SVT that can alternate with ventricular tachycardia** (VT). The other main clue to the diagnosis is **worsening of SVT after the use of calcium blockers or digoxin.**

Diagnostic Testing

WPW is diagnosed with finding a **delta wave on the EKG.** The most accurate test is **electrophysiologic studies.**

Treatment

Treatment is as follows:

- Best initial therapy *if* the patient is described as being in SVT or VT from WPW: **Procainamide**
- Best long-term therapy: **Radiofrequency catheter ablation**

Basic Science Correlate

Mechanism of WPW

There is an abnormal piece of neutralized cardiac muscle going around the AV node in WPW. This can result in either atrial or ventricular arrhythmia. The slowest conduction in the heart is the AV node. Conduction in the aberrant tract is faster; that is why the PR is short (< 120 mSec) and there is a delta wave on EKG. Calcium channel blockers and digoxin block conduction more in the normal AV and force the conduction down the abnormal conduction tract.

Ventricular Tachycardia (VT)

VT can present as **palpitation, syncope, chest pain, or sudden death.**

Diagnostic Testing

You cannot determine that VT is present without an **EKG.** If the EKG does not detect VT, then **telemetry monitoring** should be ordered. The most accurate diagnostic test is **electrophysiologic studies.**

Treatment

The table below shows therapy options for persistent VT:

Hemodynamically Stable	Hemodynamically Unstable
• Amiodarone • Lidocaine • Procainamide • Magnesium	• Synchronized cardioversion

Torsade de pointes is ventricular tachycardia with an undulating amplitude. **Magnesium** should always be given in addition to **medical or electrical therapy.**

Ventricular Fibrillation (V-Fib)

V-fib presents as **sudden death.**

Diagnostic Testing

You cannot tell what caused the loss of pulse without an **EKG.**

Treatment

Treatment of V-fib is *always* with **unsynchronized cardioversion** first. Do *not* answer intubation first. Dead people are never breathing. If you shock them back to life, they are more likely to breathe!

	Unsynchronized	**Synchronized**
When to deliver electricity:	At any point in cycle	*Not* during the T-wave
Indications:	V-fib, pulseless VT	Everything except V-fib and pulseless VT

Basic Science Correlate

Mechanism of Need for Synchronization

The T-wave represents the refractory period. An electrical shock delivered during the T-wave can set off a worse rhythm—specifically, asystole and ventricular fibrillation are worse than ventricular tachycardia. Do not deliver a shock during the refractory period.

Unsynchronized cardioversion (defibrillation) is administered as follows:

1. Continue CPR
2. Reattempt defibrillation
3. Administer IV epinephrine or vasopressin
4. Reattempt defibrillation
5. Administer IV amiodarone or lidocaine
6. Reattempt defibrillation
7. Repeat several cycles of CPR between each shock

Syncope Evaluation

The management of syncope is based on 3 criteria:

1. Was the loss of consciousness sudden or gradual?
2. Was the regaining of consciousness sudden or gradual?
3. Is the cardiac exam normal or abnormal?

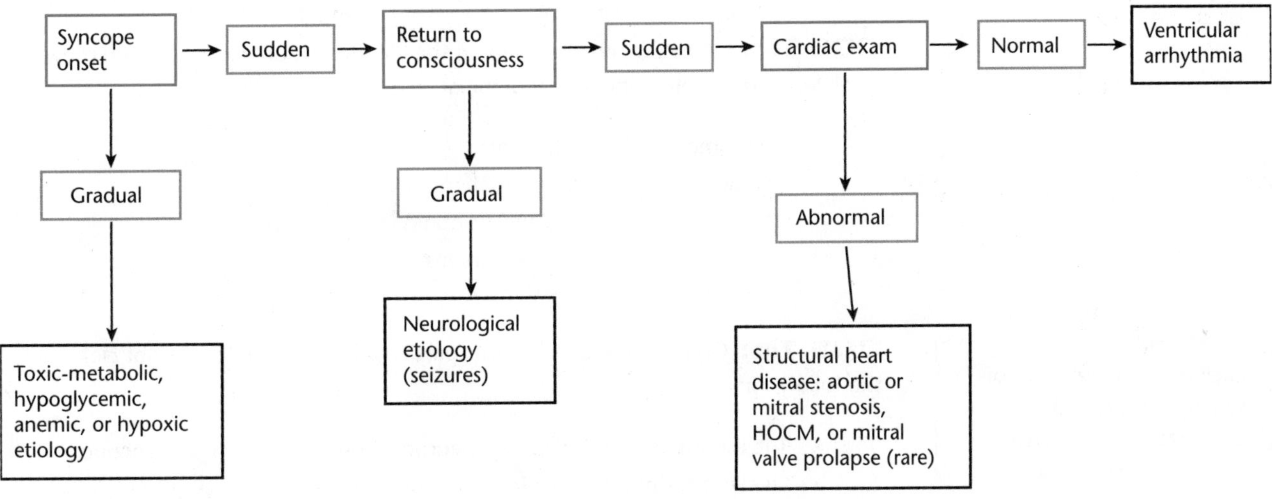

Diagnostic Testing

On the initial screen, order the following:

- Cardiac and neurological examination
- EKG
- Chemistries (glucose)
- Oximeter
- CBC
- Cardiac enzymes (CK-MB, troponin)

CCS Tip: Treat special circumstances as follows:

- If a **murmur** is present, order an echocardiogram.
- If the **neurological exam is focal** or there is a **history of head trauma due to syncope,** order head CT.
- If a **headache** is described, order head CT.
- If a **seizure** is described **or suspected,** order head CT and EEG.

> Carotid Dopplers are not useful in syncope. A patient cannot pass out from a carotid embolus.

Basic Science Correlate

Mechanism of Syncope: Caused by Brainstem Stroke Only

The brainstem controls sleep and wake in the brain. Only stroke or TIA of the posterior circulation can cause syncope. Vertebral/basilar circulation is synonymous with the posterior or brainstem circulation. There is no place in the circulation of the middle cerebral artery that can cause syncope.

CCS Tip: On further management, if the diagnosis is not clear after you move the clock forward to obtain the results of initial tests, order the following:

- Holter monitor on outpatients
- Telemetry monitoring for inpatients
- Repeat check of CK-MB and troponin levels 4 hours later
- Urine and blood toxicology screens

Exclude cardiac causes of syncope. More than 80% of mortality from syncope is from cardiac causes.

CCS Tip: On further management, particularly if the etiology is not clear, order the following:

- **Tilt table testing** to diagnose neurocardiogenic (vasovagal) syncope
- **Electrophysiological testing**

The Holter monitor is a 24- to 72-hour continuous ambulatory EKG. This is routine for most patients with syncope requiring admission.

Treatment

Treatment of syncope is based on the etiology. The majority of cases never get a specific diagnosis. The *most* important thing to do in syncope is to **exclude a cardiac etiology, such as an arrhythmia.** The majority (> 80 percent) of mortality from syncope involves a cardiac etiology.

If a ventricular dysrhythmia is diagnosed as the etiology of syncope, **an implantable cardioverter/defibrillator** is indicated.

CCS Tip: Bottom line, order the following for syncope:

- EKG
- Enzymes: Troponin/CKMB
- Echocardiogram
- Head CT

Endocrinology

4

Diabetes

Diabetes	Type 1	Type 2
Onset	Juvenile	Adult
Body type	Thin	Obese
Diabetic ketoacidosis (DKA)	Frequent	Rare
Treatment	Insulin	Lifestyle management, oral agents, or insulin

Diagnosis is made with *one* of the following:

1. **Two fasting glucose ≥ 126**
2. **One random glucose ≥ 200 with symptoms** (polyuria, polydipsia, polyphagia)
3. **Abnormal glucose tolerance test** (2-hour glucose tolerance test with 75 g glucose load)
4. Hemoglobin A1c > 6.5%

The strongest indication for screening for diabetes is hypertension.

HgA1c > 6.5% diagnoses diabetes.

Basic Science Correlate

Mechanism of Type 2 Diabetes

Adipose tissue must have insulin to permit entry of glucose and free fatty acids (FFAs). Excess fat creates a deficiency of insulin. Insulin receptors are a tyrosine kinase, which is neither a peptide nor a steroid hormone receptor. Tyrosine kinase is also a mechanism for many forms of protein production.

Type 2 Diabetes

Treatment

Diet, exercise, and weight loss are the best initial therapy for type 2 diabetes. Of patients with type 2, 25 percent can be controlled with exercise and weight loss alone.

The best initial medical therapy is **metformin.** Metformin is particularly beneficial in obese patients, because it does not lead to added weight gain. Sulfonylurea medications lead to increased weight gain because they increase the release of insulin.

A 65-year-old Hispanic man is seen in the office for follow-up. He was placed on metformin for type 2 diabetes after not responding to modifications of diet and exercise several months ago. Despite maximal doses of metformin, his blood glucose is > 150 mg/dL, and his HgA1c is above 7 percent. What is the next best step in management?

a. Add glyburide
b. Add insulin subcutaneously
c. Add insulin pump
d. Add rosiglitazone
e. Add acarbose or miglitol
f. Switch to a sulfonylurea

Answer: **A.** If a patient with type 2 diabetes cannot be adequately controlled with metformin, then add a second medication. The greatest efficacy and safety is with a **sulfonylurea.** If the question describes a patient originally placed on a sulfonylurea but not adequately controlled, then add metformin. There are several options before having to start insulin.

- **Metformin:** This agent works by **blocking gluconeogenesis.** The following are the main advantages of starting with metformin:
  - No risk of hypoglycemia
  - Does not increase obesity
- Metformin is *contraindicated* with the following:
  - **Renal insufficiency:** The metformin may accumulate and increase the risk of lactic acidosis.
  - **Use of contrast agents** for any radiologic or angiographic procedure: The contrast agents may lead to acute renal failure and, therefore, to the accumulation of metformin.
- **Sulfonylureas:** These are **glyburide, glimepiride, and glipizide.** These agents work by causing the **increased release of insulin** from the pancreas. Following are the *adverse effects* of sulfonylureas:
  - Hypoglycemia
  - SIADH

> Rosiglitazone is contraindicated with congestive heart failure.

- **Dipeptidyl peptidase IV (DPP-IV) inhibitors:** These are sitagliptin, linagliptin, alogliptin, and saxagliptin. These agents can be added as a second agent to metformin. DPP-IV inhibitors block metabolism or incretins such as glucagon-like peptide (GLP).

DPP-IV inhibitors (saxagliptin, linagliptin, alogliptin, and sitagliptin) increase insulin release and block glucagon.

Basic Science Correlate

Mechanism of Incretins

The incretins are also called glucagon-like peptides (GLPs) and glucose insulinotropic peptides (GIPs). GIP was in the past known as gastric inhibitory peptide. Incretins increase insulin release and decrease glucagon secretion from the pancreas. DPP-IV metabolizes GLP and GIP. Inhibiting DPP-IV maintains high levels of GLP and GIP.

GLP is a confusing misnomer: Glucagon raises glucose and FFA levels. **GLP *decreases* glucagon.**

- **Thiazolidinediones:** These are **rosiglitazone and pioglitazone.** These agents work by **increasing peripheral insulin sensitivity.** They may worsen congestive heart failure. Do not use with CHF.
- **Alpha-glucosidase inhibitors:** These are **acarbose and miglitol.** These agents **block the absorption of glucose at the intestinal lining.** They can lead to diarrhea, abdominal pain, bloating, and flatulence in much the same way as lactose intolerance.

Basic Science Correlate

Mechanism of Diarrhea with Glucosidase Inhibitors

When acarbose and miglitol block glucose absorption, the sugar remains in the bowel, available to bacteria. When bacteria eat the glucose, they cast off gas and acid. Using glucosidase inhibitors is like making a person lactose intolerant.

- **Insulin secretagogues:** These are **nateglinide and repaglinide.** These agents work in a **very similar fashion as sulfonylureas.** They are short acting and can cause hypoglycemia.
- **SGLT inhibitor:** Canagliflozin, dapagliflozin, and empagliflozin. These agents lead to urinary tract infections.

If other agents do not sufficiently control the level of glucose, then the patient is switched to **insulin.** A **long-acting insulin,** such as insulin glargine, which is a once-a-day injection with an extremely steady-state level of insulin, is used in combination with a **very short-acting insulin** at mealtime.

- **GLP analogs:** These agents increase insulin and decrease glucagon. GLP analogs such as exenatide and liraglutide promote weight loss and lower glucose.
- **Long-acting insulin**
  - **Glargine (Lantus):** Once a day
  - **Detemir**
  - **NPH:** Twice a day
- **Short-acting insulin:** Both of the following medications are given at mealtime and last about 2 hours. Regular insulin is given at mealtime but lasts longer, as much as 6 hours.
  - **Aspart**
  - **Lispro**
  - **Glulisine**

GLP analogs (e.g., exenatide) slow gastric emptying and promote weight loss.

Type 1 Diabetes (Juvenile Onset)

Type 1 diabetes always results from **underproduction of insulin.** The **pancreas is destroyed** during childhood on an autoimmune/genetic basis.

These patients are thin and do *not* respond to weight loss, exercise, or oral hypoglycemic agents. Sulfonylureas do *not* work, because there is no functioning pancreas to stimulate to increase insulin release.

Type 1 diabetics are more prone to developing **diabetic ketoacidosis** because of severe insulin deficiency.

Diabetic Ketoacidosis (DKA)

DKA presents as an extremely ill patient with **hyperventilation** as compensation for the **metabolic acidosis** (low bicarbonate). The patient also has a **"fruity" odor of the breath** from acetone and possibly **confusion** from the hyperosmolar state.

Diagnostic Testing

- Best initial test: **Serum bicarbonate** is the best way to determine the severity of illness. If the glucose level is high, this does *not* tell you that the patient has become acidotic. The patient may just have hyperglycemia. A **low serum bicarbonate** implies an elevated anion gap, and this is the marker for severe DKA.
- **Beta hydroxybutyrate** can also be obtained as a marker of ketone production. As you correct the ketoacidosis, the beta hydroxybutyrate level should decrease.

Lab findings in DKA are as follows:

Very high glucose artificially drops sodium level.

- **Hyperglycemia (> 250)**
- **Hyperkalemia:** Initially there will be *hyper*kalemia. If there is no insulin, potassium builds up outside the cell. The hyperkalemia will quickly translate into *hypo*kalemia as you treat the DKA. So it is very important to make sure you **supplement with potassium.**

Basic Science Correlate

Hyperkalemia is from transcellular shift of potassium out of the cell in exchange for hydrogen ions going into the cell. The cells "suck up acid" as a way of compensating for the severe metabolic acidosis and release potassium in exchange. Also, insulin drives potassium into cells with glucose.

- **Decreased serum bicarbonate**
- **Low pH,** with low pCO_2 as respiratory compensation
- **Acetone, acetoacetate, and beta hydroxybutyrate levels elevated**
- **Elevated anion gap**
- Pseudohyponatremia caused by high glucose

Acidosis = Hyperkalemia
Alkalosis = Hypokalemia

Basic Science Correlate

Mechanism of Increased Anion Gap

In order to use glucose as fuel, most cells need insulin. In the absence of insulin, glucose can't enter, and cells look for an alternate fuel source. The alternate fuel is FFA and ketones. Ketones are negatively charged acids, so using them as fuel drives down the level of bicarbonate.

Treatment

On this initial screen, order both the **labs** (chemistry, arterial blood gas, acetone level) and **fluids** (bolus of normal saline).

Once the high glucose and the low serum bicarbonate are found, order **IV insulin.** CCS does not require you to know doses, and, in fact, there is no way for you to write in a dose.

- **High glucose** + **Low bicarb** = **DKA** → Give bolus saline and IV insulin

> In a patient with DKA, the total body level of potassium is low. Chronic hyperkalemia depletes the body of potassium.

As you move the clock forward, you will notice that the potassium level drops into the normal range. Insulin drives potassium into cells, and as the acidosis corrects, the potassium level drops. At this point, you should **add potassium to the IV fluids.**

Complications of Diabetes

This is an excellent choice for an "office-based" setting of follow-up management on CCS.

Hypertension

The goal of management of hypertension in diabetes is a **BP < 140/90 mm Hg.** BP control is critical in diabetes to prevent long-term complications to the heart, eye, kidney, and brain.

Lipid Management

Diabetes is a coronary artery disease (CAD) equivalent. The LDL goal in a diabetic is < **100.** When the patient has *both* CAD and diabetes, the LDL goal is < **70.**

Retinopathy

A **dilated eye exam** should occur yearly in diabetics to detect **proliferative retinopathy.** If this is present, **laser photocoagulation** should be performed. VEGF inhibitors, ranibizumab, or bevacizumab can be used in severe proliferative retinopathy.

Nephropathy

Order a **urine microalbumin,** which detects minute amounts of albumin in the urine. If *any* form of protein, no matter how small, is present, give **ACE inhibitors.** Use ACE inhibitors for proteinuria even if the blood pressure is normal. ARBs have the same indication. Furthermore, use ACE inhibitors as first-line hypertensive agents in diabetics.

> **Basic Science Correlate**
>
> **Mechanism of Glomerular Damage**
>
> Uncontrolled diabetes removes the negative charge from the filtration slits of the glomerular basement membrane. Normally, negative charges repel the filtration of albumin, which is also negatively charged. Loss of negative charges allows albumin to pass through the glomerulus. ACE inhibitors decrease intraglomerular hypertension by dilating the efferent arteriole. This protects the glomerulus from the damage caused by intraglomerular hypertension.

Neuropathy

Foot examination yearly for diabetic neuropathy is indicated. If neuropathy is present, diagnostic testing is *not* necessary; go straight to treatment. Use **gabapentin** or **pregabalin.** Tricyclic antidepressants and carbamazepine are not as effective.

> **Basic Science Correlate**
>
> **Mechanism of Neuropathy in Diabetes**
>
> Nerves have a supply of blood vessels. Diabetes damages small blood vessels, starving off the nerves.

Erectile Dysfunction

There is no routine screening test for this condition except to **ask about its presence.** Treat with sildenafil and other phosphodiesterase inhibitors as usual. Remember: *No* sildenafil with nitrates!

Gastroparesis

The major stimulant for gastric motility is "stretch." In patients with longstanding diabetes, there is impaired ability to perceive stretch in the GI tract and impaired motility. Look for "bloating," constipation, abdominal fullness, and diarrhea. Treat with **metoclopramide** or **erythromycin.** Erythromycin increases the release of "motilin," a promotility GI hormone. You can also confirm the diagnosis with a gastric-emptying scan, but this is often unnecessary.

A 63-year-old man with longstanding diabetes comes to the office with a "pins and needles" sensation in both his feet. He is also chronically bloated and constipated. On review of systems, you find he cannot maintain erection sufficiently to complete intercourse. Urinalysis shows microalbuminuria. His LDL is 147. What is the best management for this patient?

a. HgA1c
b. Nerve conduction studies
c. Hydralazine and sildenafil
d. Ramipril, erythromycin, atorvastatin, and pregabalin
e. Gastric-emptying study and penile tumescence studies

Answer: **D.** Prescribe ACE inhibitors for the proteinuria, erythromycin for the diabetic gastroparesis and to increase GI motility, atorvastatin to decrease the LDL level to < 100 for a patient, and pregabalin for diabetic neuropathy. No further specific diagnostic tests are required when you see this collection of abnormalities.

Thyroid Disease

The following table shows the clinical presentation of hypo- and hyperthyroidism.

	Hypothyroidism	Hyperthyroidism
Weight	Gain	Loss
Intolerance	Cold	Heat
Hair	Coarse	Fine
Skin	Dry	Moist
Mental	Depressed	Anxious
Heart	Bradycardia	Tachycardia, tachyarrhythmias such as atrial fibrillation
Muscle	Weak	Weak
Reflexes	Diminished	
Fatigue	Yes	Yes
Menstrual changes	Yes	Yes

Basic Science Correlate

Thyroid hormone controls the metabolic rate of almost every cell in the body. Low thyroid hormone means reduced use of glucose and FFAs as fuel. This is why glucose intolerance and hyperlipidemia occur in hypothyroidism.

Low thyroid = Decreased metabolic rate = Weight gain

Hypothyroidism

This condition arises most often from "burnt out" Hashimoto's thyroiditis. It presents as a slow, tired, fatigued patient with weight gain.

Following are the best initial tests:

- **T4:** Decreased
- **Thyroid-stimulating hormone (TSH):** Increased

Treat with **T4** or **thyroxine replacement.** T4 will be converted in the local tissues to T3 as needed.

Hyperthyroidism

All forms of hyperthyroidism give an **elevated T4 level.** Almost all give a **suppressed TSH level.**

The table below summarizes the presentation and treatment of 4 forms of hyperthyroidism.

	Graves'	Silent	Subacute	Pituitary adenoma
Physical findings	Eye, skin, and nail findings	None	Tender gland	None
RAIU	Elevated	Low	Low	Elevated
Treatment	Radioactive iodine ablation	None	Aspirin	Surgical removal

RAIU = radioactive iodine uptake

Graves' Disease

In addition to the findings of hyperthyroidism described above, Graves' disease has several unique physical findings:

- **Ophthalmopathy:** The symptoms of ophthalmopathy include exophthalmos (eyes are bulging) and proptosis (lid is retracted).

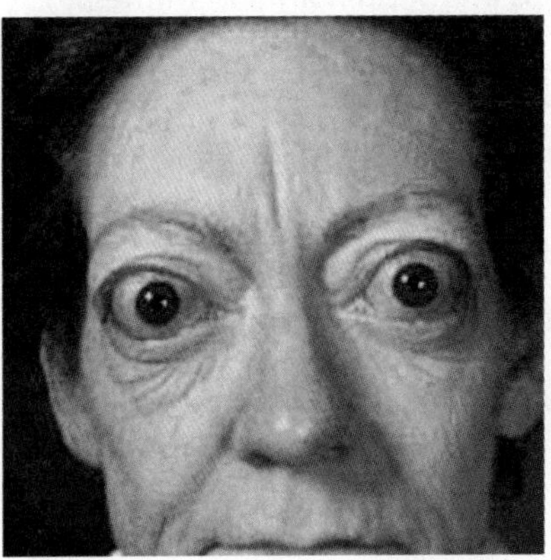

Basic Science Correlate

Mechanism of Ophthalmopathy

The levator palpebrae superioris is the muscle that lifts the eyelid, innervated by the third cranial nerve. Hyperthyroidism stimulates the beta receptors of the third cranial nerve. High thyroid levels pull up the eyelid by stimulating the levator muscle. Graves' disease also deposits mucopolysaccharides behind the eye. This pushes the eye forward, causing the exophthalmos.

- **Dermopathy:** This is thickening and redness of the skin just below the knee.
- **Onycolysis:** Occurring in only 10 percent of cases, this is separation of the nail from the nailbed.
- The radioactive iodine uptake (RAIU) level is elevated.

Treatment

- Use **propylthiouracil (PTU)** or **methimazole** acutely to bring the gland under control.
- Then use **radioactive iodine** to ablate the gland.
- Use **propranolol** to treat sympathetic symptoms, such as tremors, palpitations, etc.

Basic Science Correlate

Mechanism of PTU and Methimazole

These agents inhibit thyroperoxidase. Peroxidase will:

1. Oxidize iodine;
2. Put iodine on the tyrosine molecule to make monoiodotyrosine and diiodotyrosine; and
3. Couple up mono- and diiodotyrosine to make T4 and T3.

PTU and methimazole inhibit all of these steps in thyroid hormone synthesis.

"Silent" Thyroiditis

This condition is an autoimmune process with a **nontender gland and hyperthyroidism.** There are *no* eye, skin, or nail findings.

Unlike Graves' disease, the radioactive iodine uptake (RAIU) test is normal, since this is not a hyperfunctioning gland; it is just "leaking." **Antibodies to thyroid peroxidase and antithyroglobulin antibodies** may be present.

Treatment

None.

Subacute Thyroiditis

This condition has a viral etiology (we think!) and presents with a **tender gland.**

Diagnostic testing shows the following:

- **RAIU is low.**
- **T4 is high.**
- **TSH is low,** but that is not specific to this form of hyperthyroidism.

Treatment

Aspirin to relieve pain.

Pituitary Adenoma

This condition is rare. It is the *only* cause of hyperthyroidism with an **elevated TSH.**

Treatment

- **MRI** of the brain.
- **Remove adenoma.**

Exogenous Thyroid Hormone Abuse

The **T4 is up** and the **TSH suppressed.** However, the **thyroid gland will atrophy** to the point of nonpalpability on examination.

Thyroid "Storm"

Acute severe, life-threatening hyperthyroidism is also known as "thyroid storm."

Treatment

- **Iodine:** Blocks uptake of iodine into the thyroid gland and blocks the release of hormone.
- **Propylthiouracil or methimazole:** Blocks production of thyroxine.
- **Dexamethasone:** Blocks peripheral conversion of T4 to T3.
- **Propranolol:** Blocks target organ effect.

> PTU blocks conversion of T4 to T3.

Goiter

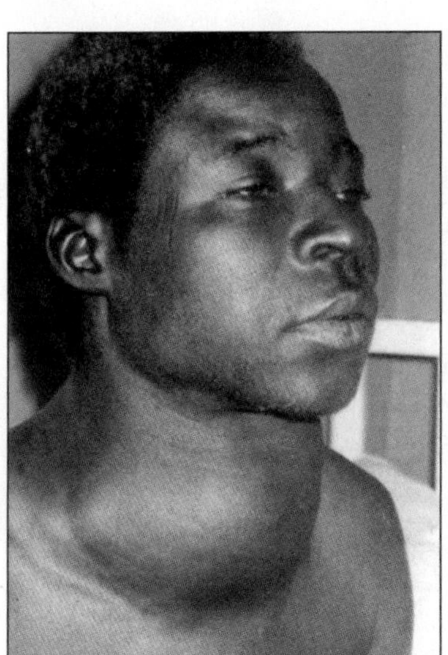

You *cannot* determine etiology only from the presence of a goiter. An enlarged gland can be associated with hyperthyroidism, hypothyroidism, or normal function of the thyroid.

Solitary Thyroid Nodule

Perform a **fine needle aspiration.** The *wrong* answers are ultrasound, radioactive iodine scan, something that says "sample" the gland, or anything that is not a "fine needle aspiration." Ultrasound is used to help place the needle.

If the nodule is cancer, an expert must remove it surgically. Do not biopsy lesions with increased thyroid function.

Calcium Disorders

Hypercalcemia

The most common cause of hypercalcemia in outpatients, by far, is **primary hyperparathyroidism.** An enormous number of people are walking around with hyperparathyroidism with no symptoms. Other causes of hypercalcemia are the following:

- **Malignancy:** Produces a parathyroid hormone–like particle
- **Granulomatous disease:** Sarcoid granulomas actually make vitamin D
- **Vitamin D intoxication**
- **Thiazide diuretics:** These increase tubular **reabsorption of calcium**
- **Tuberculosis**
- **Histoplasmosis**
- **Berylliosis**

Basic Science Correlate

Mechanism of Parathyroid Hormone (PTH) Effect

- Reabsorbs calcium at distal tubule
- Excretes phosphate at proximal tubule
- Activates vitamin D from 25 to the 1,25 dihydroxy form
- Reabsorbs both calcium and phosphate from bone

Hyperparathyroidism

The vast majority of cases present as **asymptomatic hypercalcemia.** Target organ damage is as follows:

- **Kidney stones**
- **Osteoporosis/osteomalacia/fractures**
- **Confusion**
- **Constipation and abdominal pain**

Basic Science Correlate

Mechanism of Neural Inhibition in Hypercalcemia

High calcium levels make it harder for excitable tissue such as nerves to depolarize. High calcium moves the threshold for depolarization away from the resting membrane potential. Bowels are a long muscular tube. High calcium inhibits smooth muscle contraction.

Low calcium = Hyperexcitable

Diagnostic Testing

Increased parathyroid hormone (PTH) level with hypercalcemia

Treatment

Surgical removal. Remember: Hyperparathyroidism may be a part of multiple endocrine neoplasia (MEN) syndrome. The nature of cases is as follows:

- Solitary adenoma: 80 percent
- Four-gland hyperplasia: 19 percent
- Cancer: 1 percent

When is the answer to a question about hyperparathyroidism surgical removal of the parathyroid gland?

Answer: Remove the gland under any of the following circumstances:

- Any symptomatic disease ("stones, bones, psychic moans, GI groans")
- Renal insufficiency, no matter how slight
- Markedly elevated 24-hour urine calcium
- Very elevated serum calcium (> 12.5)

Diuretics are **not** used if hydration increases urine output.

Acute, Severe Hypercalcemia

This condition presents with the following:

- **Confusion**
- **Constipation**
- **Polyuria and polydipsia** from nephrogenic diabetes insipidus
- **Short QT syndrome** on the EKG
- **Renal insufficiency, ATN, kidney stone**

Treatment

1. **Hydration:** High volume (3–4 liters) of normal saline
2. **Bisphosphonate** (pamidronate) is very potent but slow, taking a *week* to work. It inhibits osteoclasts.
3. **Furosemide:** Only *after* hydration has been given. Loop diuretics increase calcium excretion by the kidney if urine is not being produced through hydration alone.
4. **Calcitonin:** *If* hydration and furosemide do not control the calcium and you need something faster than a bisphosphonate, then calcitonin is the answer.
5. **Steroid:** Use if the etiology is **granulomatous disease.**

Basic Science Correlate

Mechanism of Volume Depletion in Hypercalcemia

High calcium levels inhibit the effect of ADH on the collecting duct, inducing nephrogenic diabetes insipidus. High calcium filtration also promotes osmotic diuresis.

Hypocalcemia

Hypocalcemia may be caused by the following:

- **Surgical removal of parathyroid glands**
- **Hypomagnesemia:** Magnesium is needed to release PTH from the gland.
- **Vitamin D deficiency**
- **Acute hyperphosphatemia:** Phosphate binds with the calcium and lowers it.
- **Fat malabsorption:** This binds calcium in the gut.
- **PTH resistance:** Pseudohypoparathyroidism that accompanies short fourth finger, round face, and mental retardation

Diagnostic Testing

Severe hypocalcemia presents with the following:

- **Seizures**
- **Neural twitching** (Chvostek's sign, Trousseau's sign)
- **Arrhythmia-prolonged QT** on EKG

Treatment

Replace the calcium. If there is vitamin D deficiency or hypoparathyroidism, then **give vitamin D and calcium.**

Adrenal Disorders

Cushing Syndrome (Hypercortisolism)

Any form of hyperadrenalism or hypercortisolism, no matter what the cause, has a common clinical presentation consisting of the following:

- **Fat redistribution:** Truncal obesity, "moon face," buffalo hump, thin arms and legs
- **Easy bruising and striae:** Loss of collagen from the cortisol thins the skin
- **Hypertension:** From fluid and sodium retention (look for hypokalemia in hyperaldosteronism)
- **Muscle wasting**
- **Hirsutism:** From increased adrenal androgen levels

Basic Science Correlate

Cortisol increases glucose levels by increasing gluconeogenesis. Cortisol breaks down proteins so the freed amino acids can be used to make sugar. Specifically, bone and skin proteins are broken down and made into sugar. This leads to bruising, striae, muscle wasting, and osteoporosis.

The following table summarizes the characteristics of the 3 sources of Cushing disease.

	Pituitary Tumor	Ectopic ACTH Production	Adrenal Adenoma
ACTH	High	High	Low
High-dose dexamethasone	Suppression	No suppression	No suppression
Specific test	MRI Petrossal vein sampling	Scan chest and abdomen	Scan adrenals
Treatment	Removal	Removal	Removal

Diagnostic Testing

Lab abnormalities are as follows:

- **Hyperglycemia, hyperlipidemia**
- **Osteoporosis**
- **Leukocytosis**
- **Metabolic alkalosis** caused by increased urinary loss of H+

Basic Science Correlate

Mechanism of Metabolic Alkalosis

Cortisol has both mineralocorticoid or aldosterone effects on the kidney. Excess adrenal steroids increase hydrogen ion excretion at the alpha-intercalated cell of the late distal/early collecting duct. Hypokalemia results from potassium excretion through the principal cell.

Following are the best initial diagnostic tests:

- **1 mg overnight dexamethasone suppression testing:** A normal person will suppress the 8:00 A.M. level of cortisol if given dexamethasone at 11:00 P.M. the night before. A normal 1 mg overnight dexamethasone suppression test excludes hypercortisolism of all kinds. An abnormal test can still be falsely elevated from various stresses, such as these:
  - Depression
  - Alcoholism
  - Emotional or physical stress
- **24-hour urine cortisol:** This test is done to confirm that an overnight dexamethasone suppression test is not falsely abnormal. The 24-hour urine cortisol adds specificity to the overnight test. If the overnight dexamethasone test is abnormal (fails to suppress), then get the 24-hour urine cortisol to confirm hypercortisolism (Cushing syndrome).

24-hour cortisol testing is more accurate (gives fewer false positives) than 1 mg overnight testing.

The overnight dexamethasone suppression and the 24-hour urine cortisol test are to **diagnose** the presence of Cushing syndrome. They do *not* determine the etiology or cause.

Treatment

Treatment is always removal of the cause.

"I have Cushing syndrome. Where is it coming from?"

"After the 1 mg overnight test and the 24-hour urine test confirm the presence of hypercortisolism, then we must determine the location or origin to treat it."

Following are indicators of the source of the hypercortisolism:

- **ACTH level low:** This means the origin is in the **adrenal gland. Scan the gland** with a CT or MRI and **remove the adenoma** that you find.
- **ACTH level high:** This means the origin is either in the **pituitary gland** or from the **ectopic production of ACTH.**

The next step is a high-dose dexamethasone suppression test.

Why bother with all this complex testing for Cushing syndrome? Why not just scan the brain and adrenals and remove what you find?

Answer: Many people have incidental adrenal and pituitary lesions. If you start with a scan, you might remove the wrong part of the body, and you cannot put it back!

A man with hypercortisolism is found to have an elevated ACTH level that suppresses with high-dose dexmethasone. MRI of this pituitary shows no visible lesion. What is the next best step in management?

a. Remove the pituitary
b. Repeat the dexamethasone suppression test
c. Use ketoconazole
d. Do petrosal venous sinus sampling
e. Order a PET scan of the brain

Answer: **D.** MRI and CT of the brain lack both sensitivity and specificity in diagnosing endocrine disorders. It is important to confirm the identity of an adrenal disorder functionally prior to scanning the patient. This patient has high cortisol with a high ACTH, indicating either the pituitary or an ectopic source of hyperadrenalism. The fact that the ACTH levels suppress with high-dose dexamethasone indicates a **pituitary adenoma,** which is the cause of Cushing syndrome in about 45 percent of patients. If the tests point to a pituitary source but the scanning is indeterminant, inferior petrosal sinus sampling is used to confirm it. Petrosal sinus sampling is also used **to localize the lesion,** as well to see which half of a pituitary should be removed.

24-hour urine cortisol is the best initial test of hypercortisolism.

If high-dose dexamethasone suppresses the ACTH, the origin is the **pituitary. Scan the pituitary. Remove the adenoma** if it is visible.

If high-dose dexamethasone does not suppress the ACTH, the origin is an **ectopic production of ACTH** or a **cancer that is making ACTH. Scan the chest** for lung cancer or carcinoid. **Remove the cancer** if possible.

Addison Disease (Adrenal Insufficiency)

The majority of cases of Addison are of autoimmune origin. It presents with the following:

- **Fatigue, anorexia, weight loss, weakness with hypotension**
- **Thin patient with hyperpigmented skin**

Diagnostic Testing

Laboratory abnormalities are as follows:

- **Hyperkalemia** with a **mild metabolic acidosis** from the inability to excrete either H^+ or K^+ because of the loss of aldosterone.
- **Hyponatremia**
- May have hypoglycemia and neutropenia: Glucocorticoids increase glucose and white cell levels.

Basic Science Correlate

Glucocorticoids increase glucose by blocking the uptake at peripheral tissues such as muscle, fat, and lymph. Glucocorticoids also have a permissive effect on glucagon, increasing its ability to break down glycogen from the liver. Glucocorticoids increase gluconeogenesis and break down protein for amino acid substrate.

The most accurate diagnostic tests are these:

- **Cosyntropin (synthetic ACTH) stimulation test:** You measure the level of cortisol before and after the administration of cosyntropin. If there is adrenal insufficiency, there will be no rise in cortisol level.
- **CT scan of the adrenal gland**

Treatment

Hydrocortisone provides both glucorticoid and mineralocorticoid effects on the kidney.

1. **Steroid replacement:** For **acute** addisonian (hypoadrenal) crisis, draw a cortisol level and give fluids and hydrocortisone. Hydrocortisone provides both glucocorticoid and mineralocorticoid activity.
2. **Prednisone: Stable** (nonhypotensive) patients are treated with prednisone.
3. **Fludrocortisone** is the steroid highest in mineralocorticoid content. Fludrocortisone is used for patients with adrenal insufficiency who are still hypotensive *after* initial replacement with prednisone.

Hyperaldosteronism

This condition presents with **hypertension, hypokalemia, and metabolic alkalosis.**

- Hypertension + Low renin + Low potassium = Hyperaldosteronism

Basic Science Correlate

The hypokalemia may lead to **motor weakness** from the inability to have normal motor contraction with the low potassium level. **Nephrogenic diabetes insipidus** can occur from hypokalemia. Hence, the case may feature "polyuria and polydipsia"; however, in primary hyperaldosteronism, the glucose level will be normal.

Diagnostic Testing

- **Low renin**
- **Hypertension**
- **Elevated aldosterone level** *despite* salt loading with normal saline

Confirm the diagnosis with a **CT scan** of the adrenal glands.

Treatment

- Solitary adenoma: **Surgical resection**
- Hyperplasia: **Spironolactone**

Pheochromocytoma

The patient presents with headache, palpitations, tremors, anxiety, and flushing. However, these symptoms are relatively nonspecific. Blood pressure that goes up in episodes is as close a clue as we get to knowing the diagnosis prior to testing.

- Pheochromocytoma = Episodic hypertension

Diagnostic Testing

- Best initial tests:
  - **High plasma and urinary catecholamine levels**
  - **Plasma-free metanephrine and VMA levels**
- Most accurate test:
  - **CT or MRI of the adrenal glands**
  - Metastatic disease is detected with an **MIBG scan,** which is a nuclear isotope scan to detect occult collections of pheochromocytoma.

Pheochromocytoma is part of MEN II.

Treatment

1. **Phenoxybenzamine (alpha blockade)** *first* to control blood pressure. Without alpha blockade, patients' blood pressure can significantly rise intraoperatively.
2. **Propranolol** is used *after* an alpha blocker like phenoxybenzamine.
3. **Surgical or laparoscopic resection.** Metastatic disease cannot be treated with surgery.
4. Metastatic disease is treated medically.

Congenital Adrenal Hyperplasia (CAH)

All forms of CAH have the following characteristics:

- **Elevated ACTH.**
- **Low aldosterone and cortisol levels.**
- Treatable with **prednisone,** which inhibits the pituitary.

The different kinds of CAH:

- **21 hydroxylase deficiency:** This is the most common type.
  - Hirsutism caused by increased adrenal androgens and *hypo*tension
  - Diagnose with **increased 17 hydroxyprogesterone level**
- **11 hydroxylase deficiency**
  - Hirsutism caused by increased adrenal androgens and *hyper*tension
- **17 hydroxylase deficiency**
  - **Hypertension** with *low* adrenal androgen levels

	Hypertension	Virilization
21	No	Yes
11	Yes	Yes
17	Yes	No

Basic Science Correlate

In CAH, hypertension is caused by increased 11-deoxycorticosterone, which acts like a mineralocorticoid. Because 11- and 17-hydroxylase deficiencies involve an increased level of 11-deoxycorticosterone, there is hypertension. Virilization is caused by increased adrenal androgens, DHEA, and androstenedione.

Prolactinoma

Prolactinoma is the most common pituitary tumor. It presents differently in men and women:

- **Men**
  - Presents with **impotence, decreased libido, and occasionally gynecomastia.** Presents *late.* No man rushes to the doctor in a panic to yell, "I can't get an erection and my breasts are big, too!"
  - Men are more likely to have the signs of mass effect of a tumor, such as **headache and visual disturbance.**
- **Women**
  - **Amenorrhea and galactorrhea in the absence of pregnancy** has women presenting *early.*

Basic Science Correlate

Prolactin inhibits GNRH. If there is no GNRH, the body cannot release LH and FSH.

Prolactinoma should *only* be investigated under the following conditions:

- Pregnancy has been excluded.
- Drugs such as metoclopramide, phenothiazines, or tricyclic antidepressants have been excluded as the cause of the high prolactin level.
- Prolactin level is *very* high (> 200).
- Other causes of hyperprolactinemia have been excluded:
  - Hypothyroidism: High thyrotropin-releasing hormone level stimulates prolactin
  - Nipple stimulation, chest wall irritation
  - Stress, exercise

Diagnostic Testing

The most accurate diagnostic test is an **MRI of the brain.**

Treatment

- Best initial therapy: **Dopamine agonist** agents, such as **bromocriptine** or **cabergoline.** Most prolactinomas respond to dopamine agonists.
- **Surgical removal** is performed for the small number of patients in whom medical therapy does *not* work.

Acromegaly

Acromegaly is the excess production of growth hormone from a growth hormone-secreting adenoma in the pituitary. It presents with **enlargement of the head** (hat size), **fingers** (ring size), **feet** (shoe size), **nose, and jaw.** In addition, there is **intense sweating** from enlargement of the sweat glands. It also causes the following:

- **Joint abnormalities:** These arise from unusual growth of the articular cartilage
- **Amenorrhea:** Growth hormone is frequently cosecreted with prolactin
- **Cardiomegaly and hypertension**
- **Colonic polyps**

Diabetes is common because growth hormone acts as an anti-insulin.

Diagnostic Testing

- Best initial test: **Insulinlike growth factor (IGF)** is done *first* to confirm a diagnosis of acromegaly. Growth hormone (GH) level is *not* done first, because GH has its maximum secretion in the middle of the night during deep sleep. GH also has a short half-life. IGF is the "best initial test" because it has a much longer half-life.

Basic Science Correlate

IGF is "insulinlike" because it works through the tyrosine kinase receptor, which is also how growth hormone (GH) builds protein. GH has a direct effect of increasing glucose and free fatty acids (FFAs). The protein effect results entirely from the increase in DNA polymerase brought about by IGF stimulation of tyrosine kinase. Insulin also helps build proteins.

- Most accurate test: Normally GH should be suppressed by glucose. GH raises glucose levels because it is a stress hormone. If the glucose level is high, this should suppress the level of GH. **Suppression of GH by giving glucose excludes acromegaly.**
- **MRI** will show a lesion in the pituitary, but it is essential to know the function of a pituitary tumor *before* anatomic visualization happens with an MRI.

Treatment

- **Surgical resection with transphenoidal removal** cures 70 percent of cases.
- **Octreotide:** Somatostatin has some effect in preventing the release of growth hormone.
- **Cabergoline or bromocriptine:** Dopamine agonists inhibit growth hormone release.
- **Pegvisomant:** This is a growth hormone receptor antagonist.

Hormones of Reproduction

Amenorrhea

Primary amenorrhea is caused by a genetic defect, such as the following:

1. **Turner's syndrome:** Look for short stature, webbed neck, wide-spaced nipples, and scant pubic and axillary hair. The **XO karyotype** prevents menstruation.
2. **Testicular feminization:** This is a genetically male patient who looks, feels, and acts as a woman. Socially the patient is female. The absence of testosterone receptors results in no penis, prostate, or scrotum. The patient does not menstruate.

Testicular feminization presents as a girl who does not menstruate. The girl has breasts but no cervix, tubes, or ovaries, and she is missing the top third of the vagina. She also does not have a penis, prostate, or scrotum.

Secondary amenorrhea is caused by the following:

- **Pregnancy, exercise, extreme weight loss, hyperprolactinemia**
- **Polycystic ovary syndrome (PCOS):** Obesity, amenorrhea, and hirsuitism are associated with large cystic ovaries. There are increased adrenal androgens. PCOS is an idiopathic disorder that presents as infertility and hirsutism. Why androgen levels such as DHEA increase is unknown. The mechanism of diabetes and glucose intolerance is likewise unknown. Treat PCOS with metformin. Treat the virilization with spironolactone, which has anti-androgenic effects.

Male Hypogonadism

Klinefelter's Syndrome

Patients with this syndrome are **tall men** with the following characteristics:

- **Insensitivity of the FSH and LH receptors on their testicles**
- **XXY on karyotype**
- The **FSH and LH levels are very high,** but *no* testosterone is produced from the testicles.

Treatment is with **testosterone.**

Kallman's Syndrome

This syndrome results in **anosmia with hypogonadism.** This is a problem originating at the hypothalamus, so there is **low GnRH, FSH, and LH. Anosmia** is the key to the diagnosis.

Pulmonology

5

Asthma

Asthma presents as a patient who is short of breath with **expiratory wheezing.** In severe cases, there is use of accessory muscles, and the patient is unable to speak in complete sentences.

> Remember: To wheeze, one must have airflow. If the asthma exacerbation is severe, there may *not* be any wheezing. This is an ominous sign.

The most important features of a *severe* asthma exacerbation are the following:

- **Hyperventilation/increased respiratory rate**
- **Decrease in peak flow**
- **Hypoxia**
- **Respiratory acidosis**
- **Possible absence of wheezing**

Diagnostic Testing

Patient with Unclear Diagnosis of Asthma

If a patient is admitted with **acute shortness of breath** and it is unclear if the diagnosis is asthma, **pulmonary function testing (PFT)** should be performed before and after inhaled bronchodilators. Asthma and reactive airway disease are confirmed with an **increase in the FEV_1 of > 12 percent.**

Asymptomatic Patient

A young man comes to the clinic for evaluation of intermittent episodes of shortness of breath. Currently he is not short of breath. What is the best test to determine a diagnosis of reactive airway disease?

a. Chest x-ray
b. Diffusion capacity of carbon monoxide (DLCO)
c. High-resolution CT scan
d. Methacholine stimulation testing
e. Pre- and postbronchodilation pulmonary function testing (PFT)

Answer: **D.** Methacholine stimulation testing looks for a decrease in FEV_1 in response to synthetic acetylcholine. Methacholine will decrease FEV_1 if the patient has asthma. The DLCO is a good test of interstitial lung disease, in which it is decreased. Asthmatic patients may have an increased DLCO from hyperventilation. High-resolution CT scanning is a test for interstitial lung disease and for bronchiectasis. Pre- and postbronchodilation PFTs are an appropriate assessment if the patient is currently short of breath to see if there is improvement, but they are of no value in an asymptomatic patient. Chest x-ray is not specific enough to be the "most accurate test."

Treatment

All patients with shortness of breath should receive the following:

- Oxygen
- Continuous oximeter
- Chest x-ray
- Arterial blood gas (ABG)

The best initial therapies, which should be ordered with the first screen on CCS, are the following:

- **Inhaled bronchodilators (albuterol):** There is no maximum dose of inhaled bronchodilators.
- **Bolus of steroids (methyl prednisolone):** Steroids need 4–6 hours to be effective.
- **Inhaled ipratropium**
- **Oxygen**
- **Magnesium**

Any patient with asthma and **respiratory acidosis with CO_2 retention** should be placed in the **ICU.** *Persistent* respiratory acidosis is an indication for **intubation and mechanical ventilation.**

Acute Asthma

The following therapies have *no* benefit for acute asthma exacerbation:

- Theophylline
- Cromolyn and nedocromil
- Montelukast
- Inhaled corticosteroids
- Omalizumab (anti-IgE)
- Salmeterol and long-acting beta agonists
- Epinephrine: Subcutaneously administered epinephrine has *no* benefit in addition to inhaled bronchodilators.
- Terbutaline: Terbutaline is less efficacious than inhaled albuterol. Terbutaline is always a *wrong* answer choice.

If there is an indication for beta blockers that decreases mortality in an asthmatic, then use the beta blocker.

Basic Science Correlate

Omalizumab is an IgG against IgE. Decreasing IgE decreases activation and release of mast cells.

Nonacute Asthma

1. Best initial therapy: **Inhaled bronchodilator** (albuterol)
2. If the patient is not controlled, add a chronic controller medication, such as an **inhaled steroid.**
3. If inhaled albuterol and inhaled steroids do not control symptoms, add a **long-acting inhaled beta agonist,** such as salmeterol or formeterol.
4. Oral steroids are used *only* as a last resort because of adverse effects.

Efficacy of beta blockers for mortality (MI, CHF) is more important than adverse effects (asthma, COPD).

The following table shows alternate long-term controller medications besides inhaled steroids.

Cause	Medication
Extrinsic allergies, such as hay fever	Cromolyn or nedocromil
Atopic disease	Montelukast
Chronic obstructive pulmonary disease (COPD)	Tiotropium, ipratropium
High IgE levels, no control with cromolyn	Omalizumab (anti-IgE antibody)

Basic Science Correlate

Mechanism of Antimuscarinic Medications

Because they are inhaled, ipratropium and tiotropium inhibit muscarinic receptors predominantly on respiratory mucosae. Antimuscarinic activity dries the secretions of goblet cells, decreases bronchoconstriction, and inhibits excess fluid production in bronchi. These agents are especially effective in COPD.

Exercise-Induced Asthma

Exercise-induced asthma is best treated with an **inhaled bronchodilator** prior to exercise.

Chronic Obstructive Pulmonary Disease (COPD)/Emphysema

This condition presents in a **long-term smoker with increasing shortness of breath and decreased exercise tolerance.**

In cases of COPD, order *arterial blood gas (ABG).* ABG is critical in acute shortness of breath from COPD because there is no other way to assess for CO_2 retention.

Acute episodes of shortness of breath should be handled as follows:

- **Oxygen and arterial blood gas (ABG)**
- **Chest x-ray**
- **Albuterol,** inhaled
- **Ipratropium,** inhaled
- **Bolus of steroids** (e.g., methyl prednisolone)
- **Chest, heart, extremity, and neurological examination**
- If fever, sputum, and/or a new infiltrate is present on chest x-ray, add ceftriaxone and azithromycin for community-acquired pneumonia.

For mild respiratory acidosis, answer *CPAP* or *BiPAP* and move the clock forward 30–60 minutes. If the CO_2 retention and hypoxia are improved, the patient is spared from intubation.

CCS Tip: On CCS, move the clock forward 15–30 minutes and reassess the patient. Oxygen administration in COPD may *worsen* the shortness of breath by eliminating hypoxic drive.

Do *not* intubate patients with COPD for CO_2 retention alone. These patients often have **chronic CO_2 retention.** *Only* intubate if there is a worsening drop in pH indicative of a worse **respiratory acidosis.** Serum bicarbonate is often elevated due to metabolic alkalosis as compensation for chronic respiratory acidosis.

Office/Clinic-Based Cases Emphasizing "Further Management"

CCS and single best answer questions on Step 3 often emphasize chronic conditions needing "further management." Although one should perform a complete physical examination in all of these cases, the important findings are the following:

- Physical findings:
  - Barrel-shaped chest
  - Clubbing of fingers
  - Increased anterior-posterior diameter of the chest
  - Loud P2 heart sound (sign of pulmonary hypertension)
  - Edema as a sign of decreased right ventricular output (the blood is backing up due to the pulmonary hypertension)
- Laboratory testing:
  - **EKG:** Right axis deviation, right ventricular hypertrophy, right atrial hypertrophy
  - **Chest x-ray:** Flattening of the diaphragm (due to hyperinflation of the lungs), elongated heart, and substernal air trapping
  - **CBC: Increased hematocrit** is a sign of chronic hypoxia. Reactive erythrocytosis from chronic hypoxia is often **microcytic.** An erythropoietin level is not necessary.

In moderate to severe cases of COPD, patients may become members of the 50/50 club—the pCO_2 is 50 mm Hg and the pO_2 is also 50 mm Hg. Here's an example ABG for a patient with COPD:

- pH: 7.35
- pCO_2: 49
- pO_2: 52
- HCO_3: 32

- **Chemistry: Increased serum bicarbonate** is metabolic compensation for respiratory acidosis.
- **ABG:** Should be done even in office-based cases to assess CO_2 retention and the need for chronic home oxygen based on pO_2 (you expect the pCO_2 to rise and the pO_2 to fall).

Basic Science Correlate

Mechanism of Right Heart Enlargement in COPD

Hypoxia in the lungs causes capillary constriction, in which precapillary sphincters in the lungs constrict to shunt blood away from hypoxic areas of the lung. Since the hypoxia of COPD is global throughout the lung, this diffuse vasoconstriction increases pressure in the right ventricle and right atrium. Over time, the result is hypertrophy of both chambers, leading to cor pulmonale, or right heart failure.

- **Pulmonary function testing (PFT):** You should expect to find the following:
  - Decrease in FEV_1
  - Decrease in FVC from loss of elastic recoil of the lung
  - Decrease in the FEV_1/FVC ratio
  - Increase in total lung capacity from air trapping
  - Increase in residual volume
  - Decrease in diffusion capacity lung carbon monoxide (DLCO) caused by destruction of lung interstitium

PFT Results: COPD

FEV_1	FVC	FEV_1/FVC ratio	Total Lung Capacity	Residual Volume	DLCO
↓	↓	↓	↑	↑	↓

Chronic Medical Therapy of COPD

- **Tiotropium** or **ipratropium inhaler**
- **Albuterol inhaler**
- **Pneumococcal vaccine:** Heptavalent vaccine, Pneumovax
- **Influenza vaccine:** Yearly. Inactivated injections only.
- **Smoking cessation**
- **Long-term home oxygen** if the $pO_2 < 55$ or the oxygen saturation is < 88 percent

Almost all patients with COPD can tolerate beta-1-specific blockers.

Which of the following lowers mortality in COPD?

a. Smoking cessation
b. Home oxygen therapy (continuous)

Answer: Both of these therapies reduce mortality in COPD.

Basic Science Correlate

Mechanism of Bicarbonate Increase in COPD

COPD generates CO_2 retention. CO_2 retention generates respiratory acidosis. Chronic respiratory acidosis increases new bicarbonate generation at the distal tubule of the kidney.

COPD = Bicarbonate increase

Alpha-1 Antitrypsin Deficiency

This is a genetic disorder that presents with a combination of cirrhosis and COPD. Look for a case of COPD at an **early age (< 40)** in a **nonsmoker** who has bullae at the bases of the lungs.

Diagnostic Testing

- **Chest x-ray:** Findings of COPD (bullae, barrel chest, flat diaphragm)
- **Blood tests:** Low albumin level and elevated prothrombin time (caused by **cirrhosis**)
- **Alpha-1 antitrypsin level is low**
- **Genetic testing**

Treatment

Treatment is with alpha-1 antitrypsin infusion.

Bronchiectasis

Bronchiectasis is caused by an **anatomic defect** of the lungs, usually from an infection in childhood. This results in **profound dilation of bronchi.**

It presents as chronic resolving and recurring **episodes of lung infection** that give a very **high volume of sputum** that can be measured by the cupful. **Hemoptysis and fever** occur as well. Clubbing is seldom present.

Diagnostic Testing

A **chest x-ray** shows dilated bronchi with **"tram tracking,"** which are parallel lines consistent with dilated bronchi. The most accurate diagnostic test is a **high-resolution CT scan of the chest.**

Treatment

There is *no* curative therapy. Treat the infectious episodes as they occur.

- **Chest physiotherapy** with "cupping and clapping" will help dislodge secretions.
- **Rotating antibiotics** are tried to avoid the development of resistance.

Interstitial Lung Disease (ILD)

ILD can be idiopathic, such as a form of pulmonary fibrosis secondary to occupational or environmental exposure and medications (e.g., trimethoprim/sulfamethizole [Bactrim], or nitrofurantoin). If no cause is found, the diagnosis is "idiopathic pulmonary fibrosis" by exclusion.

Nitrofurantoin is associated with lung fibrosis.

The following table shows the causes of interstitial lung disease:

Cause	Disease
Asbestos	Asbestosis
Glass workers, mining, sandblasting, brickyards	Silicosis
Coal worker	Coal worker's pneumoconiosis
Cotton	Byssinosis
Electronics, ceramics, fluorescent light bulbs	Berylliosis
Mercury	Pulmonary fibrosis

ILD presents with **shortness of breath with a dry, nonproductive cough and chronic hypoxia.** ILD is a long-term disease and is often punctuated by episodes of bronchitis and pneumonia.

Physical findings are the following:

- **Dry, "Velcro" rales**
- **Loud P2 heart sound as a sign of pulmonary hypertension**
- **Clubbing**

In ILD, the EKG will show pulmonary hypertension with right atrial and right ventricular hypertrophy.

ILD does *not* give fever or systemic findings.

Basic Science Correlate

Pulmonary hypoxia causes vasoconstriction of the lungs. Chronic vasoconstriction causes increased pressure in the pulmonary artery. Pulmonary hypertension kills patients.

Diagnostic Testing

- **Chest x-ray:** Interstitial fibrosis
- **High-resolution CT scan:** Shows more detail on interstitial fibrosis
- **Lung biopsy**
- **Pulmonary function testing (PFT):** Shows decreased FEV_1 and decreased FVC with a normal ratio, decreased total lung capacity, and decreased DLCO. All the measures are decreased, but they are decreased proportionately.

PFT Results: ILD

FEV_1	FVC	FEV_1/FVC Ratio	Total Lung Capacity	Residual Volume	DLCO
↓	↓	Normal / ↑	↓	↓	↓

DLCO = diffusion capacity lung carbon monoxide

Treatment

There is *no* specific therapy to reverse any of the forms of ILD.

The most common type of cancer in asbestosis is *lung cancer,* not mesothelioma.

- If the biopsy shows an inflammatory infiltrate, a **trial of steroids** is used. The only form of ILD that definitely responds to steroids is **berylliosis,** because it is a granulomatous disease.
- There is definitely no therapy for silicosis, mercury vapor-induced fibrosis, asbestosis, or byssinosis.

BOOP/COP

Bronchiolitis obliterans organizing pneumonia (BOOP), also known as cryptogenic organizing pneumonia (COP), is a rare bronchiolitis or inflammation of small airways with a chronic alveolitis of unknown origin, although a few cases are associated with rheumatoid arthritis.

Although BOOP/COP has many similarities to ILD, the presentation is more acute over weeks to months. In addition to **cough, rales, and shortness of breath,** there is **fever, malaise, and myalgias.** (These systemic findings are *absent* from ILD.) Also, there is **no occupational exposure** in the history.

Diagnostic Testing

- **Chest x-ray:** Shows bilateral patchy infiltrates
- **Chest CT:** Shows interstitial disease and alveolitis
- Most accurate diagnostic test: **Open lung biopsy** is the only definitive way to make the diagnosis of BOOP/COP.

Treatment

Treat BOOP/COP with **steroids.** There is *no* response to antibiotics.

The following table compares BOOP/COP and ILD.

BOOP/COP	ILD
Fever, myalgias, malaise (clubbing uncommon)	No fever, no myalgias
Presents over days to weeks	Six months or more of symptoms
Patchy infiltrates	Interstitial infiltrates
Steroids effective	Rarely responds to steroids

Sarcoidosis

This condition presents in an **African-American woman** under 40 with **cough, shortness of breath,** and **fatigue** over a few weeks to months. Physical examination shows **rales.** Although sarcoidosis can involve many organs, the vast majority of cases present with lung findings only.

Rare physical findings and presentation include the following:

- **Eye:** Uveitis that can be sight threatening
- **Neural:** Seventh cranial nerve involvement is the most common.
- **Skin:** Lupus pernio (purplish lesion of the skin of the face), erythema nodosum
- **Cardiac:** Restrictive cardiomyopathy, cardiac conduction defects
- **Renal and hepatic involvement:** Occurs without symptoms
- **Hypercalcemia:** This occurs in a small number of patients secondary to vitamin D production by the granulomas of sarcoidosis.

Diagnostic Testing

- Best initial test: **Chest x-ray,** which always shows **enlarged lymph nodes.** There may be interstitial lung disease in addition to the nodal involvement.
- Most accurate diagnostic test: **Lung or lymph node biopsy** showing **noncaseating granulomas**

- Calcium and ACE levels may be elevated, but these are not specific enough to lead to a specific diagnosis.
- **Bronchoalveolar lavage** shows increased numbers of helper cells.

Treatment

Steroids are the undisputed best therapy.

Pulmonary Hypertension

Primary pulmonary hypertension presents as an idiopathic cause of **shortness of breath, more often in young women,** from overgrowth and obliteration of pulmonary vasculature, leading to decreased flow out of the right ventricle. Pulmonary hypertension can occur secondary to the following:

- Mitral stenosis
- COPD
- Polycythemia vera
- Chronic pulmonary emboli
- Interstitial lung disease

Physical findings are as follows:

- **Loud P2**
- **Tricuspid regurgitation**
- **Right ventricular heave**
- **Raynaud's phenomenon**

Diagnostic Testing

- **Transthoracic echocardiogram (TTE):** Shows right ventricular hypertrophy and enlarged right atrium
- **EKG:** Shows the same findings as well as right axis deviation
- Most accurate test: **Right heart catheterization** (Swan-Ganz catheterization) **with increased pulmonary artery pressure**

Treatment

- **Bosentan** is an endothelin inhibitor that prevents growth of the vasculature of the pulmonary system.
- **Epoprostenol** and **treprostinil** are prostacyclin analogs that act as pulmonary vasodilators.
- **Calcium channel blockers** (weak efficacy)
- **Sildenafil**

Pulmonary Embolism (PE)

PE presents with the **sudden onset of shortness of breath** and **clear lungs** in patients with risk factors for deep venous thrombosis (DVT). The following are risk factors for DVT:

- Immobility
- Malignancy
- Trauma
- Surgery, especially joint replacement
- Thrombophilia, such a factor V mutation, lupus anticoagulant, or protein C and S deficiency

There are *no specific physical findings* for PE.

Diagnostic Testing

- **Chest x-ray:** The most common result is **normal.** The most common abnormality found is **atelectasis.** Wedge-shaped infarction and pleural-based humps are rare.
- **EKG:** The most common showing is **sinus tachycardia.** The most common abnormality is **nonspecific ST-T wave changes.** Right axis deviation and right bundle branch block are uncommon.
- **ABG:** This shows hypoxia with an increased A-a gradient and mild respiratory alkalosis.

Basic Science Correlate

Mechanism of Right Heart Strain

PE blocks blood flow. Blood flow block causes a severe pressure increase in the pulmonary artery and right ventricle. The increase in pressure from increased pressure in PE, not as much the hypoxia-induced vasoconstriction of COPD. Right heart strain occurs only with the most severe, large emboli that kill.

Right heart strain + Hypotension = Thrombolytics

A patient who has recently undergone hip fracture repair develops the sudden onset of shortness of breath. His pulse is 110 per minute. The chest is clear to auscultation. Chest x-ray is normal, and the EKG shows sinus tachycardia. ABG shows pH 7.48, pCO_2 28, pO_2 75. What is the next best step in management?

a. Heparin
b. V/Q scan
c. Spiral CT scan
d. D-dimers
e. Lower extremity Doppler
f. Angiography

Answer: **A.** When the case so clearly suggests a pulmonary embolus with sudden onset of shortness of breath and clear lungs in a patient with a risk factor, the first thing to do after the chest x-ray and blood gas is to start heparin. Do not wait for the results of V/Q scan or spiral CT to start heparin.

Confirmatory Testing

CT Angiogram

A CT angiogram is standard to confirm the presence of a pulmonary embolus. The CT angiogram is excellent if it is positive because of its specificity. The sensitivity of CT angiogram is excellent, and the test can miss some emboli if they are small and in the periphery. The CT angiogram is clearly the **test of choice if the x-ray is abnormal.**

V/Q Scan

For a V/Q scan to be accurate, the chest x-ray *must* be normal. The less normal the x-ray, the less accurate the V/Q scan. This is still a good test for PE. The problem is that *only* a truly normal scan excludes a PE. Of patients with low-probability scans, 15 percent still have a PE, and 15 percent of those with of high-probability scans don't have a PE.

Lower Extremity Doppler

These are excellent tests *if* they are positive; if positive, no further diagnostic testing is necessary. The problem is that 30 percent of PEs originate in pelvic veins, and the Doppler scan is normal even in the presence of a PE. Hence, the sensitivity of lower extremity Doppler is about 70 percent.

D-Dimer Testing

This is a very sensitive test with poor specificity. If the D-dimer is negative, PE is extremely unlikely. The best use of D-dimer testing is in a patient with a **low probability of PE in whom you want a single test to exclude PE.**

Basic Science Correlate

D-dimers are a metabolic breakdown product of fibrin. Plasmin chops up fibrin into D-dimers, but it is only effective with fresh, new clots that have formed over the last day. Older clots have been stabilized with factor XIII or clot stabilizing factor, which make them impervious to dissolution by plasmin.

D-dimers = Plasmin chopped up fresh clot

Angiography

Angiography is the single most accurate test for PE. Unfortunately, angiography is **invasive with a significant risk of death** of about 0.5 percent. CT angiography makes angiography with a catheter rarely ever the best answer.

A 45-year-old man comes to the emergency department after a motor vehicle accident resulting in a liver hematoma. On the third hospital day, he becomes suddenly short of breath. His chest x-ray is normal, and he is diagnosed with a pulmonary embolus. What is the next best step in management?

a Angiography
b. Embolectomy
c. Heparin
d. Inferior vena cava filter

Answer: **D.** When a patient has a pulmonary embolism and there is a contraindication to anticoagulation, a vena cava interruption filter should be placed. This patient has a liver hematoma, so a filter should be placed.

Treatment

- **Heparin and oxygen:** This is the standard of care in pulmonary embolism.
- **Warfarin:** Should be used for **at least 6 months** *after* the use of heparin.
- **Venous interruption filter:** This should be placed in all patients who have **a contraindication to anticoagulation.**
- **Thrombolytics:** These are used in patients who are **hemodynamically unstable.** Hemodynamic instability can be defined as *hypotension.* Thrombolytics essentially replace embolectomy, which is rarely performed because of the high operative mortality.

Basic Science Correlate

Thrombolytics activate plasminogen to plasmin. Plasmin dissolves only fresh clots, not clots stabilized by factor XIII. This is part of why thrombolytics are only useful within 12 hours post-MI. In PE, clots are older than the coronary clots of MI, but when they have formed is unclear. This is why there is no precise time frame for using thrombolytics in PE.

Pleural Effusion

Diagnostic Testing

- Best initial test: **Chest x-ray.** Decubitus films with the patient lying on one side should be done next to see if the fluid is freely flowing.
- **Chest CT** may add a little more detail to a chest x-ray.
- Most accurate test: **Thoracentesis**

Exudate	Transudate
Cancer and infection	Congestive failure
Protein level **high** (> 50 percent of serum level)	Protein level **low** (< 50 percent of serum level)
LDH level **high** (> 60 percent of serum level)	LDH level **low** (< 60 percent of serum level)

- Order the following tests on pleural fluid:
  - Gram stain and culture
  - Acid-fast stain
  - Total protein (also order serum protein)
  - LDH (also order serum LDH)
  - Glucose
  - Cell count w/differential
  - Triglycerides
  - pH

Treatment

- Small pleural effusions do *not* need therapy. **Diuretics** can be used, especially for those caused by congestive heart failure (CHF).
- For larger effusions, especially those caused by infection (empyema), a **chest tube** for drainage is placed.
- If the effusion is large and recurrent from a cause that cannot be corrected, **pleurodesis** is performed.

Basic Science Correlate

Pleurodesis is the infusion of an irritative agent, such as bleomycin or talcum powder, into the pleural space. This inflames the pleura, causing fibrosis so the lung will stick to the chest wall. When the pleural space is eliminated, the effusion cannot reaccumulate.

- If pleurodesis fails, **decortication** is performed. Decortication is the stripping off of the pleura from the lung so it will stick to the interior chest wall. This is an operative procedure.

Sleep Apnea

Look for an **obese patient** complaining of **daytime somnolence.** The patient's sleep partner will report **severe snoring.** In addition, there will be hypertension, headache, erectile dysfunction, and a fat neck.

The majority (95 percent) of cases are obstructive sleep apnea from fatty tissues of the neck blocking breathing. A small number of patients will have central sleep apnea, which is decreased respiratory drive from the central nervous system.

Diagnostic Testing

Sleep apnea is diagnosed with a sleep study, **polysomnography.** The patient is observed for periods of apnea lasting > 10 seconds each. The patient's oxygen saturation is also monitored. Mild sleep apnea is defined as 5–20 apneic periods an hour. Severe sleep apnea is defined as > 30 periods an hour.

Treatment

Obstructive Disease

- Treat with **weight loss** and **continuous positive airway pressure (CPAP)** or **BiPAP.**
- If this is not effective, **surgical resection of the uvula, palate, and pharynx** can be performed.

Central Sleep Apnea

- Central sleep apnea is managed by **avoiding alcohol and sedatives.**
- It may respond to **acetazolamide,** which causes a metabolic acidosis. This may help drive respiration.
- Some patients respond to **medroxyprogesterone,** which is also a central respiratory stimulant.

Basic Science Correlate

Mechanism of Acetazolamide

Acetazolamide is an inhibitor of carbonic anhydrase. This enzyme is needed for reabsorption of bicarbonate that has been filtered at the glomerulus. In the absence of carbonic anhydrase, the bicarbonate is urinated off and the body becomes acidotic. Acidosis acts as a stimulant to the medulla to drive respiration.

Allergic Bronchopulmonary Aspergillosis (ABPA)

This presents as an **asthmatic patient with worsening asthma symptoms** who is coughing up **brownish mucous plugs with recurrent infiltrates.** There is **peripheral eosinophilia. Serum IgE is elevated. Central bronchiectasis is visible.**

Diagnostic Testing

- **Aspergillus skin testing**
- Measurement of **IgE levels, circulating precipitins, and *A.* fumigatus-specific antibodies**

Inhaled steroids **do not** help ABPA.

Treatment

Treatment is with **oral corticosteroids** and, in patients with refractory disease, **itraconazole.**

Acute Respiratory Distress Syndrome (ARDS)

ARDS is a **sudden, severe respiratory failure syndrome** resulting from diffuse lung injury secondary to a number of **overwhelming systemic injuries** such as these:

- Sepsis
- Aspiration of gastric contents
- Shock
- Infection: pulmonary or systemic
- Lung contusion
- Trauma
- Toxic inhalation
- Near drowning
- Pancreatitis
- Burns

Diagnostic Testing

- **Chest x-ray:** This shows diffuse patchy infiltrates that become confluent. May suggest congestive failure.
- Normal wedge pressure
- **pO_2/FIO_2 ratio < 200,** with the FIO_2 expressed as a decimal (e.g., room air is 0.21). For example, if the pO_2 is 100/0.21, the ratio is 476.

Treatment

- **Ventilatory support** with **low tidal volume** of 6 mL per kg
- **Positive end expiratory pressure (PEEP)** to keep the alveoli open
- **Prone positioning** of the patient's body
- Possible use of **diuretics** and **positive inotropes,** such as dobutamine
- Transfer the patient to the **ICU** if not already there

Steroids are *not* effective in cases of ARDS.

Basic Science Correlate

Mechanism of PEEP

Positive-end expiratory pressure (PEEP) keeps the alveoli open. When the alveoli are thus expanded, more surface area is available for gas exchange. Without PEEP, there is more atelectasis and less surface area for gas exchange.

Swan-Ganz (Pulmonary Artery) Catheterization

Use the measurements below when a case is described and the question says: Which of the following will most likely be found in this patient?

Type	Cardiac Output	Wedge Pressure	Systemic Vascular Resistance (SVR)
Hypovolemia	Low	Low	High
Cardiogenic Shock	Low	High	High
Septic Shock	High	Low	Low

Pneumonia

Pneumonia presents with **fever, cough, and often sputum.** Severe illness also presents with **shortness of breath.** Following are the most likely organisms involved:

- **Community-acquired pneumonia (CAP):** *Pneumococcus*
- **Hospital-acquired pneumonia (HAP):** Gram-negative bacilli

PPI use increases the risk of hospital-acquired pneumonia.

What is the strongest indication for admission?

a. Respiratory distress
b. Hypotension, tachycardia
c. Confusion
d. Fever
e. Leukocytosis, hyponatremia, hyperglycemia

Answer: **A.** Patients who are older (> 65) with chronic diseases of the lungs, liver, or kidney are more prone to respiratory failure. Other risks for a poor prognosis are diabetes, HIV, steroid use, and lack of a spleen. The pneumonia severity index (PSI) is used to risk-stratify patients with pneumonia. You do not need to memorize the criteria for Step 3, but suffice it to say that **elderly, hypoxic patients with or without a fever should be admitted.** You should consider the ICU, depending on the severity of the hypoxia. Decide whether to use outpatient versus inpatient monitoring; then, if inpatient, ICU or no ICU.

Diagnostic Testing

- Best initial diagnostic test: **Chest x-ray**
- Most accurate test: **Sputum Gram stain and culture**

Order tests as follows:

- *All* cases of respiratory disease (fever, cough, sputum) should have a **chest x-ray and oximeter** ordered with the first screen.
- If there is shortness of breath, also order **oxygen** with the first screen.
- If there is shortness of breath and/or hypoxia, order an **ABG.**

Treatment

Treat **outpatient** pneumonia with:

- **Macrolide** (azithromycin, doxycycline, or clarithromycin)
- **Respiratory fluoroquinolone** (levofloxacin, moxifloxacin)

Treat **inpatient** pneumonia with:

- Ceftriaxone and azithromycin
- **Fluoroquinolone** as a single agent

A positive sputum culture is **not** pneumonia.

Treat **ventilator-associated pneumonia (VAP)** with:

- Imipenem or meropenem, piperacillin/tazobactam or cefepime;
- Gentamicin; *and*
- Vancomycin or linezolid

Specific Associations

Presentation	Cause
Recent viral syndrome	*Staphylococcus*
Alcoholics	*Klebsiella*
Gastrointestinal symptoms, confusion	*Legionella*
Young, healthy patients	*Mycoplasma*
Persons present at the birth of an animal	*Coxiella burnetii*
Arizona construction workers	Coccidioidomycosis
HIV with < 200 CD4 cells	Pneumocystis (PCP)

An HIV-positive man comes to the emergency department with shortness of breath and a dry cough. His LDH is elevated and the chest x-ray shows bilateral interstitial infiltrates. His pO_2 is 65. What is the next best step in management?

a. Sputum induction
b. Respiratory isolation
c. Trimethoprim/sulfamethoxazole and prednisone
d. Pentamidine
e. Bronchoalveolar lavage

Answer: **C.** PCP is best managed with trimethoprim/sulfamethoxazole. This has better efficacy than pentamidine. Bronchoalveolar lavage needs to be done and is the most accurate test, but it is more important to start specific therapy. Steroids are indicated if the $pO_2 < 70$ or the A-a gradient > 35. Sputum induction is not as important as starting treatment. Also, it is only positive in 50–70 percent of patients.

VAP is:
- Fever
- Hypoxia
- New infiltrate
- Increasing secretions

Tuberculosis (TB)

TB occurs in **specific risk groups,** such as immigrants, HIV-positive patients, homeless patients, prisoners, and alcoholics. TB presents with **fever, cough, sputum, weight loss, and night sweats.**

Diagnostic Testing

- Best initial test: **Chest x-ray**
- **Sputum acid-fast stain and culture** should be done to confirm the presence of TB.

Treatment

Once the acid-fast stain is positive, treatment with 4 antituberculosis medications should be started. Six months of therapy is the standard of care.

1. Isoniazid (INH): 6 months
2. Rifampin: 6 months
3. Pyrazinamide: Stop after 2 months
4. Ethambutol: Stop after 2 months

All of these medications can lead to **liver toxicity.** TB medications should be stopped if the transaminases reach 5 times the upper limit of normal. Specific toxicities are the following:

- Isoniazid: Peripheral neuropathy
- Rifampin: Red/orange-colored bodily secretions
- Pyrazinamide: Hyperuricemia
- Ethambutol: Optic neuritis

The following conditions require treatment for **more than 6 months:**

- Osteomyelitis
- Meningitis
- Miliary tuberculosis
- Cavitary tuberculosis
- Pregnancy

Latent Tuberculosis

Diagnostic Testing and Treatment

The **PPD is a screening test for those in risk groups,** such as the homeless, immigrants, alcoholics, health care workers, and prisoners. A **positive test** is as follows:

- 5 mm: Close contacts, steroid users, HIV-positive
- 10 mm: Those in the risk groups described above
- 15 mm: Those without an increased risk

If a patient has never been tested or it has been several years since the last test, **2-stage testing** is recommended. This means that if the first test is negative, a second test should be performed in 1–2 weeks to make sure the first test was truly negative.

Bacille-Calmette Guerin (BCG) administration in the past has *no* effect or influence on these recommendations for treatment of latent TB. It does not matter if a patient has had BCG in the past; the patient must still take isoniazid if the PPD is positive. If BCG is an answer choice, it is *always* wrong according to current guidelines.

Interferon gamma release assay (IGRA) (Quantiferon) is an in-vitro blood test that is used for the detection of latent tuberculosis. The indication for an IGRA is the same as for a PPD. The main difference is that the IGRA is more specific than a PPD. There are no false positives on an IGRA with previous BCG infection.

IGRAs have a 90 percent sensitivity for previous TB exposure. A positive test is treated with INH alone. A positive IGRA does not mean active infection. As with a PPD, a positive IGRA confers only a 10 percent lifetime risk of TB.

If the PPD is **positive,** proceed as follows:

1. A **chest x-ray** should be performed to make sure occult active disease has not been detected.
2. If the chest x-ray is abnormal, **sputum staining for tuberculosis** is performed.
3. If this is positive, then **full-dose, 4-drug therapy** is used.

Isoniazid alone is used for 9 months to treat a positive PPD. This reduces the 10 percent lifetime risk of developing tuberculosis to 1 percent. Once a PPD is positive, the test should never be repeated.

Rheumatology

6

Rheumatoid Arthritis (RA)

Rheumatoid arthritis presents most often in **women > 50.** Patients have **joint pain and morning stiffness** that is **symmetrical** and in **multiple joints of the hands** lasting for **more than 1 hour in the morning** with the symptomatic episode going on for **at least 6 weeks.** There is often a prodrome of malaise and weight loss, but this is *not* enough to make a clear diagnosis.

RA is defined as having 4 or more of the following present for diagnosis:

- **Morning stiffness lasting more than 1 hour**
- **Wrist and finger** involvement **(MCP, PIP)**
- **Swelling of at least 3 joints**
- **Symmetric** involvement
- Rheumatoid **nodules** (not necessary to diagnose RA)
- **X-ray abnormalities showing erosions** (not necessary to diagnose RA)
- **Positive rheumatoid factor or anti-CCP**
- **C-reactive protein (CRP) or ESR**

Other findings in RA include the following:

- **Cardiac:** Pericarditis, valvular disease
- **Lung:** Pleural effusion with a very low glucose level, lung nodules
- **Blood:** Anemia with normal MCV
- **Nerve:** Mononeuritis multiplex
- **Skin:** Nodules

Diagnostic Testing

Rheumatoid arthritis is diagnosed with a **constellation of physical findings, joint problems, and lab tests.** There is *no* single diagnostic criteria to confirm the diagnosis. There is *no* single therapy to control and treat the disease.

A 34-year-old woman presents with pains in both hands for the last few months and stiffness that improves as the day goes on. Multiple joints are swollen on exam. X-rays of the hands show some erosion. What is the single most accurate test?

a. Rheumatoid factor
b. Anti-cyclic citrullinated peptide (anti-CCP)
c. Sedimentation rate
d. ANA
e. Joint fluid aspirate

Answer: **B.** Rheumatoid factor (RF) is present in only 75–85 percent of patients with rheumatoid arthritis (RA). It can also be present in a number of other diseases; hence, the RF is rather nonspecific. Anti-cyclic citrulinated peptide (anti-CCP) is the single most accurate test for RA. It is > 95 percent specific for RA, and it appears earlier in the course of the disease than the RF. There is nothing specific on joint aspiration to determine a diagnosis of RA.

Joint findings in RA are the following:

- **Metacarpophalangeal (MCP) swelling and pain**
- **Boutonniere deformity:** Flexion of the proximal interphalangeal (PIP) with hyperextension of the distal interphalangeal (DIP)
- **Swan neck deformity:** Extension of the PIP with flexion of the DIP
- **Baker's cyst** (outpocketing of synovium at the back of the knee)
- **C1/C2 cervical spine subluxation:** check before intubation
- **Knee:** Although the knee is commonly involved, multiple small joints are involved more commonly over time.

Felty's syndrome consists of the following:
- Rheumatoid arthritis
- Splenomegaly
- Neutropenia

New alternate diagnostic criteria for RA include:
- Synovitis (a single joint is enough to diagnose RA)
- RF or anti-CCP
- ESR or CRP
- Prolonged duration (beyond 6 weeks)

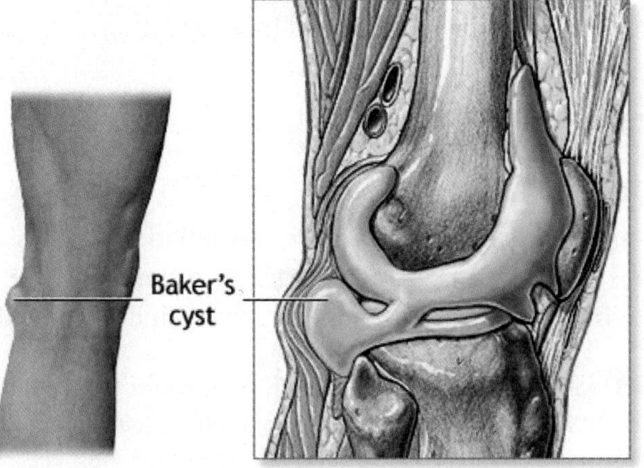

Normocytic, normochromic anemia is very characteristic of RA.

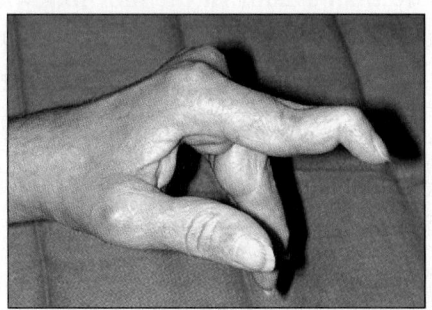

CCS Tip: In addition to x-rays, RF, and anti-CCP, you should also order a **CBC, sedimentation rate,** and C-reactive protein. If the case describes a swollen joint with an effusion, **aspiration of the joint** should also be done to establish the initial diagnosis.

Which of the following will have the lowest glucose level on pleural effusion?

a. CHF
b. Pulmonary embolus
c. Pneumonia
d. Cancer
e. Rheumatoid arthritis
f. Tuberculosis

Answer: **E.** Rheumatoid arthritis has the lowest glucose level of all the causes of pleural effusion described here.

The sacroiliac joint is *spared* in rheumatoid arthritis.

Treatment

NSAIDs combined with a disease-modifying antirheumatic drug (DMARD) is the standard of care in patients with RA. There is *no* therapeutic difference among NSAIDs, and you may use ibuprofen for any of the rheumatological diseases described. There is *no* point in waiting to use a DMARD in a patient with severe RA or anyone with joint erosions. NSAIDs will *not* delay the progression of the disease.

Eliminating an abnormal x-ray as a criterion for diagnosis allows earlier treatment with DMARDs.

DMARDs

The best initial DMARD is methotrexate. Add others if it is not effective.

- **Methotrexate:** This is the best-tolerated and most widely used DMARD. Adverse effects are bone marrow suppression, pneumonitis, and liver disease.
- **Biological agents (infliximab, adalimumab, etanercept):** All of these block the activity of tumor necrosis factor (TNF). Methotrexate *and* these biological agents can be used in combination. Anti-TNF agents are added if methotrexate fails.
- **Hydroxychloroquine:** Use with **mild disease.** The patient will need a regular **eye exam** to check for retinopathy. Anti-TNF agents are added if methotrexate fails.
- **Sulfasalazine:** This is the same drug that was used in the past for ulcerative colitis. It can suppress the bone marrow.

DMARDs are started to prevent x-ray abnormalities.

The following are alternate DMARDs:

- **Rituximab:** Anti-CD-20 antibody
- **Anakinra:** IL-1 receptor antagonist
- **Tocilizumab:** IL-6 receptor antagonist. Added to methotrexate if it is ineffective.
- **Leflunomide:** Pyrimidine antagonist that is similar in effect to methotrexate, with less toxicity
- **Abatacept:** Inhibits T-cell activation
- **Gold salts:** Rarely used because of toxicity, such as nephrotic syndrome

Steroids

Glucocorticoids, such as prednisone, are *not* disease modifying. However, steroids do enable quick control of the disease and allow time for the other DMARDs to take effect. Steroids are a **bridge to DMARD therapy.** They are the answer for an **acutely ill patient with severe inflammation.** Long-term glucocorticoid use should be avoided if at all possible.

Seronegative Spondyloarthropathies

This group of inflammatory arthritic conditions consists of:

- **Ankylosing spondylitis**
- **Reactive arthritis** (formerly known as Reiter's syndrome)
- **Psoriatic arthritis**
- **Juvenile rheumatoid arthritis** (adult-onset Still's disease)

These conditions all have the following characteristics:

- **Negative test for rheumatoid factor**
- Predilection for the **spine**
- **Sacroiliac joint** involvement
- Association with **HLA-B27**

Ankylosing Spondylitis (AS)

AS presents in a **young (< 40) male patient with spine or back stiffness.** Peripheral joint involvement is less common. The pain is **worse at night** and is **relieved by leaning forward.** This can lead to **kyphosis** and **diminished chest expansion.** Rare findings are these:

- Uveitis (30 percent)
- Aortitis (3 percent)
- Restrictive lung disease (2–15 percent)

Diagnostic Testing

A 27-year-old man presents with months of back pain that is worse at night. He has diminished expansion of this chest on inhalation and flattening of the normal lumbar curvature. What is the most accurate of these tests?

a. X-ray
b. MRI
c. HLA-B27
d. ESR
e. Rheumatoid factor

Answer: **B.** MRI of the SI joint is more sensitive than an x-ray, detecting edematous, inflammatory changes years before an x-ray in ankylosing spondylitis (AS). HLA-B27 can be present in 8 percent of the general population and is not necessary to confirm a diagnosis of AS. The ESR is not always elevated and is a nonspecific test. The rheumatoid factor will be negative in AS. In a CCS case, all of these tests should be performed, with the x-ray done first and then going on to the MRI if the x-ray is negative.

The most common **wrong answer** for ankylosing spondylitis treatment is steroids. They do not work.

Treatment

- NSAIDs
- Biological agents, such as infliximab or adalimumab
- Sulfasalazine

Methotrexate does not work well on the spine and sacroiliac joints.

Do not use steroids.

Reactive Arthritis

Reactive arthritis (formerly known as Reiter's syndrome) presents with an **asymmetric arthritis with a history of urethritis or gastrointestinal infection.** There may be constitutional symptoms, such as **fever, fatigue, or weight loss.**

- **Arthritis:** May be monoarticular, oligoarticular, or more diffuse
- **Genital lesions:** Circinate balanitis (around head of penis); urethritis or cervicitis in women
- **Conjunctivitis**
- **Keratoderma blenorrhagicum:** A skin lesion characteristic of reactive arthritis

Diagnostic Testing

There is *no* specific diagnostic test. Look for the triad of **knee (joint), pee (urinary), and see (eye)** problems with a history of *Chlamydia, Shigella, Salmonella, Yersinia,* or *Campylobacter.*

Treatment

Treat with **NSAIDs.**

Psoriatic Arthritis

Psoriatic arthritis presents as **joint involvement with a history of psoriasis.** Rheumatoid factor is absent. The **sacroiliac spine is involved,** as it is in all seronegative spondyloarthropathies. The following are key features of psoriatic arthritis:

- **Nail pitting**
- **Distal interphalangeal (DIP) involvement** (Remember: RA involves the proximal joint.)
- **"Sausage-shaped" digits** (dactylitis)
- **Enthesitis:** Inflammation of tendinous insertion sites

No single test is specific for psoriatic arthritis.

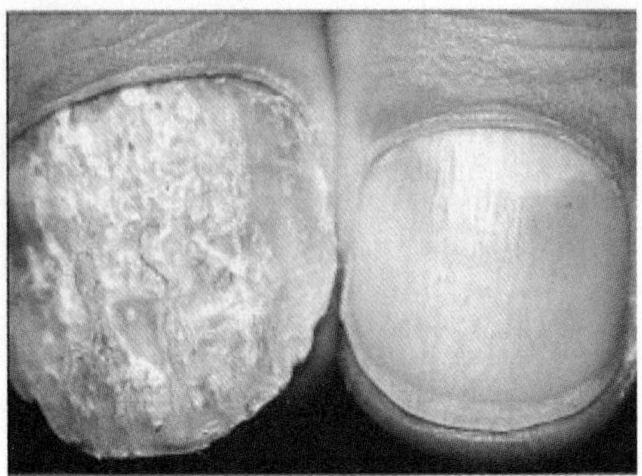

Psoriasis involvement of the nail produces pitting and yellowing, which can be mistaken for onychomycosis.

Diagnostic Testing

No single test is specific for psoriatic arthritis.

Treatment

- Best initial therapy: **NSAIDs**
- **Methotrexate is used for resistant disease.**
- **Infliximab and the other anti-TNF agents are effective.**

Basic Science Correlate

Mechanism of Anti-TNF Reactivation of TB

Most TB is reactivation TB. Old TB is encased off in granulomas. Granulomas are held together by TNF. When you start a TNF inhibitor, it breaks open granulomas and the TB escapes to reactivate.

Juvenile Rheumatoid Arthritis (JRA)

JRA, or adult-onset Still's disease, presents with:

- **Fever**
- **Salmon-colored rash**
- **Polyarthritis**
- **Lymphadenopathy**
- **Myalgias**

This can be a *very* difficult diagnosis to recognize. Additional minor criteria are the presence of **hepatosplenomegaly and elevated transaminases.**

Diagnostic Testing

There is *no* specific diagnostic test. JRA is characterized by the following:

- **Very high ferritin level**
- **Elevated white blood cell count**
- **Negative rheumatoid factor and negative ANA** are *essential* to establishing the diagnosis.

Treatment

Treat with **NSAIDs.** Unresponsive cases can be treated with **steroids**. Those with persistent symptoms need methotrexate or anti-TNF medications to get off steroids.

Whipple Disease

Although it causes **diarrhea, fat malabsorption, and weight loss,** the most common presentation of Whipple disease is with **joint pain.**

Biopsy of the bowel showing PAS positive organisms is the most specific test.

Treatment with **TMP/SMX** is curative.

Osteoarthritis (OA)

Osteoarthritis, the most common joint abnormality, is associated with aging and increased use of a joint. The **morning stiffness is < 30 minutes** in duration and there is **crepitus** on moving the joint. OA affects the **distal interphalangeal (DIP) joints** (RA does *not* affect the DIPs). Note the following:

- Heberden's nodes: DIP osteophytes
- Bouchard's nodes: PIP osteophytes

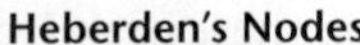

Heberden's Nodes

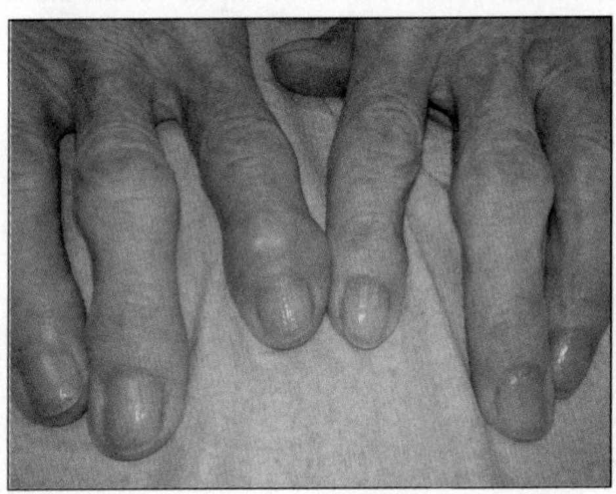

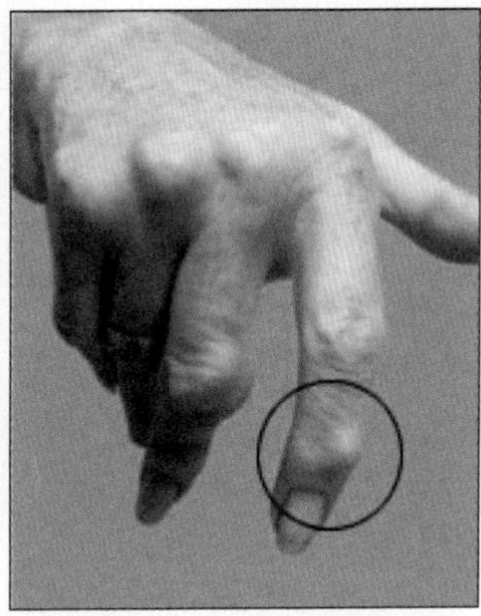

Diagnostic Testing

The best initial test is **x-ray of the joint.**

For CCS, *all* of the following should be ordered; there is *no* specific diagnostic test:

- **ANA**
- **ESR**
- **Rheumatoid factor**
- **Anti-CCP**

All other inflammatory markers will be normal. Joint fluid will have a *low* leukocyte count < 2,000/mm^3.

Treatment

Treatment is with **acetaminophen. Chondroitin sulfate** is **not** clearly useful to slow joint deterioration. Weight loss and exercise help.

The following table compares osteoarthritis with rheumatoid arthritis.

Glucosamine is a wrong answer. Glucosamine = placebo

	OA	RA
Morning stiffness	< 30 minutes	> 1 hour
DIP	Yes	No
PIP	Yes	Yes
MCP	No	Yes
RF, anti-CCP	No	Yes
Joint fluid leukocyte count	< 2,000	5,000–50,000

Systemic Lupus Erythematosus (SLE)

- Rash + Joint pain + Fatigue = Lupus

As shown in the following table, there are 11 criteria for lupus; **4 are needed** to confirm the diagnosis.

Diagnostic Criteria for SLE	
Skin	• Malar rash • Photosensitivity rash • Oral ulcers rash • Discoid rash
Arthralgias	Present in 90 percent of patients
Blood	Leukopenia, thrombocytopenia, hemolysis; any blood involvement counts as *1 criterion*
Renal	Varies from benign proteinuria to end stage renal disease
Cerebral	Behavioral change, stroke, seizure, meningitis
Serositis	Pericarditis, pleuritic chest pain, pulmonary hypertension, pneumonia, myocarditis
Serology	• ANA (95 percent sensitive) • Double-stranded (DS) DNA (60 percent sensitive) Each of the serologic abnormalities counts as 1 criterion. Hence, if the person has joint pain, a rash, and both an ANA and DS DNA, that patient would have 4 criteria.

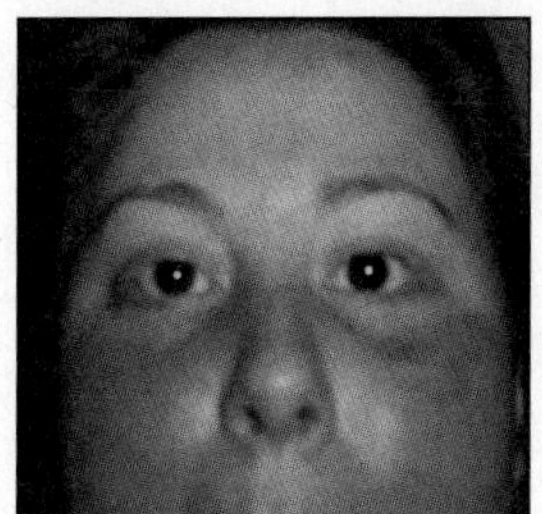

Malar Rash

Diagnostic Testing

- Best initial test: **ANA**
- Most specific test: **Anti-DS DNA** (60–70 percent) **or anti-Sm** (Smith) (10–20 percent)

SLE on CCS: Complement levels, anti-Sm, and anti-DS DNA should be performed on *all* patients.

What is the best test to follow the severity of a lupus flare-up?

Answer: **Complement levels** (drop in flare-up) and **anti-DS DNA** (rise in flare-up).

As part of prenatal care, a woman with lupus is found to have a negative test for anticardiolipin antibodies, but she is positive for anti-Ro (SSA) antibody. What is the baby at risk for?

Answer: Heart block. The presence of anti-Ro or anti-SSA antibodies is a risk for the development of heart block.

The anemia of chronic disease is more common than hemolysis in SLE.

Additionally, the following are found in SLE:

- **Joint x-ray** is normal. Lupus causes joint pain without destruction of the synovium.
- The **anemia** of chronic disease is more common than hemolysis.
- In a **lupus flare**, complement levels go down and anti-DS DNA goes up.
- **Anti-SM** is the only test more specific for lupus than anti-DS DNA.

The following are other findings in lupus that are *not* part of specific diagnostic criteria:

- **Fatigue**
- **Hair loss**
- **Antiphospholipid syndrome**
- **Elevated sedimentation rate**

Treatment

Treatment is as follows:

> Belimumab inhibits B cells as treatment of SLE.

- **Acute flare-ups:** Prednisone and other glucocorticoids
- **Joint pain:** NSAIDs
- **Rash and joint pain not responding to NSAIDs:** Hydroxychloroquine
- **Severe disease relapse upon cessation of steroids:** Belimumab, azathioprine, and cyclophosphamide
- **Nephritis:** Steroids and mycophenolate mofetil (mycophenolate or cyclophosphamide)

Drug-Induced Lupus

The most common causes of drug-induced lupus are **hydralazine, procainamide, and isoniazid.** Keep the following in mind on Step 3:

- Drug-induced lupus gives **anti-histone antibodies** and always a positive ANA.
- It **never** gives renal or CNS involvement.
- Complement level and anti-DS DNA are normal.

Sjögren's Syndrome

Look for a **woman** (9:1 female predominance) with **dry eyes, dry mouth, and a sensation of "sand under the eyelid."** There is often **loss of taste and smell** from profound mouth dryness. (You need saliva to wet the food so you can taste it.) Look for **loss of teeth at an early age,** because saliva is critical to preventing dental cavities.

Diagnostic Testing

- Most accurate test: **Lip biopsy**
- **Schirmer test:** Decreased wetting of paper held to the eye shows decreased lacrimation.
- Serologic testing:
  - **ANA:** 95 percent sensitive but least specific
  - **RF:** 70 percent sensitive
  - **Anti-Ro/SSA:** 50–65 percent sensitive but fairly specific
  - **Anti-La/SSB:** 30–65 percent sensitive but fairly specific

CCS Tip: When you see **anti-Ro (SSA) or anti-La (SSB),** think **Sjögren's syndrome.** They are present in a small number of people with lupus, and can help diagnose ANA-negative lupus.

Treatment

- **Keep the eyes and mouth moist.**
- **Pilocarpine and cevimeline** increase acetylcholine, which increases oral and ocular secretions.

Basic Science Correlate

Acetylcholine stimulation massively increase secretions from the salivary glands. Pilocarpine inhibits acetylcholine esterase everywhere and increases acetylcholine. Cevimeline is specific to the salivary glands.

Scleroderma (Systemic Sclerosis)

Scleroderma presents with 3 main symptoms:

- Tight Skin + Heartburn + Raynaud's = Scleroderma

1. **Skin:** Look for a **woman** with **tight, fibrous thickening of the skin** that gives a tight face and tight, immobile fingers known as **"sclerodactyly."**
2. **Raynaud's phenomenon:** This is a 3-phase **vascular hyperreactivity,** with the skin of the fingers becoming white, then blue, then red; it can be quite painful. **Digital ulceration** may occur from infarction of the skin. There might also be abnormal **giant capillaries in the nail folds.**
3. **Joint pain:** The pain is **mild and symmetrical.**

Diffuse scleroderma also presents with the following:

- **Lung: Fibrosis and pulmonary hypertension** (these are the leading cause of death)
- **GI:** Wide-mouthed colonic diverticula and esophageal dysmotility, leading to reflux and Barrett's esophagus. There is primary biliary cirrhosis in 15 percent of patients.
- **Heart:** Restrictive cardiomyopathy
- **Renal:** May lead to malignant hypertension

Diagnostic Testing

There is *no* single diagnostic test.

- ANA is present in 95 percent of cases but is nonspecific.
- **Antitopoisomerase (anti-Scl 70)** is only present in 30 percent of patients.

Treatment

Interstitial lung disease is treated with cyclophosphamide.

No treatment has been proven effective in stopping scleroderma. Penicillamine is *not* effective in delaying progression of this disease. One can use the following therapies:

- **Renal involvement and hypertension:** Use ACE inhibitors.
- **Pulmonary hypertension:** Use **bosentan** (endothelin antagonist), **prostacyclin analogs** (epoprostenol, treprostinil, iloprost), or **sildenafil.**
- **Raynaud's:** Use calcium channel blockers.
- **GERD:** Regular use of PPIs
- **Lung fibrosis** is treated with cyclophosphamide.

"CREST" Syndrome (Limited Scleroderma)

This form of scleroderma presents with the following:

- Calcinosis of the fingers
- Raynaud's
- Esophageal dysmotility
- Sclerodactyly
- Telangiectasia

CREST does present with primary hypertension.

It does *not* present with the following:

- Joint pain
- Heart involvement
- Lung involvement (except for pulmonary hypertension)
- Kidney involvement

Diagnostic Testing

CREST syndrome has anti-Scl70 less often, but does have anti-centromere antibodies more often.

CREST is characterized by **anticentromere antibodies.**

Eosinophilic Fasciitis

Eosinophilic fasciitis presents with **thickened skin that looks like scleroderma.** However, the following *are not present*:

- Hand involvement
- Raynaud's
- Heart, lung, or kidney involvement

There is **marked eosinophilia** and the appearance of an **"orange peel" (peau d'orange).** Symptoms are worse with exercise.

Treatment is with **corticosteroids.**

Polymyositis (PM) and Dermatomyositis (DM)

In both conditions, the patient **cannot get up from a seated position** without using the arms. There can also be **muscle pain and tenderness.**

For **polymyositis,** look for the following:

- **Proximal muscle weakness**
- Signs of **muscle inflammation** on blood tests, electromyography, and biopsy

For **dermatomyositis,** you find the same thing and **various rashes.**

- **Gottron's papules:** Over metocarpophalangeal joint surfaces
- **Heliotrope rash:** Periorbital and purplish lesion around the eyes
- **Shawl sign:** Shoulder and neck erythema

- Weakness + ↑CPK + ↑Aldolase + Biopsy = Polymyositis
- Weakness + ↑CPK + ↑Aldolase + Biopsy + **Skin rash** = Dermatomyositis

Diagnostic Testing

Testing reveals **elevated CPK and aldolase** with an **abnormal electromyogram (EMG).** For CCS, order **all the liver function tests** as well as **ANA.**

Biopsy is the single most accurate test of PM/DM.

A 50-year-old patient presents with muscle weakness of the girdle with an increased CPK and aldolase. Her anti-Jo-1 antibody is positive. Which of the following is most likely to happen to her?

a. Stroke
b. Myocardial infarction
c. Septic arthritis
d. DVT
e. Interstitial lung disease

Answer: **E.** PM/DM presents with weakness and increased markers of muscle inflammation. The presence of **anti-Jo-1** indicates a markedly increased risk of interstitial lung disease.

What is the most common serious complication of PM/DM?

a. Rhabdomyolysis
b. Hyperkalemia
c. Metabolic acidosis
d. Malignancy

Answer: **D.** For unclear reasons, the most common serious threat to life from PM/DM is malignancy. DM has a greater risk than PM. Cancer hits the cervix, lungs, pancreas, breasts, and ovaries.

Treatment

Treat polymyositis and dermatomyositis with glucocorticoids.

Fibromyalgia

Look for a **woman** (10 times more common in females) with **muscle aches and stiffness with trigger points on palpation and nonrefreshing sleep. Depression and anxiety** are common.

Diagnostic Testing

All blood tests are normal. There is *no* objective evidence of disease. This is a pain syndrome with tender trigger points.

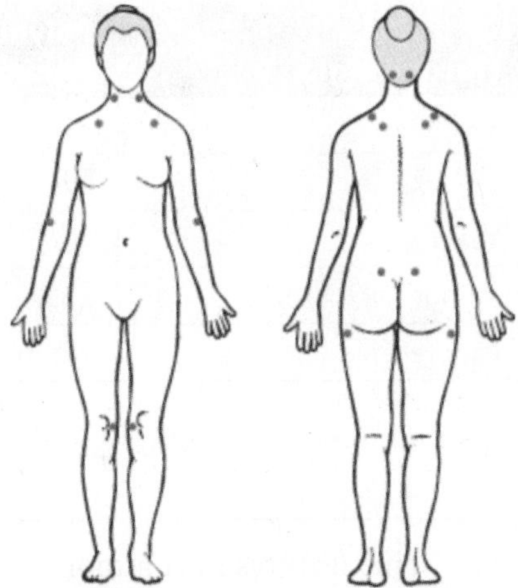
Fibromyalgia Trigger Points

Treatment

Treat symptoms with the following:

- **Exercise**
- **Milnacipran, duloxetine, or pregabalin (the best initial therapy)**
- **Tricyclic antidepressants**, such as amitriptyline, are effective but have more adverse effects.

NSAIDs are **not** first line for fibromyalgia.

Polymyalgia Rheumatica (PMR)

Presents with a **person > 50 years old** with **profound pain and stiffness of the proximal muscles,** such as shoulders and pelvic girdle. The stiffness is **worse in the morning** and is **localized to the muscles** rather than to the joints. The **ESR is elevated,** and there is an amazing response to steroids.

Pain is much more prominent than weakness in PMR.

Nonspecific features of PMR are the following:

- Fever, weight loss, and malaise
- Normocytic anemia
- *Normal* CPK, EMG, aldolase, and muscle biopsy
- *No* muscle atrophy

- Age > 50 + Proximal muscle pain + ↑ESR = PMR

The following table compares chronic fatigue syndrome, fibromyalgia, and polymyalgia rheumatica.

	Chronic Fatigue Syndrome	Fibromyalgia	Polymyalgia Rheumatica
Fatigue/malaise	+++++ > 6 months	++	++
Nonrefreshing sleep	+++++	++	No
Trigger points	No	Yes	No
Blood tests	All normal	All normal	↑ESR
Treatment	None	Pain relief	Prednisone

Vasculitis

Methotrexate causes liver and lung fibrosis.

All forms of vasculitis have some features in common:

- On presentation, they can all have:
  - **Fatigue, malaise, weight loss**
  - **Fever:** May present as a fever of unknown origin (FUO)
  - **Skin lesions:** Palpable purpura, rash
  - **Joint pain**
  - **Neuropathy:** Mononeuritis multiplex
- Common laboratory features:
  - **Normocytic anemia**
  - **Elevated ESR**
  - **Thrombocytosis**

Diagnostic Testing

Biopsy is the most accurate test for vasculitis. See also the lab features noted above.

Treatment

Best initial therapy: **Prednisone and glucocorticoids**

If steroids are not effective, alternate and/or additional therapies are the following:

- **Cyclophosphamide**
- **Azathioprine/6-Mercaptopurine**
- **Methotrexate**

Polyarteritis Nodosa (PAN)

PAN has **all of the features of vasculitis** described above. What is different enough about PAN to allow you to establish the diagnosis is:

- **Abdominal pain** (65 percent)
- **Renal involvement** (65 percent)
- **Testicular involvement** (35 percent)
- **Pericarditis** (35 percent)
- **Hypertension** (50 percent)

PAN does **not** affect the lungs.

Diagnostic Testing

- Best initial test: **Angiography of abdominal vessels**
- Most accurate test: **Biopsy (of skin, muscle, or sural nerve)**

CCS Tip: There is *no* good blood test for PAN.

Hepatitis B surface antigen is found in 30 percent of patients with PAN.

Treatment

Therapy is with **prednisone and cyclophosphamide.**

Wegener's Granulomatosis

This disorder, like PAN, can affect the majority of the body. However, look for **upper and lower respiratory findings and c-ANCA.**

The most accurate test is **biopsy.** Treatment is with **prednisone and cyclophosphamide.**

- Upper and lower respiratory findings + c-ANCA = Wegener's

Churg-Strauss

Although Churg-Strauss can affect any organ in the body, the key to recognizing it is that it involves **vasculitis, eosinophilia, and asthma.** Although the p-ANCA and anti-myeloperoxidase can be positive, too, these findings are not as uniquely suggestive as the presence of eosinophilia and asthma.

Biopsy is the most accurate test. There is an excellent response to **steroids.**

- Vasculitis + Eosinophilia + Asthma = Churg-Strauss

Temporal Arteritis

Temporal arteritis is a type of **giant cell arteritis.** It is related to polymyalgia rheumatica. **Fever, weight loss, malaise, and fatigue** can be present, as they are in all forms of vasculitis.

The most accurate test is a **biopsy.**

A patient presents with headache, jaw claudication, visual disturbance, and tenderness of the scalp. The ESR is elevated. What is the next best step in management?

Answer: **Treatment with steroids** is more important than getting a specific diagnostic test in temporal arteritis.

Takayasu's Arteritis

- Young Asian female + Diminished pulses = Takayasu's arteritis

The most accurate test for Takayasu's is *not* a biopsy.

Half of patients with Takayasu's arteritis have the usual **vasculitis** findings present *before* the **loss or decrease of pulse:**

- **Fatigue, malaise, weight loss, arthralgia**
- **Anemia, increased ESR**

The special features of this vasculitis are **TIA and stroke** from vascular occlusion.

Takayasu's is also distinctive in that it is diagnosed with **aortic arteriography** or **magnetic resonance angiography (MRA).**

Takayasu's is treated with **steroids** like all vasculitis.

Cryoglobulinemia

Cryoglobulinemia has all the usual features of vasculitis, such as **fatigue, malaise, skin lesions, and joint pain.** There is an association with **hepatitis C and renal involvement.** Sryoglobulins and rheumatoid factor are very similar.

Treat the hepatitis C with **interferon and ribavirin.** (Note that Step 3 loves this question!)

Behcet Disease

This condition presents in patients of Middle Eastern or Asian ancestry. Features are the following:

- **Oral and genital ulcers**
- **Ocular involvement** (uveitis, optic neuritis): Can lead to blindness
- **Skin lesions:** "Pathergy," which is **hyperreactivity to needle sticks,** resulting in sterile skin abscesses

There is *no* specific test for Behcet disease. Use the features described above.

Treatment is with **prednisone and colchicines.**

Inflamed Joints

To diagnose inflamed joints, you need to look at the fluid. Inflamed joints will generally have effusions. **Joint aspiration** is the most accurate test for gout, pseudogout, and septic arthritis.

The Gram stain lacks sensitivity and, even in bacterial septic arthritis, will only detect 50–60 percent of infections. The best initial test for septic arthritis is the **cell count.** There is still overlap. Infectious septic arthritis could be present with as few as 20,000 white cells, although most cases have > 50,000–100,000.

The following table compares synovial fluid cell count values.

Normal	Inflammatory (Gout/ Pseudogout)	Infectious
< 2,000 WBCs	2,000–50,000 WBCs	> 50,000 WBCs

Gout

Look for a **man** with a **sudden onset** of **severe pain** in the **toe at night.** The toe will be red, swollen, and tender, and it can look very similar to a toe with an infection.

Rasburicase and pegloticase break down uric acid to allantoin. Use if allopurinol and febuxostat are not enough.

The following can precipitate acute gouty attacks:

- **Binge drinking of alcohol**
- **Thiazides**
- **Nicotinic acid**

Diagnostic Testing

- Best initial test: **Arthrocentesis** (aspiration of joint fluid)
- Most accurate test: **Polarized light examination** of the fluid will show **negatively birefringent needles.**

- Gout = Negative birefringence
- Pseudogout = Positive birefringence

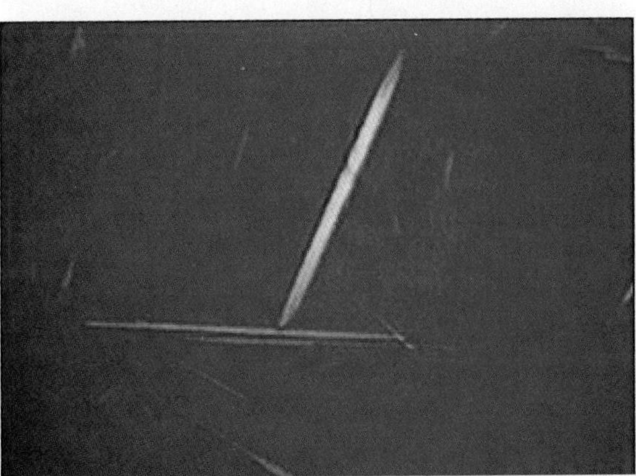

> Of all gout patients, 30 percent can have at least one *normal* uric acid level, especially during the attack, because the uric acid is being deposited into the joints from the blood. An elevated uric acid level alone is *not* an indication for treatment in an asymptomatic patient. You *must* tap the joint.

For CCS, also do the following:

- **Joint fluid examination for cell count, culture, and protein level**
- **Serum uric acid level:** However, do *not* rely on uric acid level to make an accurate diagnosis.
- **X-ray of the toe:** May show "punched-out" lesions
- **Extremity examination for tophi**

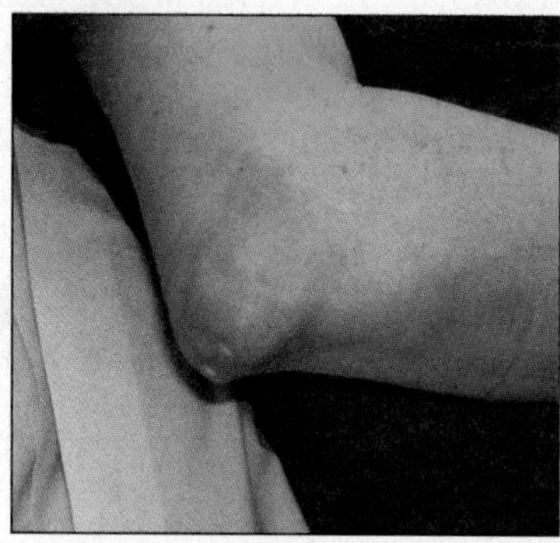

> Febuxostat is an alternative to allopurinol.

Treatment

- Best initial therapy for an acute gouty attack is **NSAIDs.**
- If there is insufficient response or a contraindication to NSAIDs, use **steroids** to treat acute gouty attacks. If a single joint is involved, give steroids by injection. If multiple joints are involved, give steroids orally or by IV. Steroids are much more the standard of care in acute gout and pseudogout than colchicine. For an acute attack of gout, *the answer is never allopurinol.*
- **Colchicine** is useful under the following conditions:
  - In the **first 24 hours** of an attack
  - When there is a **contraindication to the use of NSAIDs,** such as renal insufficiency, and a reason not to use steroids
  - As part of **preventive therapy** to decrease the risk of a gouty attack
- Colchicine has the following adverse effects:
  - Nausea and diarrhea
  - Bone marrow suppression
- Prevention:
  - **Allopurinol** lowers the level of uric acid. Allopurinol has the following adverse effects: rash, allergic interstitial nephritis, and hemolysis.
  - **Weight loss and avoiding alcohol**
  - **Febuxostat** is a xanthine oxidase inhibitor that markedly lowers uric acid levels. Febuxostat is the answer when the patient is intolerant of allopurinol.

> Treat gout with colchicine **only if** NSAIDs and steroids cannot be used.

> Do *not* start allopurinol during an acute attack of gout.

- **Uricase** (rasburicase and pegloticase) are benign drugs to break down uric acid. Use if allopurinol or febuxostat is not enough.
- Probenecid and sulfinpyrazone are *rarely used* for gout any longer. They increase urinary excretion of uric acid, which is contraindicated in those with renal insufficiency.

CCS Tip: Do not add probenecid and sulfinpyrazone for gout. They will never be the correct answer.

Calcium Pyrophosphate Deposition Disease (Pseudogout)

In pseudogout, the **knee and wrist are involved** but *not* the toes. Pseudogout is much slower in onset than gout, and the patient will *not* wake up with severe pain.

CCS Tip: In a case of pseudogout, expect hemochromatosis, hyperparathyroidism, acromegaly, or hypothyroidism in the history.

Diagnostic Testing

Tap the joint and look for **positively birefringent rhomboid-shaped crystals.**

Treatment

NSAIDS are the best initial therapy. Colchicine is used but is not as effective. Acute management is the same as gout: NSAIDs or steroids.

Septic Arthritis

The more abnormal the joint, the more likely a patient is to have septic arthritis: prosthetic joint > rheumatoid arthritis > osteoarthritis > normal joint.

Any arthritic joint or prosthetic joint is a risk factor for septic arthritis.

Septic arthritis presents with a **swollen, red, immobile, tender joint.**

The etiology is as follows:

- *Staphylococcus aureus* (40 percent)
- *Streptococcus* (30 percent)
- Gram-negative bacilli (20 percent)

CCS Tip: Call an **orthopedic surgery consult** when you suspect a septic joint. The consultation won't offer much on the CCS, but it needs to be done.

Disseminated gonorrhea is diagnosed by culture of:

- Joint fluid (50 percent positive)
- Pharynx (10–20 percent positive)
- Rectum (10–20 percent positive)
- Urethra (10–20 percent positive)
- Cervix (20–30 percent positive)

Diagnostic Testing

- Best initial test: **Tap the joint (arthrocentesis).** A finding of > 50,000 white cells is consistent with infection.
- Gram stain has a 50–60 percent sensitivity.
- Most accurate test: **Culture** is > 90 percent sensitive but is *never* available when you must make an acute treatment decision.

Treatment

Empiric therapy with **ceftriaxone and vancomycin intravenously** is effective. This is the choice for CCS when you have to write in one answer.

The following table shows other possible answers for multiple-choice questions. These are used **in combination:** one for *Staphylococcus/Streptococcus* and one for Gram-negative bacilli.

Staph and Strep Drug	Gram-Negative Bacilli Drug
• Oxacillin • Nafcillin • Cefazolin	• Ceftriaxone • Ceftazidime • Gentamicin
Penicillin allergy: Anaphylaxis • Vancomycin • Linezolid • Daptomycin • Clindamycin	Penicillin allergy: Anaphylaxis • Aztreonam • Fluoroquinolone

Paget's Disease of Bone

This condition is often **asymptomatic.** It may lead to **pain, stiffness, aching, and fractures.** Soft bones lead to **bowing of the tibias. Sarcoma** arises in 1 percent of patients.

In cases of Paget's, osteolytic lesions will be found initially. These may be replaced with osteoblastic lesions.
So on Step 3,
- if osteo*lytic,* then think Paget's or osteoporosis; *but*
- if osteo*blastic,* think about metastatic prostate cancer in the differential diagnosis.

Diagnostic Testing

- Best initial test: **Alkaline phosphatase level.** It will be elevated.
- Most accurate test: **x-ray**
- For CCS, also order the following:
  - **Urinary hydroxyproline**
  - **Serum calcium level**—It will be normal
  - **Serum phosphate level**—It will be normal
  - **Bone scan**

Treatment

Treat with **bisphosphonates and calcitonin.**

Baker's Cyst

A Baker's cyst is a **posterior herniation of the synovium of the knee.** Look for a patient with **osteoarthritis or rheumatoid arthritis** with a **swollen calf.** A ruptured Baker's cyst is a "pseudo-phlebitis." Unruptured cysts can be palpated.

Diagnostic Testing

Exclude a deep vein thrombosis with **ultrasound.**

Treatment

Treat with **NSAIDs** and, occasionally, with steroid injection.

Plantar Fasciitis and Tarsal Tunnel Syndrome

The following table compares these 2 conditions.

Do not order a foot x-ray for plantar fasciitis or tarsal tunnel syndrome. Heel spurs make no difference.

Plantar Fasciitis	Tarsal Tunnel Syndrome
Pain on bottom of foot	Pain on bottom of foot
Very severe in the morning, better with walking a few steps	More painful with more use; like carpal tunnel of the foot; may have numbness of the sole, too
Stretch the foot and calf	Avoid boots and high heels; may need steroid injection
Resolves spontaneously over time	May need surgical release

Morton Neuroma

This condition presents with the following:

- **Painful burning sensation** in the interdigital web space between the 3rd and 4th toes
- **Tenderness** when pressure is applied between the heads of the 3rd and 4th metatarsals
- **Sharp, intermittent pain** radiating into the toes that feels better when shoes are taken off

Hematology

7

Anemia

All forms of anemia lead to **fatigue** and a subjective sense of **loss of energy.** The case will use words such as *tired, fatigue, malaise,* or *loss of energy.* You will be able to recognize more severe anemia when the question says *short of breath, lightheadedness,* or *confusion.* Other diseases may also present with fatigue or shortness of breath, similar to anemia.

If the question describes a **craving for ice or dirt** (i.e., forms of pica), think anemia. Step 3 loves to use pica as a lead in to anemia.

Diseases with presentations similar to those of anemia:

- Hypoxia
- Carbon monoxide poisoning
- Methemoglobinemia
- Ischemic heart disease

Physical Examination

On CCS, choose the following physical exams: general appearance, CV, chest, extremities, and HEENT.

Potential positive findings are **pallor, flow murmur** described as I/VI or II/VI systolic murmur, and **pale conjunctiva.** Hemolysis will also give jaundice and scleral icterus (yellow eyes). The chest exam is chosen routinely in any patient with shortness of breath, even though there are no positive findings in anemia, to exclude other causes of shortness of breath. In severe anemia, an ECG is needed to exclude ischemia. Anemia kills through myocardial ischemia.

CCS Tip: There are *no* unique physical findings in anemia to allow you a specific diagnosis. For CCS cases, you find one anyway. For single best answer questions, go straight for the CBC.

Diagnostic Testing

- Best initial test: **CBC with peripheral smear** (pay special attention to the MCV/MCHC)
- Additional initial tests: **Reticulocyte count, haptoglobin, LDH, total and direct bilirubin, TSH with T4, B12/folate levels, iron studies**
- Also order **urinalysis with microscopic analysis**

Categorizing Anemia

Based on the MCV, determine whether the anemia is microcytic, macrocytic, or normocytic. The MCHC may indicate whether there is a problem with the synthesis of hemoglobin. Based on this measurement, anemia can be further categorized as hypochromic, hyperchromic, or normochromic.

Basic Science Correlate

Mechanism of Dyspnea in Anemia

Dyspnea occurs when there is no oxygen delivery to tissues. If there is low hemoglobin, there is no ability to transport oxygen to tissues. Anemia is perceived the same way as hypoxia. Carbon monoxide poisoning does not release the oxygen from hemoglobin. All of these cause light-headedness and ultimately myocardial ischemia. Anemia kills via left ventricular ischemia and infarction.

Microcytic Anemia

Diagnostic Testing and Treatment

Specific Diagnostic Tests and Treatments				
When this is in the history/ physical...	Blood loss Elevated platelet count	Rheumatoid arthritis End-stage renal disease or Any chronic infectious, inflammatory, or connective tissue disease	Very small MCV with few or no symptoms Target cells	Alcoholic Isoniazid Lead exposure
...this is the diagnosis.	Iron deficiency	Anemia of chronic disease	Thalassemia	Sideroblastic anemia
What is the best initial diagnostic test?	Iron studies: • Low ferritin • High TIBC • Low Fe • Low Fe sat • Elevated RDW	Iron studies: • High ferritin • Low TIBC • Low Fe • Normal or low Fe sat	Iron studies: • Normal	Iron studies: • High Fe
What is the most accurate diagnostic test?	Bone marrow biopsy (do not do this on CCS)	No specific diagnostic test	Hemoglobin Electrophoresis Beta: Elevated HgA2,HgF Alpha: Normal	Prussian blue stain
What is the best initial therapy?	Prescribe ferrous sulfate orally	Correct the underlying disease	No treatment for trait	Major: Remove the toxin exposure Minor: Prescribe pyridoxine replacement

> Alpha thalassemia is most accurately diagnosed by DNA sequencing.

A 62-year-old-man with a history of anemia from a bleeding peptic ulcer comes for evaluation. He is constipated and has black stool. His medications are omeprazole, oral ferrous sulfate, and occasional liquid antacids. What would you do next?

a. EGD
b. Colonoscopy
c. Guaiac testing/hemoccult
d. Discontinue omeprazole
e. Increase the dose of ferrous sulfate

Answer: **C.** Oral ferrous sulfate can turn the stool black, but elemental iron such as this does not make the stool guaiac positive. Only the iron in hemoglobin or myoglobin can make the stool guaiac card positive.

Diagnostic testing is as follows:

- Most important test: **Iron studies/profile** (Fe level, Fe saturation, ferritin, TIBC)
- Most accurate test: **Bone marrow biopsy**

HgH has Beta-4 tetrads with 3-gene deleted alpha thalassemia.

Only iron deficiency is associated with an elevated red cell distribution of width (RDW). This is because the newer cells are progressively smaller and smaller; therefore, the red cell width changes over time. **Prussian blue** is an iron stain. **Sideroblastic anemia** is associated with iron building up inside the mitochondria of the red cell.

A 68-year-old woman is found on routine CBC to have a hematocrit of 32 percent (normal 37–42) and an MCV of 70 (normal 80–100). Her stool is heme negative. What should you do next?

a. Colonoscopy
b. Sigmoidoscopy
c. Barium enema
d. Upper endoscopy
e. Two more stool tests now
f. Repeat the stool testing in a year
g. Capsule endoscopy

Answer: **A.** Colonoscopy is indicated in all patients > 50 simply as routine screening. Hence, in this case, the patient needs colonoscopy anyway, regardless of what the stool tests show. Another reason to go straight to colonoscopy is the presence of microcytic anemia. Unexplained microcytic anemia in a patient above 50 is most likely caused by colon cancer. Sigmoidoscopy will do nothing to evaluate the right side of the colon and would miss nearly 40 percent of cancers. No matter what a sigmoidoscopy showed, you would need to inspect the right side of the colon. Capsule endoscopy is done to evaluate bleeding when the upper and lower endoscopy are normal and the source of bleeding is likely to be in the small bowel.

The only microcytic anemia with a high reticulocyte count is HgH.

A patient comes with end stage renal disease for evaluation of shortness of breath. After dialysis, he is found to have a hematocrit of 28 with an MCV of 68. Iron studies are performed. What do you expect to find?

	Iron	Total Iron Binding Capacity	Ferritin	RDW
a.	Low	High	Low	High
b.	Low	Low	Normal	Normal
c.	Normal	Normal	Normal	Normal
d.	High	High	Normal	Normal

Answer: **B.** The anemia of chronic disease, such as that found in patients with end stage renal disease, is associated with normal or increased amounts of iron in storage (ferritin/TIBC) but the inability to process the iron into usable cells and hemoglobin. The only form of anemia of chronic disease that reliably responds to erythropoietin is caused by end stage renal disease.

Macrocytic Anemia

"Extravascular" hemolysis occurs in spleen and liver, so you **cannot** see it on the smear.

All anemia presents with **fatigue,** including macrocytic anemia, which is caused by **vitamin B12 or folate deficiency.**

- **Vitamin B12 deficiency** presents with **neurological findings** as well.
  - The most common is **peripheral neuropathy,** but *any* form of neurological abnormality can develop at any part of the peripheral or central nervous system.
  - The least common neurological problem is dementia.
  - Neurological problems resolve with treatment if they have been present for a short period of time.
- **B12 deficiency** also causes a **smooth tongue (glossitis) and diarrhea.**
- **Folate deficiency:** This does not present with neurological problems.

> Metformin blocks B12 absorption.

Diagnostic Testing

- Best initial test: **CBC with peripheral blood smear** (look for hypersegmented neutrophils and oval cells). The average number of lobes in the normal white cell is 3.5. If the average is > 4 if more than 5 percent of the cells have > 5 lobes, the patient has **megaloblastic anemia** as well as macrocytosis. *Macrocytosis* means "big cells" (i.e., large MCV). Megaloblastic anemia means the presence of hypersegmented neutrophils as well. For CCS cases you should also order a **bilirubin level and LDH,** which are commonly elevated. The **reticulocyte count will be decreased. Oval cells** will be visible on the peripheral smear as well. The 3 images below show hypersegmented neutrophils (megaloblastic anemia).

> Reticulocytes are low in B12 deficiency.

Basic Science Correlate

B12 deficiency raises LDH and indirect bilirubin by destroying red cells early, as they come out of the bone marrow. This phenomenon is called "ineffective erythropoiesis," and it is why the reticulocyte count is low. Although the marrow itself is hypercellular, B12 deficiency creates a molecular defect that breaks down the cells just as they leave the marrow.

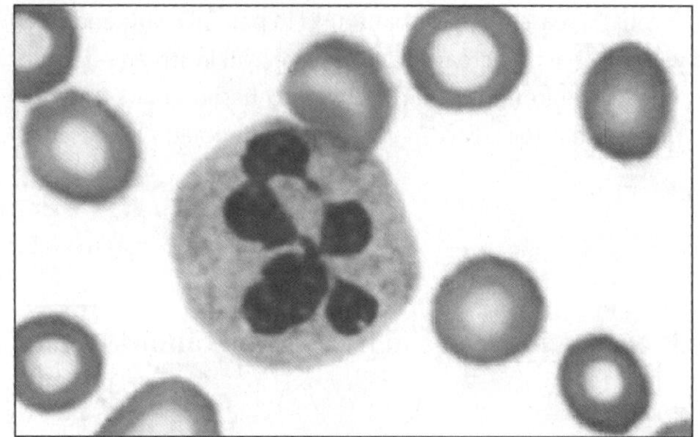

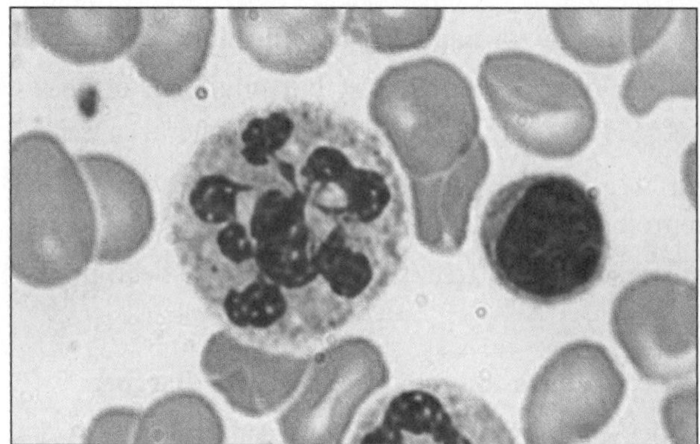

After B12 replacement therapy:

- Reticulocytes improve first.
- Neurological abnormalities improve last.

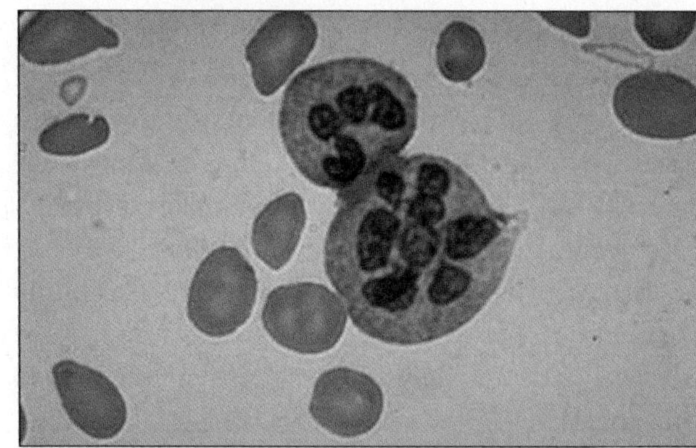

- Most accurate tests: **Low B12 level** (for B12 deficiency) and **folate level** (for folate deficiency). Note: Up to 30 percent of those with B12 deficiency can have a *normal* B12 level, because transcobalamin is an acute phase reactant and any form of stress can cause its elevation. If you suspect B12 deficiency but the B12 level is normal, order a **methylmalonic acid level.** Homocysteine levels go up in *both* vitamin B12 deficiency and folate deficiency.
- When asked, *after* finding a low B12 level or elevated methylmalonic acid level, "What is the next best test to confirm the etiology of the B12 deficiency?"

answer **antiparietal cell antibodies** and **anti-intrinsic factor antibodies.** Antiparietal cell antibodies and anti-intrinsic factor antibodies confirm pernicious anemia as the etiology of the B12 deficiency. Essentially, **pernicious anemia** is an allergy to parietal cells; it is a kind of autoimmune disorder against this part of the stomach.

- Schilling's test is an older, rarely done method of confirming the etiology and is not necessary if the antibodies are present.

> Folate will correct the blood problems in B12 deficiency, but not the neurological problems.

Treatment

B12 deficiency and folate deficiency are treated with **replacement.**

Hemolytic Anemia

All forms of hemolytic anemia present **with the sudden onset of weakness and fatigue** associated with anemia. The first thing to improve is the reticulocyte count and LDH.

Diagnostic Testing

Hemolysis shows the following:

- Elevated indirect bilirubin level
- Elevated reticulocyte count
- Elevated LDH level
- Decreased haptoglobin level
- Spherocytes on smear

> Autoimmune hemolysis also gives spherocytes.

Basic Science Correlate

Mechanism of Lab Abnormalities in Hemolysis

When cells are destroyed, they release indirect (lipid-soluble) bilirubin. The liver has limited capacity to glucuronidate it into direct (water-soluble) bilirubin. Indirect bilirubin never goes into the urine, because it is attached to albumin and cannot be filtered. Haptoglobin is a transport protein for newly released indirect bilirubin and is rapidly used up during hemolysis. LDH increases from any form of tissue breakdown and is extremely nonspecific.

CCS Tip: In a case of hemolysis, order a peripheral smear, LDH, bilirubin level, reticulocyte count, and haptoglobin level on the first CCS screen.

> Watch for low potassium after treating B12 deficiency!

Intravascular hemolysis *also* shows the following:

- Abnormal peripheral smear (schistocytes, helmet cells, fragmented cells)
- Hemoglobinuria
- Hemosiderinuria (metabolic, oxidized product of hemoglobin in the urine)

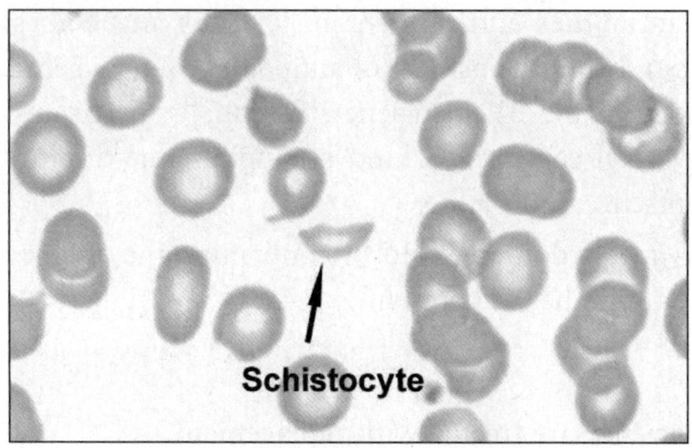

Microangiopathic Intravascular Hemolysis

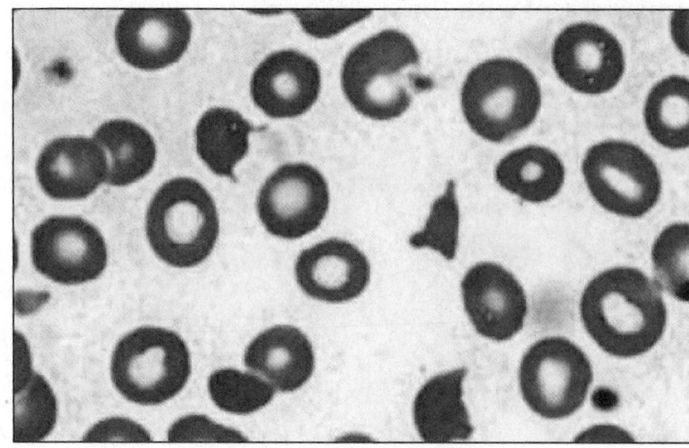

Sickle Cell Anemia

The *most* likely hemolysis question to be asked will concern sickle cell anemia. The question will describe **pain in the chest, back, and thighs that is very severe.**

Physical Exam

A **complete physical examination** is *very* important for the sickle cell case. If there is a fever *after* you give oxygen, fluids, analgesics, and antibiotics, then perform a complete physical examination.

Possible findings of the physical include the following:

- HEENT: Retinal infarction
- CV: Flow murmur from anemia
- Abdomen: Splenomegaly in children; absence of spleen in adults
- Chest: Rales or consolidation from infection or infarction
- Extremities: Skin ulcers (unclear etiology in sickle cell) and aseptic necrosis of hip. Aseptic necrosis is found on MRI.
- Neurological: Stroke, current or previous

Treatment

- Next best step: **Oxygen, hydration** with normal saline continuously, and **pain medications**
- If a fever is present: Give **ceftriaxone, levofloxacin,** or **moxifloxacin** with the first screen. Fever in a patient with sickle cell disease is an *emergency* because the patient has *no* spleen.
  - Hence, for a question of "Most urgent next step?" answer **antibiotics** when fever is present. This is *more* important than waiting for results of testing.
  - If it is a CCS question, answer **blood cultures, urinalysis, reticulocyte count, CBC, and chest x-ray** with the first screen as well, but if fever is present, do not wait for results.

When do you answer "exchange transfusion" in sickle cell disease?

- **Eye:** Visual disturbance from retinal infarction
- **Lung:** Pulmonary infarction leading to pleuritic pain and abnormal x-ray
- **Penis:** Priapism from infarction of prostatic plexus of veins
- **Brain:** Stroke

The goal of exchange transfusion is to decrease hemoglobin S to 30–40 percent.

A patient admitted for sickle cell crisis has a drop from her usual hematocrit of 34 to 26 over 2 days in the hospital. The reticulocyte count is 2 percent. What is the diagnosis? What is the most accurate test? What is the treatment?

Answer: Sudden drops in the hematocrit in sickle cell patients or those with hemoglobinopathy can be caused by **parvovirus B19** or **folate deficiency.** Sickle cell patients should universally be on **folate replacement.**

If the patient is on replacement therapy, then the diagnosis shifts to parvovirus B19, which is an **infection that invades the marrow** and stops production of cells at the level of the pronormoblast. The most accurate diagnostic test is **PCR for DNA of the parvovirus.** This is more accurate than IgM or IgG antibody testing or bone marrow.

Treat with **transfusions and intravenous immunoglobulins.**

When a patient with sickle cell anemia is ready for discharge, prescribe:

- Folate replacement
- Pneumococcal vaccination
- Hydroxyurea to prevent further crises if they happen > 4 times per year

Basic Science Correlate

Mechanism of Hydroxyurea in Sickle Cell Disease

Hydroxyurea increases the percentage of hemoglobin that is hemoglobin F, or fetal hemoglobin. Increased fetal hemoglobin dilutes the sickle hemoglobin and decreases the frequency of painful crises.

Hemoglobin Sickle Cell (SC) Disease

This condition is like a **mild version of sickle cell disease** with fewer crises. Visual disturbance is frequent. Painful crises do not occur. Renal problems are the only significant manifestation, including the following:

- Hematuria
- Isosthenuria (inability to concentrate or dilute the urine)
- Urinary tract infections

There is no specific therapy for hemoglobin SC disease.

Sickle cell trait: Renal manifestations are the only findings. They are hematuria and a concentrating defect. With hypoxia (as in scuba diving) splenic vein thrombosis can occur.

Autoimmune Hemolysis

Look for **other autoimmune diseases in the history,** such as SLE or rheumatoid arthritis. Other clues are a history of chronic lymphocytic leukemia (CLL), lymphoma, or medications such as penicillin, alpha-methyldopa, quinine, or sulfa drugs.

Diagnostic Testing

The **LDH, indirect bilirubin level, and reticulocyte count will be elevated** as with all forms of hemolysis. The **haptoglobin level can be decreased** in both intravascular and extravascular forms of hemolysis.

- Peripheral smear: May show **spherocytes**
- Most accurate diagnostic test: **Coombs test**

Basic Science Correlate

Mechanism of Spherocytes in Autoimmune Hemolysis

A normal red blood cell (RBC) is a biconcave disc. When antibodies attack the RBC membrane, they pull out pieces of it. Removing membrane decreases the surface area, which turns the RBC into a sphere. It takes more surface area to maintain biconcave disc than a sphere.

Treatment

- Best initial therapy: **Steroids,** such as prednisone
- If the case describes recurrent episodes of hemolysis, **splenectomy** is the most effective therapy. Rituximab works on both IgG and IgM.

The antibodies found in Coombs test are also called **"warm antibodies,"** which are IgG. *Only* IgG antibodies respond to steroids and splenectomy.

CCS Tip: If the case describes **severe hemolysis** not responsive to prednisone or repeated blood transfusion, use **intravenous immunoglobulins** as the best therapy to stop acute episodes of hemolysis.

A response to IVIG predicts a response to splenectomy.

Cold-Induced Hemolysis (Cold Agglutinins)

Look for the following:

- **Mycoplasma** or **Epstein-Barr virus** is in the history.
- Standard **Coombs test is negative.**
- **Complement test is positive.**
- There is **no response to steroids, splenectomy, or intravenous immunoglobulins.** Treat with rituximab.

Syphilis causes cold agglutinins with IVIG.

CCS Tip: CCS does *not* require you to know dosing. Do not memorize doses. There is no way to order doses on CCS.

Basic Science Correlate

Rituximab is an antibody against the CD20 receptor on lymphocytes. The CD20 positive cells are the ones that make antibodies, such as the IgM against red cells known as the "cold agglutinin." Rituximab's effect in both this disease and rheumatoid arthritis is to remove antibody-producing cells.

Glucose-6-Phosphate Dehydrogenase (G6PD) Deficiency

Sudden onset of hemolysis, which can be quite severe, is seen. As an **X-linked disorder,** hemolysis from G6PD deficiency is much more often described in **males.**

The most common form of oxidant stress to cause acute hemolysis with G6PD deficiency is an **infection. Oxidizing drugs,** such as sulfa medication, primaquine, or dapsone, are frequently in the history. **Fava bean ingestion** may also be in the history.

Diagnostic Testing

- Best initial test: **Heinz body test, bite cells.**

Basic Science Correlate

Heinz bodies are collections of oxidized, precipitated hemoglobin embedded in the red cell membrane. **Bite cells** appear when pieces of the red cell membrane have been removed by the spleen.

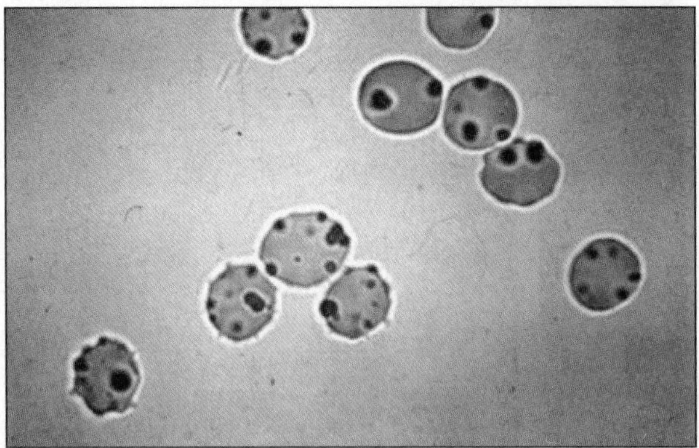

Heinz bodies

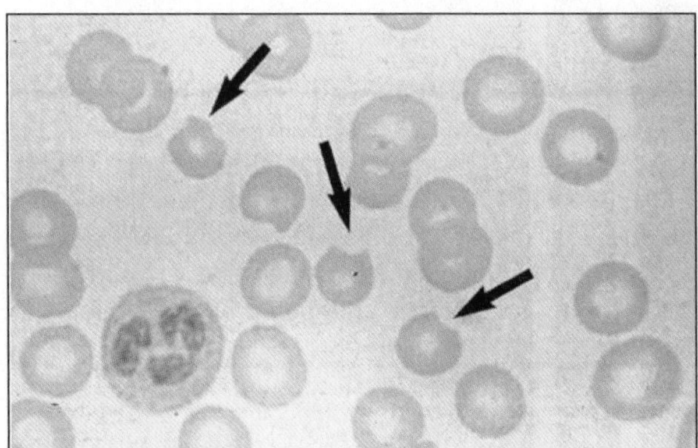

Bite cells

Test for G6PD before using dapsone.

- Most accurate test: The **level of G6PD**—but *only* after 2 months have passed. A normal level of G6PD immediately after an episode of hemolysis does *not* exclude G6PD deficiency. On the day of the hemolysis, the most deficient cells have been destroyed, and the level of G6PD is normal.

Treatment

There is *no* specific therapy for G6PD deficiency. **Avoid oxidant stress.**

Pyruvate Kinase Deficiency

Presents the **same way as G6PD deficiency in terms of hemolysis.** However, pyruvate kinase deficiency is *not* provoked by medications or fava beans; what precipitates the hemolysis with pyruvate kinase deficiency is *not* clear.

Hereditary Spherocytosis

This condition presents with:

- **Recurrent episodes of hemolysis**
- **Splenomegaly**
- **Bilirubin gallstones**
- **Elevated mean corpuscular hemoglobin concentration** (MCHC)

Diagnostic Testing

The most accurate test for hereditary spherocytosis is an **osmotic fragility test.**

Treatment

Splenectomy will prevent hemolysis since the cells are destroyed in the spleen. **Splenectomy** helps in these patients.

Basic Science Correlate

Hereditary spherocytosis is the genetic loss of both ankyrin and spectrin in the red cell membrane. Ankyrin and spectrin are the basis of the cytoskeleton that maintains the RBC membrane in its biconcave disc. Without this cytoskeleton, the RBC pops into a sphere.

Hemolytic Uremic Syndrome (HUS) and Thrombotic Thrombocytopenic Purpura (TTP)

Look for **E. coli 0157:H7** in the history for HUS. Medications such as **ticlopidine** predispose to TTP.

Diagnostic Testing

Diagnosis is based on:

- **HUS triad: ART**
  - **Intravascular hemolysis** with abnormal smear (**A:** Autoimmune hemolysis)
  - **Elevated BUN and creatinine** (**R:** Renal failure)
  - **Thrombocytopenia** (**T:** Thrombocytopenia)

Never use platelets in HUS or TTP.

- **TTP pentad (FAT RN)** *also* has the following
  - **Fever** (**F:** Fever)
  - **Neurological abnormalities** (**N:** Neurological issues)

Get an ADAMTS-13 level in TTP/HUS.

ADAMTS-13 level is down in TTP.

Treatment

Some cases **resolve on their own.** Severe cases of either TTP or HUS should be treated with **plasmapheresis.** Steroids will *not* help. Antibiotics for HUS from *E. coli* may make it worse; platelet transfusions for either will *definitely* make it worse.

Basic Science Correlate

Mechanism of HUS/TTP

ADAMTS-13 is the metalloproteinase that breaks down von Willebrand's factor (VWF) to release platelets from one another. When VWF is not dissolved, the platelets form abnormally prolonged strands that serve as a barrier to RBCs. RBCs that run into these strands break down and are destroyed. The purpose of plasmapheresis in the treatment of severe TTP is to replace the ADAMTS-13. This is why giving platelets only makes matters worse: It increases the size of the abnormal platelet strands.

Paroxysmal Nocturnal Hemoglobinuria (PNH)

Eculizumab inhibits C-5 and prevents complement activation. PNH is treated with eculizumab.

Presents with pancytopenia and recurrent episodes of dark urine, particularly in the morning. The most common cause of death is **large vessel venous thrombosis,** such as portal vein thrombosis.

PNH can transform into the following:

- Aplastic anemia
- Acute myelogenous leukemia (AML)

Diagnostic Testing

- Most accurate test: **CD 55** and **CD 59** antibody (also known as **decay accelerating factor**)

Treatment

The best initial treatment is with glucocorticoids, such as prednisone. Transfusion-dependent patients with severe illness are treated with eculizumab.

A pregnant woman comes with weakness and elevated liver function tests. She is in her 35th week of pregnancy. The prothrombin time is normal. The smear of blood shows fragmented red cells. Platelet count is low. What is the treatment?

a. Transfuse platelets
b. Plasmapheresis
c. Fresh frozen plasma
d. Delivery of the baby
e. Prednisone

Answer: **D.** Deliver the baby with the **HELLP syndrome.** HELLP syndrome stands for **h**emolysis, **e**levated **l**iver function tests, and **l**ow **p**latelets. This disorder is idiopathic and can be distinguished from DIC by the normal coagulation studies, such as the prothrombin time and aPTT.

Methemoglobinemia

The key to recognizing this condition is that the patient presents with **shortness of breath for no clear reason** with **clear lungs on exam** and a **normal chest x-ray.** Methemoglobinemia is **blood locked in an oxidized state that cannot pick up oxygen.** Look for an **exposure to drugs** such as nitroglycerin, amyl nitrate, nitroprusside, dapsone, or any of the anesthetic drugs that end in *-caine* (e.g., lidocaine, bupivicaine, tetracaine). Methemoglobinemia can occur with as little exposure as to a topical anesthetic administered to a mucous membrane. Look for **brown blood** in the case description. Treat with **methylene blue.**

Transfusion Reactions

Match the most likely diagnoses with each of the following cases:

a. ABO incompatibility
b. Transfusion-related acute lung injury (TRALI) or "leukoagglutination reaction"
c. Urticarial reaction
d. IgA deficiency
e. Febrile nonhemolytic reaction
f. Minor blood group incompatibility

Case 1: Twenty minutes after a patient receives a blood transfusion, the patient becomes short of breath. There are transient infiltrates on the chest x-ray. All symptoms resolve spontaneously.
Case 2: As soon as a patient receives a transfusion, he becomes hypotensive, short of breath, and tachycardic. The LDH and bilirubin levels are normal.
Case 3: During a transfusion, a patient becomes hypotensive and tachycardic. She has back and chest pain, and there is dark urine. The LDH and bilirubin are elevated, and the haptoglobin level is low.
Case 4: A few days after a transfusion, a patient becomes jaundiced. The hematocrit does not rise with transfusion, and he is generally without symptoms.

Case 5: A few hours after a transfusion, a patient becomes febrile with a rise in temperature of about 1 degree. There is no evidence of hemolysis.

Answers:
Case 1: B. TRALI presents with acute shortness of breath from antibodies in the donor blood against recipient white cells. There is no treatment, and it resolves spontaneously.
Case 2: D. IgA deficiency presents with anaphylaxis. In the future, use blood donations from an IgA deficient donor or washed red cells.
Case 3: A. ABO incompatibility presents with acute symptoms of hemolysis while the transfusion is occurring.
Case 4: F. Minor blood group incompatibility to Kell, Duffy, Lewis, or Kidd antigens or Rh incompatibility presents with delayed jaundice. There is no specific therapy.
Case 5: E. Febrile nonhemolytic reactions result in a small rise in temperature and need no therapy. These reactions are against donor white cell antigens. They are prevented by using filtered blood transfusions in the future to remove the white cell antigens.

Leukemia

Acute Leukemia

Presents with signs of pancytopenia, such as **fatigue, bleeding,** and **infections** from white cells that don't work. Patients have a **functional immunodeficiency.**

Diagnostic Testing

- Best initial test: **Peripheral smear showing blasts**

The most important prognostic finding in acute leukemia is **cytogenetic abnormalities,** such as specific karyotypic abnormalities. Cytogenetics tell who will relapse. If the patient is as high risk for relapse after chemotherapy, **bone marrow transplantation** should be performed as soon as chemotherapy induces remission.

Auer rods are associated with acute myeloid leukemia (AML).

Treatment

Chemotherapy with **idarubicin** (or **daunorubicin**) and **cytosine arabinoside** is the best initial therapy for acute myelogenous leukemia. Add **all trans retinoic acid (ATRA)** to the treatment of M3 (acute promyelocytic) leukemia. Add **intrathecal methotrexate** for acute lymphocytic leukemia (ALL).

M3, acute promyelocytic leukemia, is associated with disseminated intravascular coagulation (DIC). This is the most frequently tested information about acute leukemia.

A patient presents with shortness of breath, confusion, and blurry vision. His white cell count is over 100,000. What is the best initial therapy?

Answer: Acute leukemia can sometimes present with an extremely high white cell count. When the count goes above 100,000, these cells result in sludging of the blood vessels of the brain, eyes, and lungs. Chronic lymphocytic leukemia rarely does this, because lymphocytes are much smaller and do not occlude vessels. Leukostasis is treated with **leukapheresis,** which removes white cells via centrifugation of blood. **Hydroxyurea** is also added to lower the white cell count.

Myelodysplasia

This condition presents in elderly patients with **pancytopenia, elevated MCV, low reticulocyte count,** and **macroovalocytes.** There is a special neutrophil with 2 lobes called a **"Pelger-Huet cell."** Look for a **normal B12 level.** There will be a **small number of blasts** but not enough to be considered acute leukemia. Myelodysplasia is like a **mild, slowly progressive preleukemia syndrome.** Just as cervical dysplasia may sometimes progress to cervical cancer, myelodysplasia may progress to acute leukemia. The most common cause of death is not leukemia; most patients die of **infection** or **bleeding.**

Lenalidomide has tremendous efficacy in decreasing transfusion dependence in MDS.

Treatment is largely supportive with **transfusions as needed.** Azacitadine, decitabine, and lenalidomide are specific therapies for myelodysplasia (MDS). Those with the 5q minus syndrome are treated with lenalidomide. Only azacytadine increases survival.

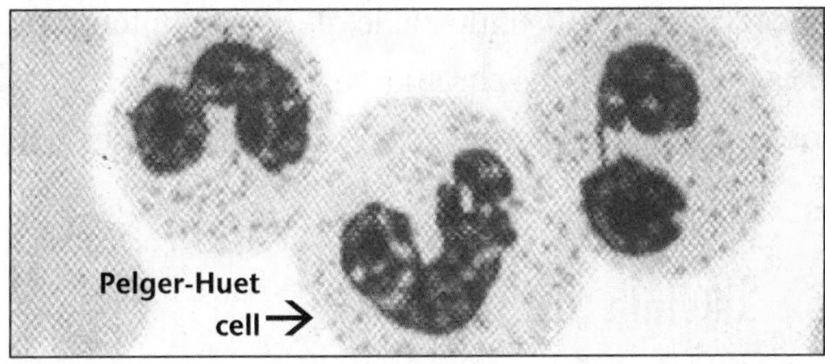

Myeloproliferative Disorders

Chronic Myelogenous Leukemia (CML)

Look for an **elevated white cell count** that is predominantly neutrophils. **Splenomegaly** is frequent.

Untreated CML has the highest risk of transformation into acute leukemia of all forms of myeloproliferative disorders.

Basic Science Correlate

Mechanism of Early Satiety in CML and CLL

The spleen is anatomically right on top of the stomach. When the spleen is enlarged, it presses on the stomach and compresses it. This stomach compression makes a person feel full right after eating.

Test for CML with
- PCR, or
- FISH

Diagnostic Testing

- An elevated neutrophils count with a low LAP score is CML. Reactive high white counts from infection give an elevated LAP score. LAP is up in normal cells, not CML.
- Most accurate test: **Philadelphia chromosome** by PCR of blood or BCR/ABL by fluorescence in situ hybridization (FISH)

Treatment

The best initial therapy is **imatinib** (Gleevec). **Bone marrow transplantation** is the only way to cure CML, but this is *never* the best initial therapy, because imatinib leads to 90 percent hematologic remission with no major adverse effects. Dasatinib and nilotinib are tyrosine kinase inhibitors. They can be used as first-line therapy or as an alternative in those not responding to imatinib.

Following are *wrong answers* for CML treatment:

- Interferon: Much less efficacy; causes uncomfortable, flulike symptoms
- Hydroxyurea: Never makes the Philadelphia chromosome negative
- Busulfan: Never right for anything, unless the exam asks what causes pulmonary fibrosis

Chronic Lymphocytic Leukemia (CLL)

CLL exclusively presents in **patients > 50 years old** with an **elevated white cell count** that is described as "normal appearing lymphocytes." CLL is often asymptomatic and is described as being found on "routine" testing.

Diagnostic Testing

- Best initial test: **Peripheral blood smear shows "smudge" cells,** which are ruptured nuclei of lymphocytes. They are like squished jelly donuts.
- Stage 0: Elevated white cell count alone
- Stage 1: Enlarged lymph nodes
- Stage 2: Spleen enlargement
- Stage 3: Anemia
- Stage 4: Low platelets

Basic Science Correlate

Mechanism of Infection and Hemolysis in CLL

The lymphocytes in CLL produce either abnormal or insufficient immunoglobulins. When the IgG produced is abnormal, it is inappropriately directed against RBCs or platelets, causing immune thrombocytopenia or hemolysis. When IgG supply is insufficient, it leads to infection.

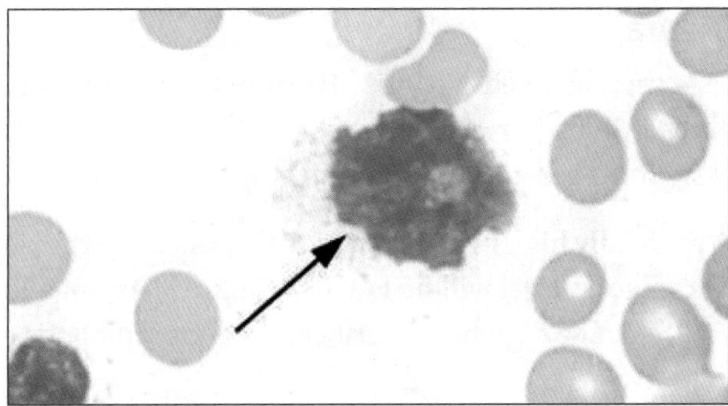

Smudge cell (found in CLL)

Treatment

Treatment for CLL is **entirely based on the stage** of the disease. Early stage disease (Stages 0 and 1) does *not* require therapy. More advanced stages of disease are treated with fludarabine combined with rituximab and cyclophosphamide. Chlorambucil is not as effective. If the questions asks, "Which therapy is most likely to extend survival?" the answer is fludarabine for advanced stage disease.

Do not treat asymptomatic elevations in white count caused by CLL.

Alemtuzumab is an anti-CD52 agent used for CLL that is better than chlorambucil. Alemtuzumab is used when fludarabine fails.

Rituximab adds significant benefit to fludarabine in CLL.

Hairy Cell Leukemia

This condition presents with the following:

- Pancytopenia
- Massive splenomegaly
- Middle-aged patient (50s)

The most accurate test is **smear showing hairy cells and immunophenotyping** (or flow cytometry).

The best initial therapy is **cladribine (2-CDA).**

Myelofibrosis

Presents in the **same way as hairy cell leukemia** (pancytopenia and splenomegaly) with a normal TRAP level. A key feature is teardrop-shaped cells on the smear. Fibrosis is found on marrow, and the JAK2 mutation is found.

Ruxolitinib inhibits Janus kinase.

Bone marrow transplantation can be curative. When transplant is not possible, the "best initial therapy" is lenalidomide or thalidomide. Ruxolitinib inhibits JAK2.

Polycythemia Vera (Pvera)

Pvera presents with **headache, blurred vision, dizziness, and fatigue. Pruritus, described as happening after a hot bath or shower,** also occurs from the release of histamine from basophils. **Splenomegaly** is common.

The key to the diagnosis is a **markedly high hematocrit in the absence of hypoxia with a low MCV. The erythropoietin level will be low.** The white cell count and platelet count can also be elevated. The high hematocrit can lead to thrombosis.

JAK2 mutation is found in Pvera and ET.

Diagnostic Testing

After the **CBC** shows a high hematocrit, order an **arterial blood gas** to exclude hypoxia as a cause of erythrocytosis. If the case is a CCS, order an **erythropoietin level,** which should be low; hematology consultation; and nuclear red cell mass test. The test for the JAK2 mutation is 97% sensitive. The B12 and LAP levels are elevated in Pvera.

Treatment

Phlebotomy is the best initial therapy. **Hydroxyurea** is also used to lower the cell count. **Daily aspirin** should also be given. **Anagrelide** is used in the context of thrombocythemia.

Essential Thrombocythemia (ET)

In Pvera on a CCS, order a B12 level and LAP in addition to the CBC. If the question is a "single best answer" question, these tests would not be the single "best initial" or "most accurate" tests.

The key feature of ET is a **markedly elevated platelet count.** ET presents with **headache, visual disturbance, and pain in the hands** referred to as erythromelalgia. The most common causes of death are **bleeding** and **thrombosis,** with thrombosis being more common.

Therapy is with **hydroxyurea** to lower the platelet count. Anagrelide is an agent specific to the treatment of ET but it is not as strong as hydroxyurea. **Daily aspirin** should also be given if patient is thrombosing.

Plasma Cell Disorders

Multiple Myeloma (MM)

The most frequent presentation of MM is with **bone pain caused by a fracture occurring under normal use.** The most common causes of death from MM are the following:

- **Infection:** Patients with multiple myeloma are effectively immunodeficient.
- **Renal failure**

Diagnostic Testing

Initial testing is as follows:

- **Skeletal survey** to detect punched out osteolytic lesions. (Osteoblastic lesions suggest metastatic prostate cancer.)
- **Serum protein electrophoresis (SPEP):** You are looking for elevated levels of monoclonal antibody (usually IgG). 20% are IgA.
- **Urine protein electrophoresis (UPEP):** Detects Bence-Jones protein.
- **Peripheral smear:** Shows "rouleaux" formation of blood cells. Mean platelet volume (MPV) is elevated because the cells stick together.
- **Elevated calcium level:** Makes sense with the osteolytic lesions.
- **Beta 2 microglobulin level:** This is a prognostic indicator.
- **BUN and creatinine:** This is to detect the frequent occurrence of renal insufficiency. Bortezomib reverses renal dysfunction.

Basic Science Correlate

Mechanism of Renal Failure in Myeloma

- Hypercalcemia leads to nephrocalcinosis.
- Hyperuricemia is directly toxic to kidney tubules.
- Bence-Jones protein clogs up glomeruli and is toxic to kidney tubules.
- Amyloid occurs in myeloma.

The single most specific test is the **bone marrow biopsy,** which detects high numbers of plasma cells (10 percent).

The B12 and LAP levels are elevated in Pvera.

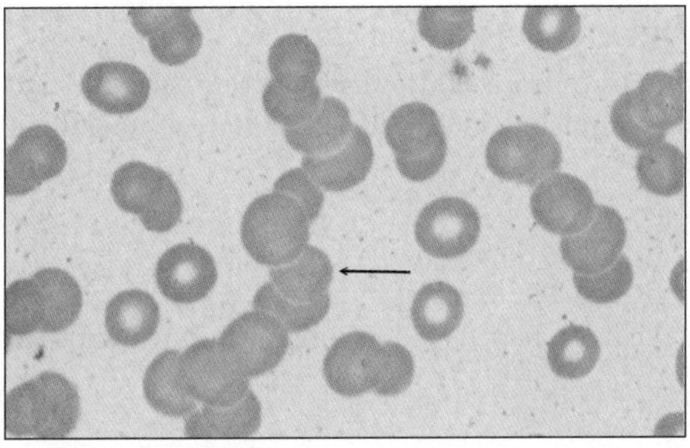

"Rouleaux" formation of blood cells

Treatment

Treat with **melphalan and steroids. Thalidomide, lenalidomide, or bortezomib** may be added: Thalidomide is an inhibitor of tumor necrosis factor that has the same efficacy as chemotherapy.

The most effective therapy is an **autologous stem cell bone marrow transplantation.** This is reserved for patients who are relatively young (<70) with advanced disease.

You should remember *also* to treat the hypercalcemia (hydration/diuresis), bone fractures (bisphosphonates), renal failure (hydration), and anemia (erythropoietin) and to prophylax against infections with vaccinations (e.g., flu, pneumovax, tetanus, etc.).

> **Basic Science Correlate**
>
> **Mechanism of Bone Marrow Transplant Success or Failure**
> Autologous transplantation can be done up to age 70, but allogeneic transplant only to age 50. Persons older than 50 have a much higher incidence of graft-versus-host disease and rejection. Autologous transplantation has no graft-versus-host disease and no rejection.

Monoclonal Gammopathy of Unknown Significance (MGUS)

MGUS presents with an **asymptomatic elevation of IgG** on an SPEP. The SPEP is done because of an elevated total protein level found in an **elderly patient,** typically over 70. There is no treatment for MGUS.

Waldenstrom's Macroglobulinemia

This presents with **hyperviscosity from IgM overproduction.** The question will describe **blurry vision, confusion, and headache. Enlarged nodes and spleen** can be found.

Diagnostic Testing

There are *no* specific findings on CBC. The best initial test is a **serum viscosity level,** which will be markedly increased, and an **SPEP,** which will show an elevated IgM level.

Treatment

- Best initial therapy: **Plasmapheresis** if symptomatic
- Further treatment: Use the agents you would use for CLL, such as **rituximab, fludarabine, chlorambucil,** or **rituximab.**

Aplastic Anemia

This condition presents with **pancytopenia** with no identified etiology.

When the patient is young (< 50) and has a match, the best possible therapy is **bone marrow transplantation.** When bone marrow transplantation is not possible (> 50 and/or no match), answer **antithymocyte globulin and cyclosporine.** Aplastic anemia never has cytogenetic abnormalities. Most are idiopathic. Chronic hepatitis B and C can cause it.

Lymphoma

Lymphoma presents with **enlarged lymph nodes,** most commonly in the cervical area. **Hodgkin's disease (HD)** spreads centrifugally away from the center, starting at the neck. **Non-Hodgkin's lymphoma (NHL)** more often presents as widespread disease.

"B" symptoms of lymphoma, which imply more widespread disease, are the following:

- Fever
- Weight loss
- Night sweats

Diagnostic Testing

- Best initial test for both HD and NHL: **Excisional lymph node biopsy.** The most common *wrong* answer is a needle biopsy. Needle biopsy is useful for infections such as tuberculosis but is *not* sufficient to diagnose lymphoma, because the visual appearance of lymphoma cells is normal; they are not grossly abnormal like acute leukemic blasts. The major difference between HD and NHL is that **HD has Reed-Sternberg cells.**
- Next tests: After the initial excisional biopsy shows the abnormal architecture of the cells, further tests **determine the stage** of the lymphoma. Staging is critical to determine therapy.
  - **Stage I:** Single lymph node group
  - **Stage II:** Two lymph node groups on one side of the diaphragm
  - **Stage III:** Lymph node involvement on both sides of the diaphragm
  - **Stage IV:** Widespread disease
- HD and NHL present with stages as follows:
  - **HD:** 80–90 percent present with Stages I and II.
  - **NHL:** 80–90 percent present with Stages III and IV.
- Staging involves the following tests:
  - **Chest x-ray**
  - **CT scans (with contrast):** Chest, abdomen, pelvis, and head
  - **Bone marrow biopsy**

Lymphoma evaluation does *not* need lymphangiogram or exploratory laparotomy of the abdomen. When these are in the choices, they are *wrong.*

Treatment

Localized disease **(Stages I and II)** without "B" symptoms is treated predominantly with **radiation and lower-dose chemotherapy.** More advanced stage disease **(Stages III and IV)** is treated exclusively with **chemotherapy:**

- HD: **ABVD** (Adriamycin [doxorubicin], bleomycin, vinblastine, dacarbazine)
- NHL: **CHOP** (cyclophosphamide, hydroxyadriamycin, Oncovin [vincristine], prednisone). Also, test for **anti-CD20 antigen;** if present, add **rituximab,** which adds efficacy to CHOP.

Coagulation Disorders

Von Willebrand's Disease (VWD)

VWD presents with **bleeding from platelet dysfunction**—superficial bleeding from the skin and mucosal surfaces, such as the gingiva, gums, and vagina. **Epistaxis** is consistent with platelet dysfunction. The question may say the bleeding is worse with the use of aspirin. The platelet count is *normal* in VWD.

A case of VWD is likely to present with epistaxis and/or petechiae.

The **aPTT can be elevated** in up to 50 percent of patients with VWD, because VWF deficiency destabilizes factor VIII.

Diagnostic Testing

- Most accurate tests: **Ristocetin cofactor assay** and **von Willebrand's factor (VWF) level.** VWF carries factor VIII in the blood.
- If the level of VWF is normal, **ristocetin testing** will tell if it is working properly.

Treatment

- First-line treatment: **Desmopressin** or **DDAVP.** This will release subendothelial stores of VWF and factor VIII, which will stop the bleeding.
- If DDAVP is not effective, the next best step in management is to use **factor VIII replacement.** Factor VIII replacement has *both* VWF and factor VIII.

Basic Science Correlate

Mechanism of Ristocetin Testing

Ristocetin acts as an artificial endothelial lining. If VWF is present, platelets will stick to it. Ristocetin is a functional test of VWF activity.

Distinguishing Types of Bleeding	
Platelet-Type Bleeding	**Factor-Type Bleeding**
• Petechiae • Epistaxis • Purpura • Gingiva • Gums • Vaginal	• Hemarthrosis • Hematoma

Idiopathic Thrombocytopenic Purpura (ITP)

ITP presents with **platelet-type bleeding** if the **platelet count < 10,000–30,000.**

Diagnostic Testing

- **Peripheral smear shows large platelets.**
- **Sonogram:** To assess for normal spleen size found in ITP
- **Bone marrow:** To find increased numbers of megakaryocytes
- **Antibodies to the glycoprotein IIb/IIIa receptor**

A generally healthy patient comes with epistaxis and petechiae. No spleen is felt on examination. The platelet count is 24,000. What is the next step in management?

a. Prednisone
b. Bone marrow biopsy
c. Antiplatelet antibodies
d. Sonogram
e. Hematology consultation

Answer: **A.** Prednisone is the most important thing to do first in mild ITP. The main point of most ITP questions is that initiating therapy is more important than determining a specific diagnosis, particularly since ITP is a diagnosis of exclusion. All of the answers listed would be given on a CCS case at the same time. In a single best answer case, however, the most important thing is to start therapy.

> Romiplostim and eltrombopag are thrombopoietin analogs.

A patient comes in with ITP and a platelet count of 5,000. The patient has epistaxis and petechiae as well as an intracranial hemorrhage and melena. What is the best initial step?

Answer: **IVIG administration.** The fastest way to raise the platelet count with ITP is to use intravenous immunoglobulins (IVIG) or RhoGAM. IVIG is the answer when the platelet count is low (< 20,000) and the case describes life-threatening bleeding, such as that into the bowel or brain.

Romiplostim and eltrombopag treat chronic ITP. They directly stimulate megakaryocytes.

Treatment

Case presents with...	Treatment
Platelet count > 50,000	No treatment
Count < 50,000 with minor bleeding	Prednisone
Count < 20,000 with serious bleeding	IVIG or Rhogam (Rho[D] immune globulin)
Recurrent episodes	Splenectomy
No response to splenectomy	Romiplostim, eltrombopag

Basic Science Correlate

Mechanism of IVIG Effect in ITP

IVIG has no direct activity against platelets. It is administered in order to prevent the action of macrophages against platelets: By stopping up all the FC receptors on the macrophages, IVIG leaves no room for the antibodies on the platelets. Thus it shuts off platelet destruction.

Uremia-Induced Platelet Dysfunction

Uremia by itself prevents platelets from working properly; **they do not degranulate.** Look for a **normal platelet count with platelet-type bleeding in a patient with renal failure.** The **ristocetin test and VWF level will be normal.**

Treatment

- Best initial therapy: **Desmopressin (DDAVP),** dialysis, and estrogen.

CCS Tip: **Mixing study** is the first test to determine the difference between a clotting factor deficiency and a factor inhibitor antibody. The aPTT will correct to normal with a clotting factor deficiency.

Clotting Factor Deficiencies

Deficiency	Factor VIII	Factor IX	Factor XI	Factor XII
Presentation	Joint bleeding or hematoma in a male child	Joint bleeding or hematoma; Less common than factor VIII deficiency	Rare bleeding with trauma or surgery	No bleeding
Diagnostic Test	Mixing study first, then specific factor level	Same	Same	Same
Treatment	Severe deficiency: (<1% activity): Factor VIII replacement Minor deficiency: DDAVP	Factor IX replacement	Fresh frozen plasma (FFP) with bleeding episodes	No treatment necessary

A woman presents with bleeding into her thigh after minor trauma. The aPTT is prolonged, and the prothrombin time is normal. Mixing study does not correct the aPTT to normal. What is the diagnosis?

Answer: **Factor VIII antibody** is the most common cause of a prolonged aPTT and bleeding that does not correct with a mixing study.

Heparin-Induced Thrombocytopenia (HIT)

HIT presents with **a drop in platelets** (at least 50 percent) a few days *after* the start of heparin. This can be from any amount of heparin, no matter how small, because HIT is an allergic reaction. **Thrombosis** is the most common clinical manifestation. Venous thromboses are 3 times more common than arterial thromboses. Although low molecular weight heparin is less likely to cause HIT, both types of heparin can do so.

Diagnostic Testing

The best initial diagnostic tests are:

- Platelet factor 4 antibodies; or
- Heparin-induced, antiplatelet antibodies.

Treatment

- Best initial therapy: **Stop the heparin** and use a **direct thrombin inhibitor,** such as argatroban, lepirudin, or fondaparinux.

Fondaparinux is safe in HIT.

If HIT happens with IV unfractionated heparin, *do not answer* "switch to low molecular weight heparin."

Thrombophilia/Hypercoagulable States

Cause	Lupus Antiphospholipid Syndromes, Anticoagulant, or Anticardiolipin Antibodies	Protein C Deficiency	Factor V Leiden Mutation	Antithrombin Deficiency
Presentation	Venous or arterial thrombosis Elevated aPTT with a normal PT Spontaneous abortion False positive VDRL	Skin necrosis with the use of warfarin Venous thrombosis	Most common cause of thrombophilia Venous thrombosis	No change in the aPTT with a bolus of IV heparin Venous thrombosis
Diagnostic Test	Mixing study first Russel viper venom test is most accurate for lupus anticoagulant	Protein C level	Factor V mutation test	Level of antithrombin III
Treatment	Heparin followed by warfarin	Heparin followed by warfarin	Heparin followed by warfarin	Large amounts of heparin or direct thrombin inhibitor followed by warfarin

Basic Science Correlate

Mechanism of Factor V Mutation

Protein C inactivates factor V—but only in its normal form. If factor V has a mutation, protein C will not inhibit it. Factor V mutation functions like protein C deficiency.

Gastroenterology

8

Esophageal Disorders

In general, esophageal disorders with any degree of anatomic damage leading to narrowing result in **dysphagia** and **weight loss.** All forms of dysphagia can lead to weight loss.

If dysphagia is present and you do not know the diagnosis, then perform a **barium study** first. In the stomach, do **endoscopy** first. The only 2 esophageal disorders for which endoscopy is indispensable in diagnosis are **cancer** and the precancerous histologic change known as **Barrett's esophagus;** biopsy is necessary to diagnose both of these.

> Remember: Dysphagia (difficulty swallowing) is different from odynophagia (painful swallowing). Odynophagia suggests an infectious process, such as HIV, HSV, *Candida,* or CMV.

Dysphagia

Achalasia

Achalasia presents in a **young nonsmoker** who has **dysphagia to both solids and liquids** at the same time. There may also be **regurgitation of food particles** and **aspiration of previously eaten material** that is regurgitated and falls into the lungs. This can be a progressive form of dysphagia in which the symptoms get worse over time.

Diagnostic Testing

- Best initial test: **Barium swallow**
- Most accurate test: **Esophageal manometry**

Endoscopy is *not* necessary to diagnose achalasia; it is done to exclude malignancy. Manometry would show absence of normal esophageal peristalsis. Achalasia presents with abnormally high pressure at the lower esophageal sphincter, since it involves a failure of the gastroesophageal sphincter to relax. There is *no* mucosal abnormality.

Treatment

- Best initial therapy: **Pneumatic dilation** or **surgical myotomy**
- Pneumatic dilation is done when surgical myotomy is unsuccessful.
- **Botulinum toxin injection** is used when the patient refuses surgery or pneumatic dilation.

> **Basic Science Correlate**
>
> **Mechanism of Botulinum Toxin**
>
> Botulinum toxin inhibits the release of acetylcholine at the neuromuscular junction. This inhibits nicotinic receptors and relaxes all skeletal muscle.

Esophageal Cancer

Esophageal cancer presents with the following:

- **Dysphagia: Solids first, liquids later**
- May have **heme-positive stool** or **anemia**
- Often found in patients > **50** who are **smokers and drinkers of alcohol**

> - Dysphagia + Weight Loss = Esophageal pathology
> - Dysphagia + Weight Loss + Heme-positive stool/ Anemia = Cancer

Diagnostic Testing

- Best initial test: **Endoscopy**
- If endoscopy is not one of the choices, then **barium swallow** can be performed.
- Manometry will *not* be useful, since cancer can *only* be diagnosed with biopsy.

CCS Tip: Just order the procedures you think you need on the CCS. Do *not* wait for a consult. If you need a consult for a procedure, the computer will tell you.

Treatment

- Best initial therapy: **Surgical resection.** Surgery is performed if there are no local or distant metastases.
- Follow surgery with **chemotherapy based on 5-fluorouracil.**

Rings and Webs

These are also known as **"peptic strictures."** They can be caused by the **repetitive exposure of the esophagus to acid,** resulting in scarring and stricture formation. Previous use of **sclerosing agents** for variceal bleeding can also cause strictures, and this is why variceal banding is a superior procedure.

Diagnostic Testing

The best initial test is a **barium study.**

Treatment

Treatment depends on the kind of stricture that presents:

- **Plummer-Vinson syndrome:** This is a **proximal stricture** found in association with **iron deficiency anemia** and is more common in **middle-aged women.** It is associated with squamous cell esophageal cancer.
  - Best initial therapy: **Iron replacement**
- **Schatzki's ring (peptic stricture):** This is a **distal ring** of the esophagus that presents with **intermittent symptoms of dysphagia.**
  - Best initial therapy: **Pneumatic dilation**
- **Peptic stricture:** This results from **acid reflux.**
  - It is treated with **pneumatic dilation.**

> **Eosinophilic Esophagitis**
> - Dysphagia
> - History of allergies
> - Scope + biopsy
> - Treat with PPTs and budesonide

Zenker's Diverticulum

Look for a patient with **dysphagia with horrible bad breath.** There is rotting food in the back of the esophagus from **dilation of the posterior pharyngeal constrictor muscles.**

The best initial test is a **barium study.** The best initial therapy is a **surgical resection.**

> To avoid perforation, do *not* do endoscopy or place a nasogastric tube with Zenker's diverticulum.

Spastic Disorders

Diffuse esophageal spasm and **"nutcracker esophagus"** are essentially the same disease. Look for a case of **severe chest pain,** often without risk factors for ischemic heart disease. The case may describe the pain as **occurring after drinking a cold beverage.** There is *always* pain, but there is *not* always dysphagia. The EKG, stress test, and possibly the coronary angiography will be presented as normal.

Diagnostic Testing

- Most accurate diagnostic test: **Manometry**
- **Barium studies** may show a **corkscrew pattern,** but *only* during an episode of spasm.

Treatment

Therapy for esophageal spasm is with **calcium channel blockers and nitrates** (the same treatment as for Prinzmetal's angina).

> Esophageal disorders can mimic **Prinzmetal's variant angina,** because the pain is sudden, severe, and not related to exercise. However, Prinzmetal's will give you ST segment elevation and an abnormality on stimulation of the coronary arteries, while esophageal spasm will not.

Scleroderma (Progressive Systemic Sclerosis)

Scleroderma presents as **symptoms of reflux.** Treat with **proton pump inhibitors.**

An HIV-positive man comes in with progressive dysphagia and odynophagia. He has 75 CD4 cells but no history of opportunistic infections. What is the next best step in management?

a. Fluconazole
b. Amphotericin
c. Barium swallow
d. Endoscopy
e. Antiretroviral therapy

Answer: **A.** Odynophagia is pain on swallowing. Dysphagia is simply difficulty swallowing (i.e., food getting "stuck" in the esophagus). When odynophagia occurs in an HIV-positive patient, particularly when there are < 100 CD4 cells, the diagnosis is most likely **esophageal candidiasis,** and giving empiric fluconazole is both therapeutic as well as diagnostic. Amphotericin is not necessary.

Esophagitis

Esophagitis presents with **pain on swallowing (odynophagia)** as the food rubs against the esophagus.

Diagnostic Testing and Treatment

- In **HIV-negative** patients, **endoscopy** is done first.
- In **HIV-positive** patients with < 100 CD4 cells, give **fluconazole.** Endoscopy in these patients is performed *only* if there is no response to the fluconazole.

Candida esophagitis causes > 90 percent of esophagitis in HIV-positive patients. Other causes of esophagitis are **pills** such as doxycycline or a bisphosphonate such as alendronate. In the case of esophagitis caused by pills, the patient should **sit up and drink more water** when taking pills and **remain upright for at least 30 minutes after taking the pill.**

Mallory-Weiss Tear

This is *not* a cause of dysphagia, although Mallory-Weiss tear is clearly an esophageal disorder. It presents as **sudden upper gastrointestinal bleeding** with **violent retching and vomiting** of any cause. There may be either hematemesis or black stool.

Diagnostic Testing

Diagnose with endoscopy.

Treatment

Most cases resolve **spontaneously.** If bleeding persists, injection of **epinephrine** can be used to stop the bleeding.

CCS Tip: How do I know I am doing the right thing on CCS?

- You may get spontaneous **nurse's notes** telling you whether the patient is doing well or not. You get these automatically as you move the clock forward.
- You can get an "interval history" as a choice under physical exam. This is a 2-minute advance of the clock that will "check in" with the patient. This often tells you how the patient is doing and, consequently, how you are doing in management.

Gastroesophageal Reflux Disease (GERD)

A patient comes with epigastric pain that is associated with substernal chest pain and an unpleasant metallic taste in the mouth. What is the next best step in management?

a. Endoscopy
b. Barium studies
c. Proton pump inhibitors (PPIs)
d. H2 (histamine) blockers
e. 24-hour pH monitor

Answer: **C.** Proton pump inhibitors (PPIs) are preferred as the first line of therapy and also serve as a diagnostic test. Using PPIs is far easier than other testing.

In addition to the epigastric pain and substernal chest pain of GERD, several other symptoms are clearly associated with acid reflux:

25 percent of chronic cough is caused by GERD.

- Sore throat
- Metallic or bitter taste
- Hoarseness
- Chronic cough
- Wheezing

Basic Science Correlate

Mechanism of Bad Taste in GERD

Sweet taste receptors are on the anterior two thirds of the tongue, and sweet taste is controlled by cranial nerve VII. The bitter taste receptors are on the back of the tongue, and bitter taste is controlled by cranial nerves IX and X.

As many as 20–25 percent of those with chronic cough are suffering from GERD.

When is reflux alarming, and when is endoscopy used in GERD? When the following symptoms are present:

- Weight loss
- Anemia
- Blood in the stool
- Dysphagia

Diagnostic Testing

PPI administration is both diagnostic and therapeutic. Further diagnostic testing, such as a 24-hour pH monitor, should *only* be done if there is no response to PPIs and the diagnosis is not clear.

Treatment

Mild disease may be controlled with **lifestyle modifications** such as:

- Losing weight
- Elevating the head of the bed
- Quitting smoking
- Limiting alcohol, caffeine, chocolate, and peppermint ingestion
- Not eating within 3 hours of going to sleep

If these do not work, **PPIs** are the next best therapy for GERD. They should control 90–95 percent of cases. All PPIs are equal in efficacy.

H2 blockers, such as ranitidine, famotidine, cimetidine, or nizatidine, control GERD in about two thirds of patients. Hence, they are *only* used if a PPI is not available. Promotility agents, such as metoclopramide, are equal to H2 blockers and much less effective than PPIs such as omeprazole; therefore, they would *not* routinely be used.

Basic Science Correlate

H2 blockers only reduce two thirds of gastric acid production. Why? Because histamine is only 1 of the 3 stimulants to acid production on the parietal cell, namely: gastrin, histamine, and acetylcholine via the vagus nerve. Histamine potentiates the other 2, resulting in a two-thirds reduction in acid. By contrast, PPI use inhibits the acid output of the cell no matter what the stimulant is.

Treatment for *Helicobacter pylori* is *not* effective or necessary for GERD. Such treatment will not tighten the LES.

If PPIs are not sufficient to control disease, then a **surgical or endoscopic procedure to narrow the distal esophagus and reconstrict the lower esophegeal sphincter** should be performed, such as a Nissen fundoplication or endoscopically suturing the lower esophageal sphincter (LES) tighter. Make sure esophageal motility is adequate before you tighten the sphincter with a surgical procedure.

Barrett Esophagus

Barrett esophagus is a **precancerous lesion.** Approximately 0.5 percent of cases per year will transform into esophageal cancer. This is why **adenocarcinoma** is an increasingly frequent histological type of esophageal cancer.

> Surgery is rarely needed for GERD anymore.

Diagnostic Testing

This condition can only be diagnosed by **endoscopy** in which you are able to visualize and biopsy the distal esophagus: Barrett esophagus is a **biopsy diagnosis.** Although the color is different, the only way to be certain that the histology has changed from squamous epithelium to columnar epithelium ("Barrett esophagus") with metaplasia is by endoscopy.

Perform endoscopy for all the symptoms described **(weight loss, anemia, heme-positive stool)** and in **anyone with symptoms of reflux disease for more than 5–10 years.**

Treatment

Endoscopic Finding	Action
Barrett esophagus	PPI and repeat endoscopy every 2–3 years
Low-grade dysplasia	PPI and repeat endoscopy in 3–6 months
High-grade dysplasia	Endoscopic mucosal resection, ablative removal, or distal esophagectomy

Epigastric Pain

A 58-year-old man comes to the office for evaluation of epigastric discomfort for the last several weeks. He is otherwise asymptomatic with no weight loss. His stool is heme-negative. What is the next best step in management?

a. Upper endoscopy
b. Serology for *Helicobacter pylori*
c. Urea breath testing for *Helicobacter pylori*
d. PPI, amoxicillin, and clarithromycin for 2 weeks
e. Ranitidine empirically

Answer: **A.** Upper endoscopy should be performed in any patient above the age of 45 with persistent symptoms of epigastric discomfort. This is, essentially, to exclude the possibility of gastric cancer. There is no way to be certain, without endoscopy, who has gastric cancer.

Non-Ulcer Dyspepsia

This is the most common cause of epigastric discomfort.

There is no proven benefit to treating *Helicobacter* for non-ulcer dyspepsia.

You can conclude that a person has non-ulcer dyspepsia *only after* **endoscopy** has excluded ulcer disease, gastric cancer, and gastritis: this is a diagnosis of exclusion. Treatment consists of symptomatic therapy with **H2 blockers, liquid antacids,** or **PPIs.** *Helicobacter* is sometimes treated in refractory disease.

Peptic Ulcer Disease

Peptic ulcer disease can be either **duodenal ulcer (DU) or gastric ulcer (GU) disease.** After ***Helicobacter,*** the most common causes of ulcers are NSAIDs, head trauma, burns, intubation, Crohn's disease, and Zollinger-Ellison syndrome. Gastric cancer occurs in 4 percent of those with GU.

There is *no* way to distinguish DU and GU by symptoms alone. The alteration of pain with food is only suggestive, not definitive. Food more often makes GU pain worse and DU pain better. However, if the patient is **above 45 and has epigastric pain,** you *must* **scope** to exclude gastric cancer.

Gastritis

Gastritis can be associated with ***Helicobacter pylori.*** If it is present, treat with a **PPI and 2 antibiotics.**

Gastritis can also be **atrophic,** caused by **pernicious anemia** and associated with **vitamin B12 deficiency.** This type of gastritis will *not* improve with treatment for *H. pylori.*

Diagnostic Testing

- Most accurate test: **Endoscopy with biopsy.** If this is done, no further testing is necessary for *Helicobacter.*
- **Serology: Very sensitive but not specific.** If the serology is negative, this excludes *Helicobacter.* A positive test *cannot* distinguish between new and previous infection.
- **Breath testing and stool antigen testing:** These are *not* standard or routinely used. They can, however, distinguish between new and old disease.

Treatment

Treat with **PPI** and **clarithromycin and amoxicillin.** *Only* treat *Helicobacter* if it is associated with gastritis or ulcer disease.

If treatment for *H. pylori* fails, proceed as follows:

1. Repeat treatment with **2 new antibiotics and a PPI.** Try **metronidazole and tetracycline** instead of clarithromycin and amoxicillin.
2. If repeat treatment fails, then **evaluate for Zollinger-Ellison syndrome** (gastrinoma).

Stress Ulcer Prophylaxis

Routine prophylactic use of a PPI or H2 blocker or sucralfate should *only* be used if one of the following is present:

- Head trauma
- Intubation and mechanical ventilation
- Burns
- Coagulopathy and steroid use in combination

NSAID or steroid use alone is *not* an indication for routine stress ulcer prophylaxis.

A 52-year-old man has epigastric discomfort. He is seropositive for *Helicobacter pylori.* Upper endoscopy reveals no gastritis and no ulcer disease. Biopsy of the stomach shows *Helicobacter.* What should you do?

a. Breath testing
b. PPI alone as symptomatic therapy
c. Repeat endoscopy after 6 weeks of PPIs
d. PPI, amoxicillin, and clarithromycin

Answer: **B.** You do not need to treat *Helicobacter pylori* unless there is gastritis or ulcer disease. This patient has epigastric pain and *Helicobacter* but no ulcer or gastritis. This is **non-ulcer dyspepsia.** Treat it symptomatically with a PPI. Enormous numbers of people are colonized with *H. pylori;* you do not need to eradicate it from the world without evidence of disease. *H. pylori* is not the cause of non-ulcer dyspepsia.

A man is found to have ulcer disease. There are 3 ulcers in the distal esophagus 1–2 cm in size. The ulcers persist despite treatment for *Helicobacter.* What should you do next?

a. Switch antibiotics
b. Breath testing
c. Gastrin level and gastric acid output
d. CT scan of the abdomen
e. ERCP

Answer: **C.** Gastrin level and gastric acid output testing should be done when there is the possibility of **Zollinger-Ellison syndrome.** ERCP will only show the ducts of the pancreas and gallbladder; it will not reveal gastrinoma.

Remember: *Everyone* on an H2 blocker or PPI has an elevated gastrin level.

Most ulcers have the following characteristics:
- Single
- < 1 cm
- Proximal near the pylorus
- Easily resolve with treatment

Zollinger-Ellison Syndrome (ZES) or Gastrinoma

ZES is diagnosed through a finding of **elevated gastrin level and elevated gastric acid output.**

Test the gastrin level and gastric acid output when the following present:

- Large ulcer (> 1 cm)
- Multiple ulcers
- Distal location near the ligament of Treitz
- Recurrent or persistent despite *Helicobacter* treatment

If the gastrin level and acid output are both elevated, the next step is to localize the gastrinoma.

Diagnostic Testing

Following are the most accurate tests of ZES:

- **Endoscopic ultrasound:** An endoscopic ultrasound is like a transesophageal echocardiogram. It is much more sensitive than a surface ultrasound.
- **Nuclear somatostatin scan:** The nuclear somatostatin scan is very sensitive, because patients with ZES have an enormous increase in the number of somatostatin receptors.
- **Secretin suppression** is the most accurate test of ZES.

What is the normal effect of infusing secretin intravenously?

- **Normal people decrease gastrin levels and acid output.**
- **Patients with ZES show no change or an increase in gastrin levels and no decrease in acid levels.**

The Effect of Infusing IV Secretin		
	Normal	**Zollinger-Ellison**
Gastrin secretion	Decreases	No change
Gastric acid output	Decreases	No change

Treatment

- **Local disease:** Surgical resection
- **Metastatic disease:** Lifelong PPIs

Hypercalcemia is the clue to the presence of a parathyroid problem with ZES and, therefore, is the clue to a **multiple endocrine neoplasia (MEN) syndrome**.

Inflammatory Bowel Disease (IBD)

Both **Crohn's disease (CD) and ulcerative colitis (UC)** can present with **fever, abdominal pain, diarrhea, blood in the stool, and weight loss.** UC most often presents with abdominal pain and bloody diarrhea.

The **extraintestinal manifestations of IBD** are as follows:

- Joint pain
- Eye findings (iritis, uveitis)
- Skin findings (pyoderma gangrenosum, erythema nodosum)
- Sclerosing cholangitis

Features more common to **Crohn's disease** are the following:

- Masses
- Skip lesion
- Involvement of the upper GI tract
- Perianal disease
- Transmural granulomas
- Fistulae
- Hypocalcemia from fat malabsorption
- Obstruction
- Calcium oxalate kidney stones
- Cholesterol gallstones
- Vitamin B12 malabsorption from terminal ileum involvement

Both Crohn's disease (CD) that involves the colon and ulceratative colitis (UC) can lead to **colon cancer. Screening colonoscopy** should be performed every 1–2 years after 8–10 years of colonic involvement.

Diagnostic Testing

Endoscopy is diagnostic in both CD and UC. **Barium studies** are also diagnostic in both. When the diagnosis is *not* clear from endoscopy or barium studies, **blood tests** are helpful.

Crohn's Disease

- Antisaccharomyces cerevisiae (ASCA): **Positive**
- Antineutrophil cytoplasmic antibody (ANCA): **Negative**

Ulcerative Colitis

- ASCA: **Negative**
- ANCA: **Positive**

	CD	UC
ASCA	Positive	Negative
ANCA	Negative	Positive

Treatment

Treatment for inflammatory bowel disease is as follows:

- Best initial therapy for *both* CD and UC: **Mesalamine**
- Sulfasalazine is *not* the best initial therapy for either CD or UC because of the following adverse effects:
  - Rash
  - Hemolytic anemia
  - Interstitial nephritis
- **Steroids: Budesonide** is a glucocorticoid that can be used to control acute exacerbations of IBD. It has extensive first-pass effect in the liver and, therefore, has limited systemic adverse effects.
- **Azathioprine and 6-mercaptopurine:** These are used in patients with **severe disease** who have **recurrent symptoms when the steroids are stopped.** Azathioprine and 6MP are used to wean a patient off of steroids.
- **Infliximab:** This is a **TNF inhibitor** that is most useful in controlling CD that is associated with fistula formation. TNF is what maintains a granuloma in place. Plant a PPD and give isoniazid if the PPD is positive prior to the use of infliximab. Remember to **screen for tuberculosis;** infliximab can reactivate tuberculosis by releasing dormant TB from granulomas.
- **Metronidazole and ciprofloxacin:** These antibiotics are used for **perianal involvement in CD.**
- **Surgery:** This can be **curative in UC by removing the colon.** However, CD will recur at the site of the surgery. Occasionally, you must do surgery in CD, despite the risk of recurrence, *if* there is a stricture and obstruction.

Infliximab reactivates tuberculosis. Screen with a PPD prior to its use in fistulizing CD.

Diarrhea

Infectious Diarrhea

The most important feature of infectious diarrhea on presentation is the **presence of blood.** Blood means the presence of invasive bacterial pathogens, such as the following:

- **Campylobacter:** This is the most common cause of food poisoning. It can be associated with Guillain-Barre syndrome and reactive arthritis.
- **Salmonella:** This is transmitted by chickens and eggs.
- ***Vibrio parahaemolyticus:*** This is associated with seafood.
- **E. coli:** This can have several variants, some of which are associated with blood.
  - ***E. coli*** **0157:H7** is most commonly associated with **hemolytic uremic syndrome** (via effects of verotoxin). Look for undercooked beef in the history. Do not give platelet transfusions or antibiotics, which can make it worse.
- ***Vibrio vulnificus:*** Look for shellfish (oysters, clams) in a person with liver disease and skin lesions.
- ***Shigella:*** Secretes Shiga toxin. This bacteria is also associated with reactive arthritis.
- ***Yersinia:*** Rodents (rarely other mammals) are the natural reservoir of this bacteria. Transmission is via vegetables, milk-derived products, and meat (case may describe pork) that is contaminated with infected urine or feces.
- **Amebic:** Perform 3-stool ova and parasite examinations or serologic testing. Treat with metronidazole. May be associated with liver abscesses.

If blood is not described in the case, **fecal leukocytes** should be tested. Fecal leukocytes tell you that an invasive pathogen is present and indicate the same diseases described above that are associated with the presence of blood.

Diagnostic Testing

- Best initial test: **Fecal leukocytes**
- Most accurate test: **Stool culture**

Treatment

- **Mild disease:** This will resolve on its own, and the patient should be hydrated only.
- **Severe disease: Fluoroquinolones,** such as **ciprofloxacin,** are the best initial therapy. Severe disease is defined as the presence of the following:
  - Blood
  - Fever
  - Abdominal pain
  - Hypotension and tachycardia

Nonbloody Diarrhea

All of the pathogens described above **can present without blood as well as with blood.** The presence of blood does *exclude* the following pathogens, which *never* result in blood:

- **Viruses:** Rotavirus, norovirus (also called "Norwalk virus")
- **Giardia:** Look for camping/hiking and men who have sex with men. Stool ELISA antigen is > 90 percent sensitive and specific and is more accurate than 3-stool ova and parasite exams. Look for bloating, flatus, and signs of steatorrhea. Treat with metronidazole or tinidazole.
- ***Staphylococcus aureus:*** Presents with vomiting in addition to diarrhea. It will resolve spontaneously.
- ***Bacillus cereus:*** Associated with refried Chinese rice and vomiting. It resolves spontaneously.
- **Cryptosporidiosis:** Look for an HIV-positive patient with < 100 CD4 cells. Diagnose with a modified acid-fast stain. Use antiretroviral medications to raise the CD4 count. Paromomycin is only partially effective. Nitazoxanide is used effectively.
- **Scombroid:** This is histamine fish poisoning. This has the fastest onset of diarrhea; within 10 minutes of eating an infected tuna, mackerel, or mahi-mahi, the patient has vomiting, diarrhea, wheezing, and flushing. Treat with antihistamines, such as **diphenhydramine.**

PPIs increase the risk of *C. diff* in hospitalized patients.

Antibiotic-Associated Diarrhea/*Clostridium difficile (C. diff)*

This develops several days to weeks after the use of antibiotics. Although **clindamycin** is the most common cause, antibiotic-associated diarrhea can be caused by **any antibiotic.** Recently **fluoroquinolones** have also come to be associated with *Clostridium difficile.* There can be both blood and fecal leukocytes with *C. difficile* colitis.

Diagnostic Testing

- Best initial test: **Stool toxin assay**

Treatment

When treating antibiotic-associated diarrhea, *only* use oral vancomycin if metronidazole fails or in severe cases.

- Best initial therapy: **Metronidazole**
- **Oral vancomycin** is used if there is no response to metronidazole and with severe disease. (IV vancomycin is *not* useful.)
- If antibiotic-associated diarrhea resolves with metronidazole and then recurs later, the patient should be **retreated with metronidazole,** not treated with vancomycin.
- Fidaxomicin is an alternative to vancomycin in severe, recurrent cases. Fidaxomicin does not have more efficacy than metronidazole on the first episode.

Chronic Diarrhea

Lactose Intolerance

This is probably the most common cause of chronic diarrhea and flatulence.

Diagnose and treat by **removing all milk and milk-related products** from the diet *except* yogurt. A lactose-intolerance test may also be performed.

Carcinoid Syndrome

This is associated with **flushing and episodes of hypotension.**

Diagnose with a **urinary 5-HIAA level.** Treat with the somatostatin analog **octreotide.**

Inflammatory Bowel Disease

Look for blood, fever, and weight loss. (This is discussed in more detail earlier in this chapter.)

Malabsorption

This type of chronic diarrhea is always associated with **weight loss. Fat malabsorption** is associated with **steatorrhea,** which leads to **oily, greasy stools** that float on the water in the toilet. There is a particularly **foul smell to the stool.**

The causes of fat malabsorption are as follows:

- **Celiac disease** (gluten sensitive enteropathy), or **nontropical sprue**
- **Tropical sprue**
- **Chronic pancreatitis**
- **Whipple disease**

All forms of fat malabsorption are associated with the following:

- **Hypocalcemia** from vitamin D deficiency, which may lead to osteoporosis
- **Oxalate overabsorption and oxalate kidney stones**
- **Easy bruising and elevated prothrombin time/INR** from vitamin K malabsorption
- **Vitamin B12 malabsorption** from either destruction of the terminal ileum or loss of the pancreatic enzymes that are necessary for B12 absorption

Diagnostic Testing

- Best initial test: **Sudan black stain of stool** to test for the presence of fat.
- Most sensitive test: **72-hour fecal fat**

Celiac Disease (Gluten-Sensitive Enteropathy)

Celiac disease can also present with **malabsorption of iron** and **microcytic anemia.** This does *not* happen with pancreatic insufficiency, since pancreatic enzymes are not necessary for iron absorption. **Folate malabsorption** also occurs from destruction of villi. Celiac disease is associated with a vesicular skin lesion not present on mucosal surfaces. This is called **dermatitis herpetiformis.**

Diagnostic Testing

- Best initial test: **Antigliadin, antiendomysial, and antitissue transglutaminase antibodies**
- Most accurate test: **Small bowel biopsy**
- **D-xylose testing** is abnormal in celiac disease, Whipple disease, and tropical sprue, because the villous lining is destroyed and D-xylose cannot be absorbed. However, this test is *rarely necessary,* because the specific antibody tests eliminate the need for it.
- **Bowel biopsy** is always necessary for celiac disease, even if the diagnosis is confirmed with antibody testing, to exclude bowel wall lymphoma.

Treatment

Eliminate wheat, oats, rye, and barley from the diet. It may take several weeks for symptoms to resolve. Beer, whiskey, and most vodkas are derived from wheat. Wine is okay.

Tropical Sprue

This presents in the **same way as celiac disease.** There will be a history of the patient being in the **tropics.** The serologic tests, such as antitissue transglutaminase, will be negative.

The most accurate test is a **small bowel biopsy showing microorganisms.** Treatment consists of **doxycycline** or **trimethoprim/sulfamethoxazole** (TMP/SMX) for 3–6 months.

Whipple Disease

Whipple disease has several additional findings on presentation, such as the following:

- **Arthralgia**
- **Neurological abnormalities**
- **Ocular findings**

Diagnostic Testing

- Most accurate test: **Small bowel biopsy showing PAS positive organisms**
- An alternate test is **PCR of the stool** for *Tropheryma whippelii.*

Treatment

Treat with **tetracycline** or **trimethoprim/sulfamethoxazole** (TMP/SMX) for 12 months.

Chronic Pancreatitis

Look for a **history of alcoholism** and **multiple episodes of pancreatitis.** The amylase and lipase levels will most likely be normal, since the fat malabsorption does not develop until the pancreas is burnt out and largely replaced by calcium and fibrosis. Malabsorption of fat-soluble vitamins, such as vitamin K and vitamin D, is less common than with celiac disease.

Diagnostic Testing

- Best initial tests:
  - **Abdominal x-ray** is 50–60 percent sensitive for the detection of **pancreatic calcifications.**
  - **Abdominal CT scan** (without contrast) is 60–80 percent sensitive.
- Most accurate test: **Secretin stimulation testing.**

> **Basic Science Correlate**
>
> A normal person should release a large volume of bicarbonate-rich pancreatic fluid in response to the intravenous injection of secretin.

- Iron and folate levels will be normal, since pancreatic enzymes are not necessary to absorb these. D-xylose testing will be normal. B12 levels can be low.

Treatment

Replace the pancreatic enzymes chronically by mouth. Amylase, lipase, and trypsin can be combined in one pill for chronic use.

Irritable Bowel Syndrome

Irritable bowel syndrome is a **pain syndrome with altered bowel habits.** This condition presents with the following symptoms:

- Abdominal pain relieved by a bowel movement
- Abdominal pain that is less at night
- Abdominal pain with diarrhea alternating with constipation

> Irritable bowel syndrome presents with pain. There is *no* fever, *no* weight loss, and *no* blood in the stool.

Diagnostic Testing

All the diagnostic tests will be normal. On CCS, you should order the following:

- **Stool guaiac, stool white cells, culture, ova, and parasite exam**
- **Colonoscopy**
- **Abdominal CT scan**

Treatment

- Best initial therapy: **Fiber.** Bulking up the stool helps relieve the pain. Fiber gives the guts a stretch, like sending the colon to yoga class!
- If there is no relief of pain with fiber, then you should add **antispasmodic/anticholinergic agents,** such as **dicyclomine** or **hyoscyamine,** which "relax" the bowel.
- If there is no response to the antispasmodic/anticholinergic agents, you should add a **tricyclic antidepressant,** such as **amitriptyline.**

Basic Science Correlate

Tricyclic antidepressants help IBS because they are anticholinergic; relieve neuropathic pain; and are antidepressant.

Colon Cancer

- Hamartomas and hyperplastic polyps: Benign
- Dysplastic polyps: Malignant

The most important thing for you to know about colon cancer, by far, is what **screening** to perform.

Diagnostic Testing

General Population

- Begin screening at **age 50.**
- Screen with the following:
  - **Colonoscopy every 10 years**
  - **Fecal occult blood testing yearly**
  - **Barium enema**

What is the best method of screening for colon cancer?

Answer: **Colonoscopy every 10 years** is the best method by far. All other methods are less accurate.

When is a "virtual colonoscopy" by CT scan the answer?

Answer: This is the answer when you are asked what colon cancer screening test NOT to do. It lacks both sensitivity and specificity, because you cannot biopsy and it misses small lesions.

One Family Member with Colon Cancer

- Colonoscopy starting at **age 40 or 10 years before the age of the family member** who had cancer

Three Family Members, Two Generations, One Premature (< 50)

- Colonoscopy every **1–2 years starting at age 25.** This is a "Lynch syndrome," or hereditary nonpolyposis colon cancer syndrome.

Familial Adenomatous Polyposis (FAP)

- Start screening sigmoidoscopies at age 12.
- Perform a colectomy once polyps are found.

On routine x-ray, a man is found to have several osteomas. What do you recommend?

Answer: Perform a **colonoscopy** to screen for cancer. This is **Gardner's syndrome.**

Gardner's Syndrome

This presents with **benign bone tumors known as osteomas,** as well as other soft tissue tumors.

Peutz-Jeghers Syndrome

This presents with **melanotic spots on the lips.** There are **hamartomatous polyps** throughout the small bowel and colon. The lifetime risk of colon cancer is about 10 percent, only slightly higher than the 6–8 percent risk of colon cancer in the general population. There is *no* extra screening recommended.

Juvenile Polyposis

There are multiple extra hamartomas in the bowel. Hamartomas do not bring a significant increase in the risk of colon cancer. There is *no* extra screening recommended. This is markedly different from FAP.

Dysplastic Polyp Found

Repeat colonoscopy **3–5 years after the polyp was found.**

Carcinoembryonic antigen (CEA) is *never* a screening test. CEA is used to follow response to therapy.

The following table summarizes the recommendations for colon cancer screening:

General Population	Single Family Member with Colon Cancer	Three Family Members, Two Generations, One < 50	Familial Adenomatous Polyposis	Gardner's, Peutz-Jeghers, Juvenile Polyposis, Turcot's Syndrome
Start screening at age 50. Colonoscopy every 10 years.	Start screening at age 40 or 10 years earlier than the age at which the family member contracted cancer.	Colonoscopy every 1–2 years starting at age 25.	Sigmoidoscopy every 1–2 years starting at age 12.	No extra screening recommendations.

Diverticular Disease

Diverticulosis and Diverticulitis

Diverticulosis

Diverticulosis is incredibly common in older Americans due to a low-fiber, high-fat, hamburger-filled, low-residue diet. They often present as follows:

- Left lower quadrant (LLQ) abdominal pain
- Lower GI bleeding

Diagnostic Testing

- Most accurate test: **Barium enema** is more accurate test than colonoscopy

Treatment

Treat with a high-fiber diet.

Diverticulitis

Colonoscopy and barium enema are *contraindicated* in diverticulitis because of an increased risk of perforation.

Diverticulitis is a complication of diverticulosis. It presents as:

- Left lower quadrant (LLQ) abdominal pain
- Tenderness
- Fever
- Elevated white cell count in blood

Diagnostic Testing

- Best diagnostic test: **Abdominal and pelvic CT scan**

Treatment

Antibiotics are the mainstay of treatment for diverticulitis. Combine agents against **gram-negative bacilli,** such as a quinolone or cephalosporin, with an agent against **anaerobes,** such as metronidazole. **Ciprofloxacin and metronidazole** are a standard combination.

LLQ Pain + Tenderness + Fever + Leukocytosis = Diverticu*litis*

Gastrointestinal (GI) Bleeding

GI bleeding presents in various ways:

- **Red blood:** Usually indicates **lower GI bleeding.** In about 10 percent of cases, extremely brisk/rapid or high-volume upper GI bleeding leads to red blood from the rectum.
- **Black stool:** Indicates **upper GI bleeding,** which is usually defined as that occurring proximal to the ligament of Treitz (demarcation between the duodenum and the jejunum). Black stool usually results from at least 100 mL of blood loss.
- **Heme-positive brown stool:** This can occur from as little as 5–10 mL of blood loss.
- **Coffee ground emesis:** Needs very little gastric, esophageal, or duodenal blood loss—as little a 5–10 mL.

A 74-year-old man with a history of aortic stenosis comes to the emergency department having had 5 red/black bowel movements over the last day. His pulse is 112, blood pressure 96/64. What is the next best step in management?

a. Colonoscopy
b. Consult gastroenterology
c. CBC
d. Bolus of normal saline
e. Transfer to the intensive care unit

Answer: **D.** The most urgent step in severe gastrointestinal (GI) bleeding is **fluid resuscitation.** When the systolic blood pressure is low or the pulse high, there has been at least a 30 percent volume loss. Step 3 does not allow you to order specific doses; hence, all you can order is a "bolus." It is fortunate that you do not have to spend a lot of time calculating or memorizing specific doses of fluids or specific medications. Although endoscopy, such as colonoscopy, is important, it is not as important as fluid resuscitation.

The *most* important thing to do in acute GI bleeding is to determine if there is **hemodynamic instability.** Orthostatic hypotension means a drop in blood pressure or rise in pulse when going from a lying to a standing or seated position. **Orthostasis** is defined as a drop in systolic pressure of > 20 mm Hg or a rise in pulse of > 10 beats per minute.

Orthostasis presents with one of the following:
- Systolic blood pressure < 100
- Heart rate > 100

Either of these implies more than 30% volume loss.

CCS Tip: On CCS with large-volume GI bleeding, order the following:

- Bolus of normal saline or Ringer's lactate
- CBC
- Prothrombin time/INR
- Type and cross
- Consultation with gastroenterology
- EKG

As you move the clock forward on CCS, the results of all tests will automatically pop up. You do not have to do anything for them to come. Test results on CCS are like your phone bill: you do not have to do anything for your bills to arrive; they automatically show up as time passes.

Test	Route of Administration	Time Ordered	Report Available
CBC	Applies to medications ordered	09:00	09:15

When do I transfuse packed red blood cells?

Answer:
- Hematocrit < 30 in an older person
- Hematocrit < 20–25 in younger patients with no heart disease

When do I transfuse fresh frozen plasma?

Answer: When there is elevated prothrombin time/INR and vitamin K is too slow.

When do I transfuse platelets?

Answer: If the patient is bleeding or to undergo surgery, transfuse platelets when they are < 50,000.

What is the most common cause of death in GI bleeding?

Answer: **Myocardial ischemia.** That is why you should get an EKG in older patients with severe GI bleeding. The myocytes of the left ventricle cannot distinguish between ischemia, anemia, carbon monoxide poisoning, and coronary artery stenosis. All of these lead to myocardial infarction.

When is "nasogastric tube" the answer?

Answer: Place a nasogastric (NG) tube in the occasional patient when you are unsure whether bleeding is from an upper or lower gastrointestinal source. The nasogastric tube has no therapeutic benefit; it will not stop bleeding. Iced saline lavage is worthless and is always wrong.

Why not use the NG tube to identify all bleeding?

Answer: If the NG tube shows bile, then you can be sure that the pyloric sphincter is open and that there is no blood in the duodenum. But if the pyloric sphincter is closed, no blood will be detectable in the NG tube even if it is present in the duodenum. Also, if you are going to scope the patient anyway, it does not matter what the NG tube shows.

Treatment

Gastrointestinal bleeding of large volume is managed first with **fluid resuscitation.** The most important measures of severity are the **pulse and blood pressure.** If the pulse is elevated or the blood pressure is decreased, you can always give more fluid. If you must give so much fluid to maintain blood pressure that the patient becomes **hypoxic,** then give the fluid and increase **oxygenation,** even if it means intubating the patient. **Hypotension** supersedes all other therapeutic priorities. Fluid resuscitation is *more important* than determining the specific etiology of the source of bleeding.

Correcting anemia, thrombocytopenia, or coagulopathy is *more* important than **endoscopy.** If the platelets are low, then giving platelets is *more* important than consulting gastroenterology or moving the patient to the ICU. Note that 80 percent of GI bleeding stops with adequate fluid resuscitation even *without* endoscopy. If you scope the patient but do *not* correct anemia, thrombocytopenia, or elevated prothrombin time/INR, the bleeding will *not* stop.

> Fluid resuscitation beats scoping!

Ulcer Disease

Add a **proton pump inhibitor** to the initial resuscitation of fluids, blood, platelets, and plasma. Note, however, that unnecessary stress ulcer prophylaxis with PPIs increases the risk of pneumonia and *Clostridium difficile* colitis.

Variceal Bleeding

Look for an **alcoholic with hematemesis and/or liver disease (cirrhosis).** The other clues to the presence of esophageal varices are the presence of **splenomegaly, low platelets,** and **spider angiomata** or **gynecomastia.**

Treatment

Treat variceal bleeding as follows:

- Add **octreotide** to the initial orders. This is a somatostatin analog and it decreases portal hypertension.
- **Upper endoscopy** should be performed promptly to do banding of the varices.
- If the bleeding persists with moving the clock forward, a **transjugular intrahepatic portosystemic shunt (TIPS)** procedure should be performed. This is using a catheter to place a shunt between the portal vein and hepatic vein. This essentially replaces the need for surgical shunt placement. The most common complication of a TIPS procedure is **hepatic encephalopathy.**

> Propranolol prevents future episodes of variceal bleeding.

- **Blakemore gastric tamponade balloon:** This procedure will *temporarily* stop bleeding from varices. It is rarely performed and is only a temporary measure to stop bleeding to allow a shunt to be placed.

Sources of Bleeding

Bleeding in the **upper GI** can have the following causes:

- **Ulcer disease**
- **Esophagitis, gastritis, duodenitis**
- **Varices**
- **Cancer**

Bleeding in the **lower GI** can have the following causes:

- **Angiodysplasia**
- **Diverticular disease**
- **Polyps**
- **Ischemic colitis**
- **Inflammatory bowel disease**
- **Cancer**

Diagnostic Testing

- **Technetium bleeding scan ("tagged red cell scan"):** This test is performed to detect the site of bleeding *if* endoscopy does not reveal the source. It will let you know the location but *not* the exact cause.
- **Angiography:** This test tells you the **precise vessel that is bleeding.** It can be done preoperatively in massive GI bleeding to let you know which part of the colon to resect.
- **Capsule endoscopy:** Swallowing a capsule with a camera in it can detect the **location of GI bleeding from the small bowel,** *if* upper and lower endoscopy do not reveal the answer. It gives an enormous quantity of pictures but does *not* allow a biopsy or therapeutic intervention such as you can do with endoscopy.

Acute Mesenteric Ischemia

This is an **embolus from the heart** resulting in an **infarction of the bowel.** There is a **sudden onset of extremely severe abdominal pain** and possible bleeding as well. Physical examination shows a relatively benign abdomen. Look for an **older patient** with a history of **valvular heart disease** and the very sudden onset of pain.

Diagnostic Testing

Look for **metabolic acidosis (elevated lactic acid)** on blood testing and an **elevated amylase level.** The most accurate test is **angiography.**

Treatment

If the bowel is dead, treatment is **surgical resection of the bowel.** Very ill patients should go *straight* to the operating room for surgical resection. **This is a surgical emergency.** If left undetected and untreated, the patient will die quickly. In ischemia that is not caused by emboli, treat the underlying low flow state.

> Abdominal pain out of proportion to physical exam = Mesenteric ischemia

Constipation

The vast majority of cases have **no clear etiology.** Although Step 3 seldom asks specifically for the diagnosis, the management of constipation involves correcting the underlying cause. Therefore, knowing the etiology is the key to determining the treatment. Following are possible causes of constipation:

- **Dehydration:** Look for decreased skin turgor in an elderly patient with an increased BUN-to-creatinine ratio (> 20:1).
- **Calcium channel blockers**
- **Narcotic medication use**
- **Hypothyroidism**
- **Diabetes:** Loss of sensation in the bowels leads to decreased detection of stretch in the bowel, which is one of the main stimulants of GI motility.
- **Ferrous sulfate iron replacement:** The stool is **black** and can look as though there is upper GI bleeding. Blood is cathartic and will usually produce **rapid bowel movement.** Ferrous sulfate is constipating and is also heme-negative when one tests for occult blood.
- **Anticholinergic medication:** This includes tricyclic antidepressants.

Treatment with **hydration and increased fiber** is always a good option. You may consider prescribing a bowel regimen with Senokot and docusate.

Dumping Syndrome

Dumping syndrome is a relatively rare disorder related to **prior gastric surgery,** usually done for ulcer disease. Treatment and eradication of *Helicobacter pylori* has made surgery for ulcer disease rare.

The patient presents with **shaking, sweating, and weakness.**

> **Basic Science Correlate**
>
> Dumping syndrome may involve hypotension. There are 2 causes. One is the rapid release of the gastric contents into the duodenum, which causes an osmotic draw into the bowel. The other is a rapid rise in blood glucose resulting in a reactive hypoglycemia.

Dumping syndrome is managed with **frequent small meals.**

Diabetic Gastroparesis

Longstanding diabetes impairs the neural supply of the bowel. There is impairment of normal motility. Patients present with **bloating and constipation as well as diarrhea.**

> **Basic Science Correlate**
>
> **Mechanism of Gastroparesis**
>
> The main stimulant to gastric motility is distension. Diabetes damages sensory nerves of all kinds, including those in the bowel. Vascular damage to the nerves of the digestive tract impairs a person's ability to detect stretching or distention of the stomach. With longstanding diabetes, the result is bloating and constipation.

Treat with **erythromycin** or **metoclopramide.** Erythromycin increases motilin in the gut, a hormone that stimulates gastric motility.

Acute Pancreatitis

This condition presents as **severe midepigastric abdominal pain and tenderness** in an **alcoholic** or someone with **gallstones.** Other causes are the following:

- Hypertriglyceridemia
- Trauma
- Infection
- ERCP
- Medications such as thiazides, didanosine, stavudine, or azathioprine

Other symptoms include:

- Vomiting without blood
- Anorexia
- Tenderness in the epigastric area

Severe cases involve these symptoms:

- Hypotension
- Metabolic acidosis
- Leukocytosis
- Hemoconcentration
- Hyperglycemia
- Hypocalcemia caused by fat malabsorption
- Hypoxia

Diagnostic Testing

- Best initial test: **Amylase and lipase** (Lipase has higher specificity.)
- Most accurate test: **Abdominal CT scan.** A CT scan can detect dilated common bile ducts and even comment on intrahepatic ducts.
- **Magnetic resonance cholangiopancreatography (MRCP)** detects causes of biliary and pancreatic duct obstruction not found on a CT scan.
- If there is dilation of the common bile duct *without* a pancreatic head mass, consider **endoscopic retrograde cholangiopancreatography (ERCP).** The ERCP can be used to detect the presence of stones or strictures in the pancreatic duct system. ERCP can also remove stones and dilate strictures. ERCP is predominantly a therapeutic tool.
- **Trypsinogen activation peptide:** This is a **urinary test** that can be used to determine the severity of pancreatitis. Pancreatitis seems to arise from the **premature activation of trypsinogen** while it is still within the pancreas instead of when it reaches the duodenum. Hence, the trypsin starts to digest and inflame the pancreas.

Treatment

Therapy consists of the following:

- No feeding (bowel rest)
- Hydration
- Pain medications

We do *not* have a medication to reverse pancreatitis.

Acute Pancreatitis
- Diagnose with ultrasound, CT, and MRCP.
- Treat with ERCP.

Necrotic Pancreatitis

Diagnostic Testing

In the past, Ranson's criteria were the major method of determining the severity of pancreatitis. **Ranson's criteria** are operative criteria to see **who needs pancreatic debridement.** The **CT scan** effectively replaces Ranson's criteria as the most precise method of determining severity.

Treatment

When the **CT shows > 30 percent necrosis** of the pancreas, the patient should

- receive antibiotics such as imipenem; and
- undergo CT-guided biopsy.

If the biopsy shows **infected, necrotic pancreatitis,** the patient should have **surgical debridement** of the pancreas.

Hepatitis

Patients with **acute hepatitis** will all present is a very similar way. You *cannot* accurately determine the etiology of acute hepatitis from history and presentation alone. All patients present with:

- Hepatitis B is associated with polyarteritis nodosa (PAN) in 30 percent of cases.
- Hepatitis C is associated with cryoglobulinemia.

- **Jaundice**
- **Fatigue**
- **Weight loss**
- **Dark urine caused by bilirubin in the urine**

Hepatitis B and C are more likely to present with **serum sickness-phenomena** like joint pain, urticaria, and fever.

Hepatitis E is most severe in pregnant women. It can be fatal.

Diagnostic Testing

All patients with acute hepatitis will give an **elevated conjugated (direct) bilirubin.** This will lead to bilirubin in the urine or urobilinogen. Uncon-jugated bilirubin, such as that associated with hemolysis, is not water soluble and will not pass into the urine. Unconjugated bilirubin is attached to albumin.

- Vira**l**: ↑ **AL**T
- Drug**s**: ↑ A**S**T

- **Viral hepatitis** gives an **elevated ALT level.**
- **Drug-induced hepatitis** is associated with an **increased AST.**

Most accurate tests:

- For **hepatitis A, C, D, and E,** the confirmatory test is **serology.** IgM levels acutely rise, and IgG levels rise in the recovery phase.
- **Surface antigen, core antibody, e-antigen, or surface antibodies** are not present in hepatitis A, C, D, or E. These tests are associated with **hepatitis B.**

Acute Hepatitis B

The *first* test to become abnormal in acute hepatitis B infection is the **surface antigen.** Elevation in ALT, e-antigen, and symptoms all occur *after* the appearance of hepatitis B surface antigen. The following table shows the appearance of the antigens and antibodies through the course of the disease:

	Surface Antigen	e-Antigen	Core Antibody	Surface Antibody
Acute disease (hepatitis B)	+ +	+ +	+ +	–
Window period (recovering)	–	–	+ +	–
Vaccinated	–	–	–	+ +
Healed/recovered	–	–	+ +	+ +

Chronic hepatitis B gives the same serologic pattern as acute hepatitis B, but it is based on **persistence of the surface antigen beyond 6 months.**

	Surface Antigen	e-Antigen	Core Antibody	Surface Antibody
Acute hepatitis B	+	+	+	–
Chronic hepatitis B	+	+	+	–
Resolved infection	–	–	+	+
Window period	–	–	+	–

These 3 tests are essentially *equal* in meaning. They all indicate **active viral replication:**

Hepatitis B DNA polymerase = e-Antigen = Hepatitis B PCR for DNA

No treatment is available for acute hepatitis B.

> The only acute hepatitis that can be treated is acute hepatitis C.

Acute Hepatitis C

- Best initial test: **Hepatitis C antibody.** This test *cannot,* however, tell the level of activity of the virus.
- Most accurate tests:
  - **Hepatitis C PCR** for RNA is the most accurate method of determining the degree of viral replication and activity of the disease. PCR RNA is also the most accurate way of determining response to therapy.
  - **Liver biopsy** is the most accurate way of determining the seriousness of the disease. The patient can have 10 years of active viral replication with relatively little liver damage. Use the biopsy to determine extent of damage to the liver.

Genotype predicts the response of hepatitis C to treatment.

Acute hepatitis C is treated with interferon/ribavirin and an oral protease inhibitor, the same as chronic disease.

Chronic Hepatitis B

The patient with surface antigen, e-antigen, and DNA polymerase or PCR for DNA is the patient who is most likely to benefit from **antiviral therapy.** Look for > **6 months of positive serology.**

Chronic hepatitis B is treated with one of the following single agents:

- **Lamivudine**
- **Adefovir**
- **Entecavir**
- **Telbivudine**
- **Tenofovir**
- **Interferon:** Interferon has the most adverse effects:
  - Flulike symptoms
  - Arthralgia
  - Myalgia
  - Fatigue
  - Thrombocytopenia
  - Depression

Chronic Hepatitis C

> Sofosbuvir allows treatment without interferon for hepatitis C.

Genotype 1 is easily treated with ledipasvir combined with sofosbuvir for >95% cure. Simeprevir or boceprevir works for other genotypes. The most common adverse effect of ribavirin is **anemia.**

- Oral protease inhibitors such as **ledipasvir, simeprevir, or sofosbuvir** are added to ribavirin. The only form of acute hepatitis that receives antiviral therapy is acute hepatitis C.
- Chronic hepatitis C is the most common reason to need a liver transplantation in the United States.

Vaccination

Vaccination for both **hepatitis A and B** is now done universally in **childhood.**

For **adults,** the strongest indications for vaccination for both **hepatitis A and B** are the following:

- **Chronic liver disease.** Someone with cirrhosis or another cause of liver disease who develops hepatitis A or B is at *much* greater risk of fulminant hepatitis.
- **Household contacts** of those with hepatitis A or B
- **Men who have sex with men**
- **Chronic recipients of blood products**
- **Injection drug users**

Specific indications for vaccines are as follows:

- **Hepatitis A vaccine**
  - Travelers
- **Hepatitis B vaccine**
  - Health care workers
  - Patients on dialysis
  - Diabetes

> Add boceprevir, telaprevir, or simeprevir to hepatitis C treatment.

A health care worker gets stuck with a needle contaminated with blood from a person with chronic hepatitis B. The health care worker has never been vaccinated. What is the most appropriate action?

Answer: Give hepatitis B immune globulin and hepatitis B vaccine. The same recommendation would be made for a child born to a mother with chronic hepatitis B. If the person had already been vaccinated, then you would check for levels of protective surface antibody. If hepatitis B surface antibody were already present, then no further treatment would be necessary.

> There is *no* vaccine and *no* postexposure prophylaxis for **hepatitis C.**

Cirrhosis

No matter what the cause of the cirrhosis, it will have a number of features:

- **Edema from low oncotic pressure:** Treat with spironolactone and diuretics
- **Gynecomastia**
- **Palmar erythema**
- **Splenomegaly**

- **Thrombocytopenia caused by splenic sequestration**
- **Encephalopathy:** Treat with lactulose
- **Ascites:** Treat with spironolactone
- **Esophageal varices:** Propranolol will prevent bleeding. Perform banding of the varices if they bleed.

Basic Science Correlate

Mechanism of Propranolol

Propranolol is a nonspecific beta blocker. This agent decreases pulse pressure in the esophageal varices, which is thought to be the reason it decreases the risk of variceal bleeding. Propranolol has no effect during an acute episode of bleeding. This is why all patients with cirrhosis should undergo endoscopy. Prophylactic beta blockers are very useful.

Ascites

Perform a **paracentesis** for all patients with ascites if any of the following are present:

- **New ascites**
- **Pain, fever, or tenderness**

Diagnostic Testing

- If the SAAG is < **1.1**, then portal hypertension is *not* present.
- If the SAAG is > **1.1**, then portal hypertension *is* present.

Perform an ascitic fluid **albumin level.** If the ascites fluid albumin level is low, the difference between the ascites and the serum level of albumin will be very great. This is a **serum-to-ascites albumin gradient (SAAG).** If the **SAAG is > 1.1, portal hypertension from cirrhosis** or **congestive failure** is present.

Spontaneous bacterial peritonitis (SBP) is diagnosed with a **cell count > 250 neutrophils.**

Treatment

- Treat with **cefotaxime.**

Chronic Liver Disease (Causes of Cirrhosis)

Alcoholic Cirrhosis

This is a **diagnosis of exclusion.** Exclude all the other causes of cirrhosis and look for a history of **longstanding alcohol abuse.**

Treat **as described above for cirrhosis.**

Primary Biliary Cirrhosis (PBC)

PBC presents with a **middle-aged woman** complaining of **itching. Xanthelasmas** (cholesterol deposits) may be found on examination. Also look for a history of **other autoimmune disorders.**

Diagnostic Testing

- Best initial test: **Elevated alkaline phosphatase with a normal bilirubin level.** IgM level is elevated.
- Most accurate tests: **Antimitochondrial antibody (AMA), liver biopsy**

Treatment

- **Ursodeoxycholic acid**

Primary Sclerosis Cholangitis (PSC)

Inflammatory bowel disease (IBD) accounts for 80 percent of PSC. PSC also presents with **itching** but is much more likely to give an **elevated bilirubin level.** The **alkaline phosphatase level is elevated.**

Diagnostic Testing

- **Most accurate tests:**
  - **ERCP** shows "beading" of the biliary system
  - **Antismooth muscle antibody (ASMA)**
  - **ANCA** is positive

Treatment

- **Ursodeoxycholic acid**

Wilson's Disease

Wilson's disease involves cirrhosis and liver disease in a person with a **choreiform movement disorder** and **neuropsychiatric abnormalities.** This condition also presents with **hemolysis.**

Diagnostic Testing

- **Best initial test:** Slit lamp looking for **Kayser Fleischer rings** is more sensitive and specific than a **low ceruloplasmin level.** On CCS, order *both.*
- **Most accurate test:** Liver biopsy is more accurate than a urinary copper level.

Treatment

- **Penicillamine or trientine**

The most common cause of death from hemochromatosis is **cirrhosis.** Cardiac disease occurs in only 15 percent of cases.

Hemochromatosis

Most often, hemochromatosis is caused by a **genetic disorder** resulting in the overabsorption of iron. The iron deposits throughout the body, most commonly in the liver. Other manifestations include the following:

- **Restrictive cardiomyopathy**
- **Skin darkening**
- **Joint pain** caused by pseudogout or calcium pyrophosphate deposition disease
- **Damage to the pancreas** leading to diabetes, referred to as **"bronze diabetes"**
- **Pituitary accumulation** with panhypopituitarism
- **Infertility**
- **Hepatoma**

Diagnostic Testing

- Best initial test: **Elevated serum iron and ferritin levels with a low iron-binding capacity.** The iron saturation is enormously elevated (> 45 percent).
- Most accurate test: **Liver biopsy.** However, an **MRI** of the liver and the specific genetic test, the **HFe gene mutation,** in combination are sufficiently diagnostic to spare the patient a liver biopsy.

Treatment

- Phlebotomy

Autoimmune Hepatitis

Look for a **young woman with other autoimmune diseases,** such as Coombs positive hemolytic anemia, thyroiditis, and ITP.

Diagnostic Testing

- Best initial tests: **ANA and antismooth muscle antibody test. Serum protein electrophoresis (SPEP)** shows hypergammaglobulinemia. The patient may also have positive ANA and liver/kidney microsomal antibody.
- Most accurate test: **Liver biopsy**

Treatment

Treat with **prednisone.** Other immunosuppressive agents, such as azathioprine, may be needed if one is attempting to wean the patient off steroids.

Nonalcoholic Steatohepatitis (NASH)

NASH is strongly associated with **obesity, diabetes, and hyperlipidemia. Hepatomegaly** is often present.

Diagnostic Testing

- Best initial test: **ALT > AST**
- Most accurate test: **Liver biopsy showing fatty infiltration.** The liver biopsy looks just like alcoholic liver disease.

Treatment

No specific therapy exists to reverse NASH. **Control the underlying causes** with weight loss, diabetes control, and management of the hyperlipidemia.

Neurology

9

Stroke and TIA

Strokes and transient ischemic attacks (TIAs) present with the **sudden onset of weakness on one side of the body. Weakness of half of the face and aphasia are common as well.** Cases may state that there is a **partial or total loss of vision,** which may be transient. The cause is decreased or altered cerebral blood flow.

Stroke

Strokes are discriminated from TIA based on time. **Strokes last for ≥ 24 hours.** There will be **permanent residual neurologic deficits,** caused by **ischemia** or **hemorrhage:** 80 percent are ischemic in nature, and 20 percent are hemorrhagic. Ischemic strokes can be either from emboli or from a thrombosis. Emboli present with more sudden symptoms.

> Stroke spares the upper third of the face, from the eyes up.

Transient Ischemic Attack (TIA)

TIAs present exactly the same as a stroke, except that the **symptoms last < 24 hours and resolve completely.** Cases may present only with **transient loss of vision in one eye,** known as **amaurosis fugax.** This happens during a transient ischemic attack because the first branch of the internal carotid artery is the ophthalmic artery. TIAs are always caused by **emboli** or **thrombosis.** TIAs are *never* due to hemorrhage; hemorrhages do not resolve in 24 hours.

A 67-year-old man with a history of hypertension and diabetes comes to the emergency department with a sudden onset of weakness in the right arm and leg over the last hour. On exam, he cannot lift the bottom half of the right side of his face. What is the best initial step?

a. Head CT with contrast
b. Head CT without contrast
c. Aspirin
d. Thrombolytics
e. MRI

Answer: **B.** Prior to administering thrombolytics or any anticoagulation, you need to **rule out hemorrhagic stroke,** which is a contraindication to thrombolytics. You cannot even give aspirin without doing a head CT first. Thrombolytics are indicated within the first 3 hours of the onset of the symptoms of a stroke. Remember, 20 percent of strokes are hemorrhagic. You do not need contrast to visualize blood; contrast is used to detect cancer or infection, such as an abscess.

Arterial Lesions and Symptoms

Identifying or localizing a lesion based on characteristic symptoms likely will be important during the exam.

Cerebral Artery	Symptoms
Anterior cerebral artery	• Profound lower extremity weakness (contralateral in the case of unilateral arterial occlusion) • Mild upper extremity weakness (contralateral in the case of unilateral arterial occlusion) • Personality changes or psychiatric disturbance • Urinary incontinence
Middle cerebral artery	• Profound upper extremity weakness (contralateral in the case of unilateral arterial occlusion) • Aphasia • Apraxia/neglect • The eyes deviate *toward* the side of the lesion. • Contralateral homonymous hemianopsia, with macular sparing
Posterior cerebral artery	• Prosopagnosia (inability to recognize faces)
Vertebrobasilar artery	• Vertigo • Nausea and vomiting • May be described as a "drop attack," loss of consciousness • Vertical nystagmus • Dysarthria and dystonia • Sensory changes in face and scalp • Ataxia • Bilateral findings
Posterior inferior cerebellar artery	• Ipsilateral face • Contralateral body • Vertigo and Horner's syndrome
Lacunar infarct	• There must be an *absence* of cortical deficits. • Ataxia • Parkinsonian signs • Sensory deficits • Hemiparesis (most notable in the face) • Possible bulbar signs
Ophthalmic artery	• Amaurosis fugax

Diagnostic Testing

The best initial diagnostic test for either stroke or TIA is a **CT scan of the head without contrast.** Within the first several days, all **nonhemorrhagic strokes** should be associated with a **normal head CT scan.** MRI is *not* done, because the CT is more widely available, less expensive, and more sensitive for blood.

> Add statins to all nonhemorrhagic stroke.

- **Head CT:** Extremely sensitive for blood. Needs 3–5 days to achieve > 95 percent sensitivity in the detection of nonhemorrhagic stroke.
- **MRI:** Achieves 99 percent sensitivity for a nonhemorrhagic stroke within 24 hours.
- **Magnetic resonance angiogram (MRA):** Most accurately images the brain for stroke. Can be positive within the hour of the stroke.

Treatment

- **Thrombolytics:** These should be administered within **3 hours** of the onset of the symptoms of a stroke. *Always* get a head CT without contrast before anticoagulating in order to rule out a hemorrhagic stroke. You must know the contraindications to thrombolytic therapy as well. Following are the **absolute contraindications to thrombolytic therapy:**
  - History of hemorrhagic stroke
  - Presence of intracranial neoplasm/mass
  - Active bleeding or surgery within 6 weeks
  - Presence of bleeding disorder
  - CPR within 3 weeks that was traumatic (e.g., chest compressions)
  - Suspicion of aortic dissection
  - Stroke within 1 year
  - Cerebral trauma or brain surgery within 6 months

> Thrombolytic use between 3 and 4.5 hours after the onset of stroke symptoms is not yet the standard of care.

- **Anti-platelet medication:** Aspirin **or** clopidogrel **or** aspirin combined with dipyridamole is acceptable as initial antiplatelet medication to prevent a subsequent stroke. However, at the present time, aspirin first is still the standard of care.
- **Aspirin:** Best initial therapy for **those coming too late for thrombolytics.** Also indicated *after* the use of thrombolytics.
- **Clopidogrel:** *Switch* to clopidogrel if the patient has developed a stroke on aspirin.
- **Dipyridamole:** If the patient is *already* on aspirin when a new stroke or TIA occurs, *add* dipyridamole or switch to clopidogrel.
- **Statin:** Add for all nonhemorrhagic stroke.
- **Heparin:** There is no clear evidence of heparin's benefit for stroke.
- Ticlopidine is always a *wrong* answer. It has *no* added benefit to the use of clopidogrel and has more adverse effects, such as TTP and neutropenia.

> Less than 20 percent of patients with a stroke come in time to get thrombolytics (< 3 hours).

Use MRI/MRA for the brainstem.

Anterior stroke and middle cerebral artery stroke are managed the same way.

The younger the patient, the more likely the cause of the stroke is a vasculitis or hypercoagulable state.

Further Management

Stroke

After you have done the head CT and given thrombolytics or aspirin, you should move the clock forward on CCS. On subsequent screens, the most important issue is to **determine the origin** of the stroke to prevent another one.

The following are indicated in all patients with stroke or TIA:

- **Echocardiogram:** Anticoagulation for clots, possible **surgery** for valve vegetations
- **Carotid Dopplers/duplex: Endarterectomy** for stenosis > 70 percent, but *not* if it is 100 percent
- **EKG and a Holter monitor** if the EKG is normal: **Warfarin, dabigatran, or rivaroxaban** for atrial fibrillation

Young patients (< 50) with no past medical history (diabetes, hypertension) should also have the following tests:

- **Sedimentation rate**
- **VDRL or RPR**
- **ANA, double-stranded DNA**
- **Protein C, protein S, factor V Leiden mutation, antiphospholipid syndromes**

Don't forget to control **hypertension, diabetes, and hyperlipidemia** in a patient who has had a stroke. Hypertensive urgency is a relative contraindication to thrombolytic therapy.

Condition	Goal
Hypertension	< 140/90 in a diabetic
Diabetes	Same tight glycemic control as general population
Hyperlipidemia	LDL < 100 add statins for all nonhemorrhagic strokes

TIA

The management of a TIA is the **same as for a stroke,** except that thrombolytics are not indicated. The object of administering a thrombolytic is to achieve resolution of symptoms. If the symptoms have already resolved, then there is no point in giving thrombolytics. Paradoxical emboli through a patent foramen ovale need closure with a catheter device.

Seizures

Only the management of status epilepticus is clear in seizure disorders. Status epilepticus therapy is as follows:

1. Benzodiazepines, such as Ativan (lorazepam).
2. If the seizure persists after moving the clock forward 10–20 minutes, then add fosphenytoin.
3. If the seizure persists after moving the clock forward another 10–20 minutes, then add phenobarbital.
4. If the seizure persists after moving the clock forward 10–20 minutes again, then add general anesthesia, such as pentobarbital, thiopental, midazolam, or propofol.

Diagnostic Testing

Do the following tests on a patient having a seizure:

- Sodium, calcium, glucose, oxygen, creatinine, and magnesium levels
- Head CT urgently; MRI later if the initial testing shows nothing
- Urine toxicology screening
- Liver and renal function

Potassium disorders do *not* result in seizures.

Further Management

If the initial set of diagnostic tests does *not* reveal the etiology of the seizure, then an **electroencephalogram (EEG)** should be performed. The EEG should *not* be done first.

Both liver failure and renal failure cause seizures.

Neurology consultation should be ordered in any patient with a seizure after initial testing is done. Consultations will always ask for your reason for the consultation in 10 words or less.

CCS Tip: On CCS, consultants *never* say anything. CCS is testing your knowledge of when you are expected to need help.

Treatment

Chronic antiepileptic drug therapy is generally not indicated **after a single seizure**. There are several exceptions, however. Treat chronically after the first seizure in the following circumstances:

- Strong family history of seizures
- Abnormal EEG
- Status epilepticus that required benzodiazepines to stop the seizure
- Non-correctable precipitating cause, e.g., brain tumor

> Many anti-epileptic drugs are associated with bone loss and osteoporosis.

No clear single agent is the best initial therapy **for the long-term management of seizures.**

- First-line therapies: **Valproic acid, carbamazepine, phenytoin, and levetiracetam (Keppra)** are all equal in efficacy. **Lamotrigine (Lamictal)** has efficacy equal to those agents but is associated with the development of **Stevens-Johnson syndrome** and severe skin reactions.
- Second-line therapies: **Gabapentin and phenobarbital** are considered second-line agents for long-term management.
- **Ethosuximide** is best for **absence or petit mal seizures.**
- Valproic acid is most dangerous in pregnancy.

Parkinson's Disease (PD)

Parkinson's disease presents with a **tremulous patient with a slow, abnormal "festinating" gait.** PD is predominantly a gait disorder. It is often characterized by **orthostasis.**

Physical Findings

- **"Cogwheel" rigidity**
- **Resting tremor** (resolves when patient moves or reaches for something)
- **Hypomimia** (a masklike, underreactive face)
- **Micrographia** (small writing)
- **Orthostasis**
- **Intact cognition and memory**

Diagnostic Testing

There are *no* specific diagnostic tests to prove that someone has Parkinson's disease.

Treatment

Mild Symptoms

- **Under age 60: Anticholinergic agent,** such as benztropine or hydroxyzine
- **Over age 60: Amantadine** (older patients develop far more adverse effects from anticholinergic agents, including constipation, glaucoma, and urinary retention)

> Anticholinergic agents can worsen memory.

Severe Symptoms

Severe symptoms are defined as the inability to perform activities of daily living, such as cooking, cleaning, personal grooming, and shopping. First-line treatments are as follows:

	Levodopa/Carbidopa	Dopamine Agonists (pramipexole, ropinirole, cabergoline)
Advantages	Greatest efficacy	Fewer adverse effects
Disadvantages	"On-off" phenomena with uneven long-term effects and more adverse effects	Less efficacy

If these medications cannot control the patient's symptoms, then use:

- **COMT inhibitors:** Tolcapone, entacapone. These medications **block the metabolism of dopamine** and extend the effect of dopamine-based medications. They are not effective by themselves.
- MAO inhibitors: Selegiline, rasagiline
- Deep brain stimulation is done when medical therapy does not control symptoms.

When levodopa causes psychosis, add quetiapine to control psychosis.

Tremor

Type of Tremor	Resting Tremor	Tremor with Intention (Action) Only	Tremor Both at Rest and with Intention
Diagnosis	Parkinson's disease	Cerebellar disorders	Essential tremor
Treatment	Amantadine	Treat etiology	Propranolol

Multiple Sclerosis (MS)

MS presents with **abnormalities of any part of the CNS;** these improve only to have **another defect develop several months to years later.** The most common abnormality to develop is **optic neuritis.** Other abnormalities are **motor and sensory problems and defects of the bladder,** such as an atonic bladder.

Other common features of MS are the following:

- **Fatigue**
- **Hyperreflexia**
- **Spasticity**
- **Depression**

Diagnostic Testing

- Best initial diagnostic test: **MRI**
- Most accurate diagnostic test: **MRI**
- There is *no* reason to order a CT scan of the head. The CT is far less sensitive than an MRI.

- **CSF (lumbar tap):** Presence of **oligoclonal bands** is only useful if the MRI is nondiagnostic.
- Visual and auditory evoked potential are *always* wrong answers.

Natalizumab causes PML.

Treatment

- Best initial therapy: **Steroids** are the best initial therapy for acute exacerbations to help speed resolution.
- Disease-modifying therapy:
  - **Beta interferon, glatiramer, mitoxantrone, natalizumab, fingolimod, or dalfampridine**
- Additional medications for other symptoms:
  - **Fatigue: Amantadine**
  - **Spasticity: Baclofen** or **tizanidine**

Dementia

Alzheimer's Disease (AD)

Alzheimer's presents with **slowly progressive loss of memory exclusively in older patients** (> 65). Although there are no focal deficits, such as motor or sensory problems, these patients develop apathy and, after several years, imprecise speech.

Diagnostic Testing

For all patients with **memory loss,** you *must* order:

- Head CT
- B12 level
- Thyroid function testing (T4/TSH)
- RPR or VDRL

Alzheimer's disease is a diagnosis of exclusion. The only abnormal test will be the **CT scan** of the head showing **diffuse, symmetrical atrophy.**

Treatment

Anticholinesterase medications (donepezil, rivastigmine, and galantamine) are the standard of care. **Memantine** is a medication from another class with modest benefit. Combinations are *not* effective.

Frontotemporal Dementia (Pick's Disease)

Personality and behavior become abnormal first. Then memory is lost afterward. There is *no* movement disorder.

Head CT or MRI shows **focal atrophy of the frontal and temporal lobes.** Treat **the same as Alzheimer's** with less response.

Creutzfeldt-Jakob Disease (CJD)

CJD is caused by prions, transmissible protein particles. It manifests as **rapidly progressive dementia and the presence of myoclonus.** The patient is younger than in Alzheimer's.

Although the **EEG is abnormal,** the *most* accurate diagnostic test is a **brain biopsy.** On CCS cases, an **MRI** should be performed as well, although there is nothing on MRI to suggest CJD. **CSF shows a 14-3-3 protein.** The presence of the 14-3-3 protein spares the patient the need for brain biopsy.

"Lewy Body" Dementia

Lewy body dementia is **Parkinson's disease plus dementia.** Lewy body is associated with very vivid, detailed hallucinations.

> Remember: Parkinson's disease is primarily a gait disorder.

Normal Pressure Hydrocephalus (NPH)

This condition generally presents in older males, but it can affect women as well. Symptoms can be remembered as **WWW:** **w**et, **w**eird, **w**obbly:

- Wet: Urinary incontinence
- Weird: Dementia
- Wobbly: Wide-based gait/ataxia

Diagnostic Testing

- **Head CT**
- A **lumbar puncture (LP)** will show normal pressure, and this should be done on CCS.

Treatment

- Treat with **placement of a shunt.**

Huntington's Disease/Chorea

Huntington's presents in a **young patient** (30s) *far* below the age for Alzheimer's disease. The question likely will mention family history. Symptoms are the following:

- **Dementia**
- **Psychiatric disturbance with personality changes**
- **Chorea/movement disorder**

Diagnostic Testing

Diagnose with **specific genetic testing.** Inheritance is autosomal dominant.

Treatment

Give **tetrabenazine** for movement disorder, **antipsychotics** for symptomatic control.

Dementia Syndromes

All patients have memory loss and should have a **head CT/MRI, VDRL, B12, and T4.** Conditions vary as follows:

- **Alzheimer's:** No focal deficits. Treatment is with anticholinesterases and memantine.
- **Pick's/frontotemporal:** Personality and behavior are affected first.
- **Lewy body:** Parkinsonian symptoms and sometimes hallucinations accompany dementia.
- **Huntington's:** Presents with movement (chorea) and personality disorders.
- **Normal pressure hydrocephalus:** Remember WWW: Wet, weird, wobbly.

Headache

Migraine

Of migraines, 60 percent are unilateral, and 40 percent are bilateral.

Triggers include the following:

- Cheese
- Caffeine
- Menstruation
- Oral contraceptive

The following symptoms may precede the headache:

- Aura of bright flashing lights
- Scotomata
- Abnormal smells

Diagnostic Testing

Head CT or **MRI** should be done when the headache has any of the following characteristics:

- Sudden and/or severe
- Onset after age 40
- Associated with focal neurological findings

Treatment

- Best initial (abortive) therapy: **Sumatriptan** or **ergotamine.**
- Prophylactic therapy (requires **several weeks** to take effect):
  - When 4 or more headaches occur per month, the patient should receive prophylactic therapy with **beta blockers (propranolol).**
  - Alternate prophylactic medications are **calcium channel blockers, tricyclic antidepressants,** or **SSRIs.**

Basic Science Correlate

Mechanism of Triptans

Triptans constrict vessels. Migraine is thought to be vasoconstriction followed by vasodilation, then pain. Triptans function by reconstricting the cerebral vessels. This is why they are dangerous in hypertension, pregnancy, and coronary disease. Triptans constrict vessels in the heart as well, and can provoke cardiac ischemia.

Cluster Headache

Cluster headaches are **10 times more frequent in men than in women.** Cluster headaches are **exclusively unilateral** with **redness and tearing of the eye** and **rhinorrhea.**

Treatment

- Best initial (abortive) therapy: **Triptans** or 100 percent oxygen. Triptans are generally used because they are easier to give at home. **Sumatriptan** is used in the same way as with migraine headache. **Steroids** can also be used.
- Best initial prophylactic therapy: Calcium channel blockers such as **verapamil**. By definition, cluster headaches occur multiple times in a short period and then resolve. The "cluster" is often over by the time prophylactic therapy has taken effect. Verapamil does prevent cluster headache.

Headache Type	Migraine	Cluster
Gender		Much more common in men
Presentation	• Unilateral or bilateral • Aura	• Only unilateral • Tearing and redness of eye; rhinorrhea • No aura
Abortive therapy	• Sumatriptan	• Sumatriptan • Special: 100% oxygen
Prophylactic therapy	• Propranolol	• Verapamil

Temporal Arteritis

Temporal arteritis presents with the following:

- Tenderness of the temporal area
- Jaw claudication

Diagnostic Testing

- **Sedimentation rate (ESR)**
- Most accurate test: **Temporal artery biopsy**

Treatment

Give **steroids first and fast** if these are available. A delay may result in **permanent vision loss.**

Pseudotumor = Headache plus:
- Sixth nerve palsy
- Visual field loss
- Transiently obscure vision
- Pulsutile tinnitus

Pseudotumor Cerebri

Look for an **obese young woman with a headache and double vision.** On exam, there is **papilledema,** but CT/MRI is normal. **Vitamin A use** is suggestive.

Diagnostic Testing

The most accurate test is a **lumbar puncture with opening pressure measurement,** which will show a markedly elevated pressure.

Treatment

- **Weight loss**
- **Acetazolamide**
- **Surgery** if they fail: VP shunt, optic nerve sheath fenestration

Dizziness/Vertigo

All patients with vertigo will have a subjective sensation of the **room spinning** around them. This is often associated with **nausea and vomiting.** All patients with vertigo will have **nystagmus** (horizontal). When a patient thinks the room is spinning, the eyes should naturally dart back and forth to give the feeling of looking at a single point.

Generally *all* patients with vertigo should have an **MRI of the internal auditory canal.**

The following table summarizes the presentation of a number of conditions that cause vertigo.

Disease	Characteristics	Hearing Loss/Tinnitus
Benign positional vertigo	Changes with position	No
Vestibular neuritis	Vertigo occurs without position changes	No
Labyrinthitis	Acute	Yes
Meniere's disease	Chronic	Yes
Acoustic neuroma	Ataxia	Yes
Perilymph fistula	History of trauma	Yes

Benign Positional Vertigo (BPV)

This presents as vertigo alone with no hearing loss, no tinnitus, and no ataxia. The question may describe a positive Dix-Hallpike maneuver. History may describe onset of symptoms when quickly changing positions.

There is no specific diagnostic test. BPV responds modestly to meclizine (Antivert).

Vestibular Neuritis

This is an idiopathic inflammation of the vestibular portion of the 8th cranial nerve. Because only the vestibular portion is involved, there is no hearing loss and no tinnitus. Presumably, this condition is viral. It is entirely characterized by vertigo and dizziness and is not related to changes in position.

There is no specific diagnostic test. Treat with meclizine.

Labyrinthitis

Labyrinthitis is inflammation of the cochlear portion of the inner ear. There is hearing loss as well as tinnitus. This condition is acute and self-limited and may be treated with meclizine and steroids. Acute hearing loss may respond to steroids.

Meniere's Disease

Same presentation as labyrinthitis (vertigo, hearing loss, tinnitus), but Meniere's is chronic with remitting and relapsing episodes. Treat with salt restriction and diuretics. For severe disease, ablation of 8th cranial nerve on one side may be needed.

Acoustic Neuroma

This is an 8th cranial nerve tumor that can be related to neurofibromatosis, or Von Recklinghausen's disease. Acoustic neuroma presents with ataxia in addition to hearing loss, tinnitus, and vertigo.

Diagnostic Testing

- MRI of the internal auditory canal.

Treatment

- Treat with surgical resection.

Perilymph Fistula

Head trauma or any form of barotrauma to the ear may rupture the tympanic membrane and lead to a perilymph fistula. Fix the hole surgically.

Wernicke-Korsakoff Syndrome

Wernicke-Korsakoff syndrome presents as follows:

- History of chronic heavy alcohol use
- Confusion with confabulation
- Ataxia
- Memory loss
- Gaze palsy/ophthalmoplegia
- Nystagmus

Diagnostic Testing

With memory loss, it is very important to perform the following tests:

- Head CT
- B12 level
- Thyroid function (T4/TSH)
- RPR or VDRL

Treatment

- Treat with thiamine. Acutely, give IV dose; then may switch to oral.
- Also give glucose with thiamine, but administer thiamine first, then glucose.

Central Nervous System Infections

Often when a CNS infection is suspected, a head CT should be performed before a lumbar puncture. Perform a head CT before a lumbar puncture (LP) in the following circumstances:

- A history of central nervous system disease
- Focal neurologic deficit
- Presence of papilledema
- Seizures
- Altered consciousness
- Significant delay in the ability to perform an LP

If these findings are present, get blood cultures and start empiric antibiotic therapy before ordering the head CT.

Bacterial Meningitis

A 45-year-old man comes to the emergency department with fever, headache, photophobia, and a stiff neck. What is the next best step in the management of this patient?

a. Lumbar puncture
b. Head CT scan
c. Ceftriaxone and vancomycin
d. Penicillin
e. Movement of patient to ICU

Answer: **A.** When you suspect bacterial meningitis, administer antibiotics quickly. Further, do blood cultures stat simultaneously with a lumbar puncture (LP), or immediately prior. Penicillin can never be used as empiric therapy for meningitis; it is not sufficiently broad in coverage to be effective empiric therapy. In this case, perform the LP.

Diagnostic Testing

The most accurate test for bacterial meningitis is a culture, but you cannot wait for the results of culture before starting therapy. Preliminary analysis of the **cerebrospinal fluid (CSF)** is useful.

- Gram stain shows: The Gram stain is only about 50–60 percent sensitive for bacterial meningitis. Therefore, a negative stain excludes nothing. On the other hand, a positive Gram stain is extremely useful and specific.
  - Gram-positive diplococci: Pneumococcus
  - Gram-negative diplococci: *Neisseria*
  - Gram-negative pleomorphic, coccobacillary organisms: *Haemophilus*
  - Gram-positive bacilli: *Listeria*

The Gram stain has poor sensitivity but good specificity for bacterial meningitis.

- Protein: An elevated protein level in the CSF is of marginal diagnostic benefit. Protein elevation is nonspecific; any form of CNS infection can elevate the CSF protein. A normal CSF protein level essentially excludes bacterial meningitis.
- Glucose: Glucose levels below 60 percent of serum levels are consistent with bacterial meningitis.
- CSF cell count: The best initial test for the diagnosis of meningitis is a cell count.
  - Although not as specific as a culture, it is available much sooner.
  - Cell count with a differential is much more specific than an elevated CSF protein level.
  - If thousands of neutrophils are present in the CSF, start IV ceftriaxone, vancomycin, and steroids. Steroids have been associated with a decrease in mortality in bacterial meningitis.

CSF cell count is the most important criterion to determine the need to treat a patient. Thousands of polys (neutrophils) indicate bacterial meningitis until proven otherwise.

Cryptococcus

Look for an HIV-positive patient with < 100 CD4 cells. This infection is slower than bacterial meningitis and may not give severe meningeal signs, such as neck stiffness, photophobia, and high fever, all at the same time.

Diagnostic Testing

- Best initial test: India ink
- Most accurate test: Cryptococcal antigen

Treatment

- Best initial therapy: Amphotericin and 5-flucytosine (5FC)
- Amphotericin and 5FC are followed with oral fluconazole.
  - If the patient's CD4 cells do not rise, fluconazole must be continued indefinitely.
  - If the CD4 count rises above 100, the fluconazole can be stopped.

Lyme Disease

Look for a patient who has recently been on a camping or hiking trip. Tick exposure is remembered only by 20 percent of patients.

Diagnostic Testing

There are no characteristic CSF findings to confirm a diagnosis of CNS Lyme. Specific serologic or Western blot testing on the CSF is the most accurate test. Look for a patient with a history of joint pain, 7th cranial nerve palsy, or a rash with central clearing (target lesion).

Treatment

Treat with IV ceftriaxone or penicillin.

Rocky Mountain Spotted Fever

Look for a camper or hiker with a rash that starts on the wrists and ankles and moves centripetally toward the center. Fever, headache, and malaise precede the rash. Only 60 percent at most will remember a tick bite.

Diagnose with specific serology. Doxycycline is the most effective therapy.

TB Meningitis

This is an extremely difficult diagnosis to be precise about. Look for an immigrant with a history of lung tuberculosis. The presentation is very slow over weeks to months; if the case describes fever, headache, and neck stiffness over hours then it is not TB.

Diagnostic Testing

TB meningitis has a very high CSF protein level. Acid fast (mycobacterial) stain of the CSF is positive in 10 percent or less of patients. For acid-fast culture, you need 3 high-volume taps that are centrifuged.

Treatment

Treat with rifampin, isoniazid, pyrazinamide, and ethambutol (RIPE) as you would for pulmonary TB. The only difference is that you should add steroids and extend the length of therapy for meningitis when compared with pulmonary disease.

Viral Meningitis

Viral meningitis is, in general, a diagnosis of exclusion. There is a lymphocytic pleocytosis in the CSF, and none of the other findings is present. There is no specific therapy for viral meningitis.

An elderly man comes to the emergency department with fever, headache, a stiff neck, and photophobia. He is HIV positive with < 50 CD4 cells and a history of pneumocystis pneumonia. His head CT is normal. CSF shows 2,500 white cells that are all neutrophils; Gram stain is normal. What is the best initial therapy?

a. Ceftriaxone and metronidazole
b. Cefoxitin and mefloquine
c. Ceftriaxone, ampicillin, and vancomycin
d. Fluconazole
e. Amphotericin

Answer: **C.** *Listeria monocytogenes* is a cause of meningitis that is not adequately treated by any form of cephalosporin. Ampicillin is added to the usual regimen of ceftriaxone and vancomycin to cover *Listeria*. This cannot be fungal meningitis, because the CSF is characterized exclusively by a high number of neutrophils; neutrophils are not consistent with fungal meningitis.

A 17-year-old male is brought to the emergency department with fever, headache, stiff neck, and photophobia. He has a petechial rash. CSF shows 2,499 neutrophils. Ceftriaxone and vancomycin are started. What should be done next?

a. Test for HIV
b. Wait for results of culture
c. Add ampicillin
d. Enforce respiratory isolation
e. Enforce respiratory isolation and prescribe rifampin for close contacts

Answer: **E.** When an adolescent presents with a petechial rash and increased neutrophils on CSF, it is suggestive of *Neisseria meningitidis*. These patients should be placed on respiratory isolation, and close contacts should receive prophylaxis.

Listeria

Look for elderly, neonatal, and HIV-positive patients and those with who have no spleen, are on steroids, or are immunocompromised with leukemia or lymphoma.

There will be elevated neutrophils in the CSF. Add ampicillin to therapy.

Neisseria meningitidis

The nurse or medical student taking care of a patient with *Neisseria* does not need prophylaxis. Those with kissing and other saliva-type contact do need prophylaxis.

Look for patients who are adolescent, in the military, or asplenic or who have terminal complement deficiency.

Treat as follows:

- Patient: Begin respiratory isolation.
- Close contacts: Start prophylaxis with rifampin, ciprofloxacin, or ceftriaxone for close contacts, such as household members and those who share utensils, cups, or kisses.
- Routine contacts: Routine school and work contacts do not need to receive prophylaxis.

Encephalitis

Fever + Confusion = Encephalitis

Look for a patient with fever and altered mental status over a few hours. If the patient also has photophobia and a stiff neck, you will not be able to diagnose encephalitis. Almost all encephalitis in the United States is caused by herpes. The patient does not have to recall a herpes infection in the past for the condition to be herpes encephalitis.

Diagnostic Testing

- Best initial test: Head CT scan
- Most accurate test: PCR of the CSF

The most common wrong answer on questions dealing with the diagnosis of encephalitis is "brain biopsy." A brain biopsy is not necessary. Do a PCR instead.

Treatment

- Best initial therapy: Acyclovir
- For acyclovir-resistant patients: Foscarnet

> **Basic Science Correlate**
>
> **Mechanism of Acyclovir**
>
> Acyclovir, valacyclovir, famciclovir, and ganciclovir all have the same mechanism, which is to inhibit tyrosine kinase. This is why ganciclovir cannot be used to treat acyclovir-resistant herpes and why foscarnet, which has a different mechanism, is used instead.

Brain Abscess

A brain abscess presents with fever, headache, and focal neurological deficits. A CT scan finds a "ring," or contrast-enhancing, lesion. Contrast ("ring") enhancement basically means either cancer or infection.

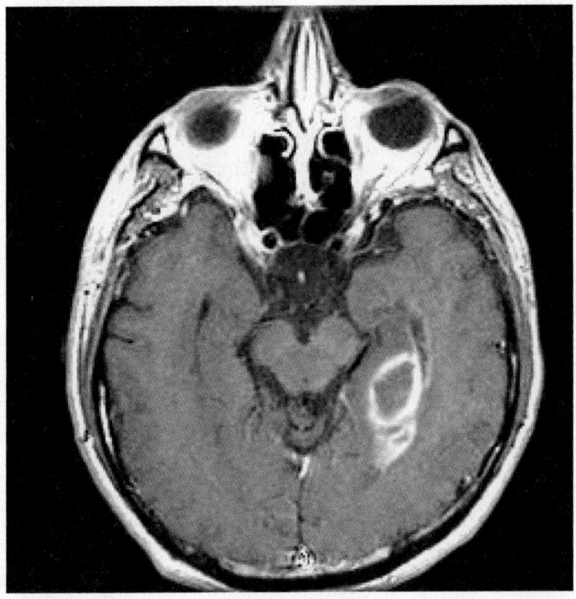

Brain Abscess

Consider HIV status in the context of a brain abscess as follows:

- HIV-negative: Brain biopsy is the next best step.
- HIV-positive: Treat for toxoplasmosis with pyrimethamine and sulfadiazine for 2 weeks and repeat the head CT.

Progressive Multifocal Leukoencephalopathy (PML)

These brain lesions in HIV-positive patients are not associated with ring enhancement or mass effect.

There is no specific therapy. Treat the HIV and raise the CD4. When the HIV is improved, the lesions will disappear.

Neurocysticercosis

Look for a patient from Mexico with a seizure.

Head CT shows multiple 1 cm cystic lesions. Over time, the lesions calcify. Confirm diagnosis with serology.

When still active and uncalcified, the lesions are treated with albendazole. Use steroids to prevent a reaction to dying parasites.

Do not use albendazole to treat if there is only calcification. Use only anti-epileptic drugs.

Head Trauma and Intracranial Hemorrhage

Do not use skull x-rays in head trauma. If the head trauma is severe, then diagnosis requires a CT scan. **LOC = CT scan.**

Diagnostic Testing

Any head trauma resulting in a loss of consciousness (LOC) or altered mental status should lead to a CT scan of the head without contrast.

The following table shows possible outcomes of head trauma that can result in a loss of consciousness and how they vary from one another.

	Concussion	Contusion	Subdural Hematoma	Epidural Hematoma
Focal deficits	Never	Rarely	Yes or no	Yes or no
Head CT	Normal	Ecchymosis	Crescent-shaped collection	Lens-shaped collection

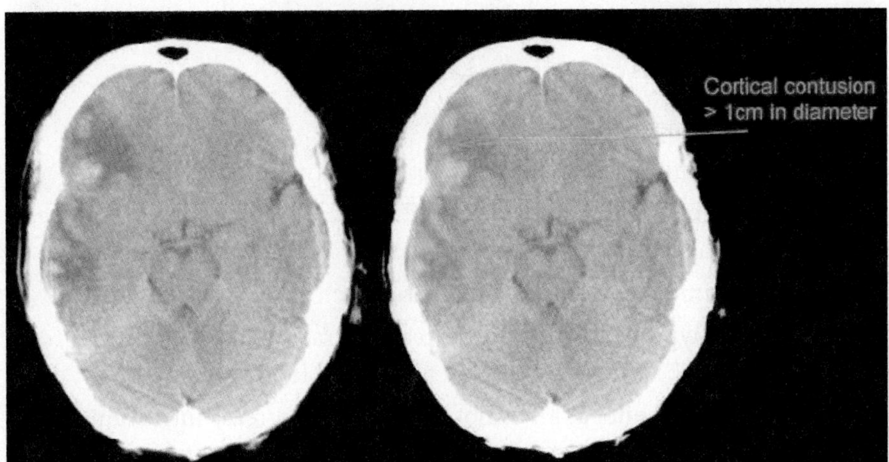

Cerebral Contusion

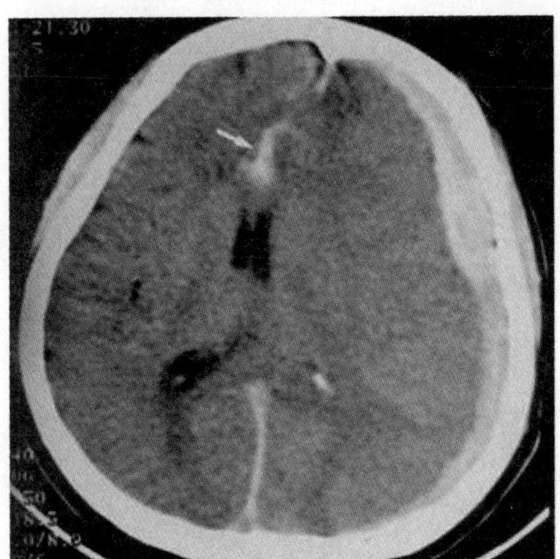

Subdural Hematoma

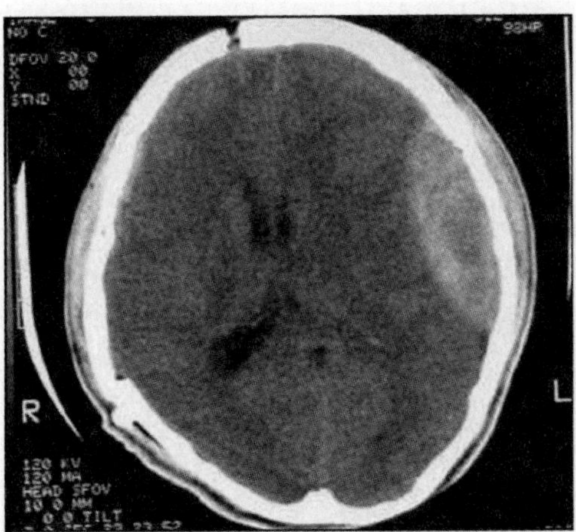

Epidural Hematoma

Treatment

Treatments for various head traumas are as follows:

- Concussion: None
- Contusion: Admit, but vast majority get no treatment.
- Subdural and epidural: Large ones are drained; small ones are left alone to reabsorb on their own.
- Large intracranial hemorrhage with mass effect:
  - Intubation/hyperventilation to decrease intracranial pressure. Decrease pCO_2 to 28–32, which will constrict cerebral blood vessels.
  - Administer mannitol as an osmotic diuretic to decrease intracranial pressure.
  - Perform surgical evacuation.

Steroids do not help intracranial hemorrhage.

Stress Ulcer Prophylaxis

Patients with any of the following conditions should receive proton pump inhibitors as prophylaxis against stress ulcer:

- Head trauma
- Burns
- Endotracheal intubation with mechanical ventilation

Subarachnoid Hemorrhage (SAH)

Look for the following symptoms:

- Sudden, severe headache
- Stiff neck
- Photophobia
- Loss of consciousness (LOC) in 50 percent of patients
- Focal neurological deficits in 30 percent of patients

SAH is like the sudden onset of meningitis with a LOC but without fever.

Basic Science Correlate

Mechanism of Blood Causing Symptoms in SAH

Blood is an irritant. It irritates the meninges in SAH and simulates meningitis. It stimulates the bowel and causes diarrhea with melena. Blood is cathartic.

Diagnostic Testing

- Best initial test: A head CT without contrast is 95 percent sensitive. If this is conclusive for an SAH, you do not need to do a lumbar puncture.
- Most accurate diagnostic test: Lumbar puncture. This is not necessary if the head CT scan shows blood.

To tell if an increased number of white cells in CSF is caused by infection or is just from blood, look for the ratio. A normal number of white cells is 1 for every 500 red cells. An infection is considered to be present only if the number of white cells is greater than the ratio of 1 to 500.

- Normal white cell count = 1 WBC:500 RBC

Treatment

1. Perform angiography to determine the site of bleeding.
2. Embolize the site of the bleeding. This is superior to surgical clipping.
3. Insert a ventriculoperitoneal shunt if hydrocephalus develops.
4. Prescribe nimodipine orally; this is a calcium channel blocker that prevents stroke.

When SAH occurs, an intense vasospasm can lead to a nonhemorrhagic stroke.

You must embolize (or clip) the source of bleeding in an SAH before it can rebleed. If it rebleeds, there is a 50 percent chance that the patient will die.

Spine Disorders

The following table summarizes some spine disorders and their symptoms:

Lumbosacral Strain	Cord Compression	Epidural Abscess	Spinal Stenosis
Nontender	Tender	Tender and fever	Pain on walking downhill

Syringomyelia

This is a defective fluid cavity in the center of the cord caused by trauma, tumors, or a congenital problem. It presents with loss of sensation of pain and temperature in the upper extremities bilaterally in a capelike distribution over the neck, shoulders, and down both arms.

Diagnose with an MRI. Treat surgically.

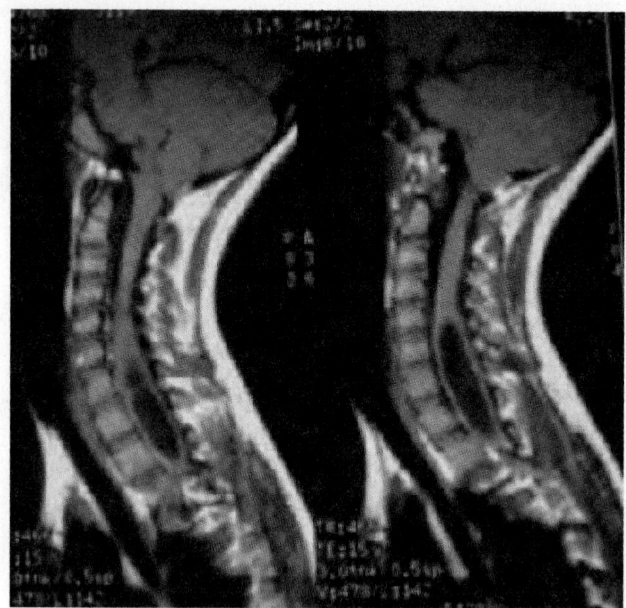

Syringomyelia

Cord Compression

Metastatic cancer presses on the cord, resulting in pain and tenderness of the spine. Lumbosacral strain does not give tenderness of the spine itself.

Scan with an MRI. Biopsy is the most accurate test if the diagnosis is not clear from the history.

The most effective therapy depends on the cause. The most urgent step in cases of cord compression is to give steroids to decrease swelling.

Spinal Epidural Abscess

A spinal epidural abscess presents with back pain with tenderness and fever.

Scan the spine with MRI. Give antibiotics against *Staphylococcus*, such as oxacillin or nafcillin. Large accumulations require surgical decompression.

Spinal Stenosis

This condition presents with leg pain on walking and can look like peripheral arterial disease. The pulses will be intact, and the pain is worse upon walking downhill, when the patient is leaning backward, but improved when walking uphill.

Diagnose with an MRI. Treat with surgical decompression.

Anterior Spinal Artery Infarction

All sensation is lost except position and vibratory sense, which travel down the posterior column. There is no specific therapy.

Brown-Sequard Syndrome

This results from traumatic injury to the spine, such as a knife wound. The patient loses ipsilateral position, vibratory sense, contralateral pain, and temperature.

A 58-year-old woman with metastatic breast cancer comes in with back pain. The spine is tender. She has hyperreflexia of the legs. What is the most urgent step?

a. X-ray
b. CT
c. MRI
d. Biopsy
e. Steroids
f. Chemotherapy
g. Radiation

Answer: **E.** The most urgent step in the management of cord compression is to administer steroids as soon as possible and to relieve pressure on the cord. Imaging studies are done after steroids are given, if the diagnosis of cord compression is clear (as it is in this case with pain, tenderness, and signs of hyperreflexia in the legs).

Amyotrophic Lateral Sclerosis

This is an idiopathic disorder of both upper and lower motor neurons; signs are listed in the table below. It is treated with riluzole, a unique agent that blocks the accumulation of glutamate.

Upper Motor Neuron Signs	Lower Motor Neuron Signs
• Hyperreflexia • Upgoing toes on plantar reflex • Spasticity • Weakness	• Wasting • Fasciculations • Weakness

Peripheral Neuropathies

Diabetes

The most common cause of peripheral neuropathy by far is diabetes. A specific test, such as an electromyogram or nerve conduction study, is not necessary in the majority of cases.

Treat with gabapentin or pregabalin. Tricyclic antidepressants are less effective and have more adverse effects.

Carpal Tunnel Syndrome

Look for pain and weakness of the first 3 digits of the hand. Symptoms may worsen with repetitive use.

Initial management is a splint. In CSS, inject steroids when you move the clock forward if symptoms persist or worsen.

Radial Nerve Palsy

Also known as "Saturday night palsy," this results from falling asleep or passing out with pressure on the arms underneath the body or outstretched, perhaps draped over the back of a chair. Radial nerve palsy results in a wrist drop.

Peroneal Nerve Palsy

This results from high boots pressing at the back of the knee. It results in foot drop and the inability to evert the foot. May see "high boots" in the case.

There is no therapy. Peroneal nerve palsy resolves on its own.

7th Cranial Nerve (Bell's Palsy)

Bell's palsy results in hemifacial paralysis of both the upper and lower halves of the face. There is also loss of taste on the anterior two thirds of the tongue, hyperacusis, and the inability to close the eye at night. Hyperacusis results in the inability to control the stapedius muscle of the middle ear, which acts as a kind of "shock absorber" for sounds. Bell's palsy is believed to result from a viral infection.

Treat with steroids. It is not clear that acyclovir helps.

Reflex Sympathetic Dystrophy

Also called chronic regional pain syndrome, reflex sympathetic dystrophy happens in a patient with previous injury to the extremity. Light touch, such as from a sheet touching the foot, results in extreme pain that is "burning" in quality.

Treat with NSAIDs, gabapentin, and occasionally nerve block. Surgical sympathectomy may be necessary.

Restless Legs Syndrome (RLS)

RLS often comes to the health care provider's attention when the bed partner comes in complaining of pain and bruises in the legs. The patient experiences an uncomfortable feeling in the legs, which is relieved by movement.

RLS is associated with iron deficiency.

Treat with pramipexole or ropinirole.

A man comes to the emergency department with weakness in his legs that has been getting markedly worse over the last few days. He has weakness and loss of deep tendon reflexes in the legs. He recalls an upper respiratory illness about 2–4 weeks prior that resolved. What is the most urgent step?

a. Steroids
b. Intravenous immunoglobulins
c. Peak inspiratory pressure
d. Intubation
e. Lumbar puncture

Answer: **C.** This case is Guillain-Barré. Ascending weakness with loss of deep tendon reflexes is characteristic. Peak inspiratory pressure is the correct answer. The peak inspiratory pressure diminishes as the diaphragm is weakened. Peak inspiratory pressure predicts who will have respiratory failure before it happens. This is the most important factor in determining the need for therapy with either intravenous immunoglobulins (IVIG) or plasmapheresis. Combinations of these medications are not effective. Steroids are not effective. Lumbar puncture will show an elevated protein level with no cells.

Myasthenia Gravis

Myasthenia gravis presents with weakness of the muscles of mastication, making it hard to finish meals. Blurry vision from diplopia results from the inability to focus the eyes on a single target. The case may classically report drooping of the eyelids as the day progresses.

Diagnostic Testing

- Best initial test: Anti-acetylcholine receptor antibodies (ACHR)
- Most accurate test: Clinical presentation and ACHR are more sensitive and specific than an edrophonium or "Tensilon" stimulation test.

Treatment

- Best initial therapy: Pyridostigmine or neostigmine
- Thymectomy: Use in patients < 60 if pyridostigmine or neostigmine do not work.
- Prednisone: If thymectomy does not work, or if there simply is no response to pyridostigmine or neostigmine.
- Azathioprine and cyclosporine are used to try to keep the patient off of long-term steroids.

Basic Science Correlate

Mechanism of Azathioprine

Cyclosporine and azathioprine inhibit the immune system. They decrease the function of T-cells, which control cellular immunity such as organ transplant rejection. The drugs do not decrease T-cell numbers, just function.

Nephrology

10

Acute Renal Failure

The first step is to **evaluate whether the renal failure is prerenal (perfusion), renal (parenchymal), or postrenal (drainage).**

- Clues to the renal failure being of **short duration** are the following:
  - Normal kidney size
  - Normal hematocrit
  - Normal calcium level
- **Chronic renal failure** will have the following effects:
  - It makes the kidneys smaller.
  - With renal failure of more than 2 weeks, the hematocrit will drop from loss of erythropoietin production.
  - Calcium levels drop from the loss of vitamin D hydroxylation (i.e., activation).

Prerenal Azotemia

Any cause of **hypoperfusion** will lead to renal failure:

- **Hypotension,** generally with a systolic pressure < 90 mm Hg
- **Hypovolemia** from dehydration or blood loss
- **Low oncotic pressure** (low albumin)
- **Congestive heart failure:** You can't perfuse the kidney if the pump doesn't work.
- **Constrictive pericarditis:** You can't perfuse the kidney if the heart cannot fill.
- **Renal artery stenosis:** Although the systemic pressure may be high, the kidney thinks the body is hypotensive because of the blockage.

Diagnostic Testing

Prerenal azotemia will have the following characteristics:

- **BUN to creatinine ratio of > 15:1 and often > 20:1**
- **Urinary sodium is low** (< 20)
- **Fractional excretion of sodium < 1 percent:** This is largely the same thing as a low urine sodium. Do not spend your time learning to do the calculation.
- **Urine osmolality > 500**
- May have hyaline casts on urinalysis.

> **Basic Science Correlate**
>
> **Mechanism of Elevation of BUN in Prerenal Azotemia**
> Low volume status increases ADH. ADH increases urea absorption at the collecting duct. There is a urea transporter that brings urea in. ADH increases the activity of the urea transporter.

Treatment

Treatment of prerenal azotemia is *entirely* based on the underlying cause.

CCS Tip: On CCS, all renal cases should have the following tests performed:

- Urinalysis
- Chemistries
- Renal ultrasound

Postrenal Azotemia (Obstructive Uropathy)

Any cause of obstruction of the kidney will lead to renal failure:

- **Stone in the bladder or ureters**
- **Strictures**
- **Cancer of the bladder, prostate, or cervix**
- **Neurogenic bladder** (atonic or noncontracting, such as from multiple sclerosis or diabetes)

> Remember: The obstruction *must* be bilateral to cause renal failure. Unilateral obstruction cannot cause renal failure.

Obstructive uropathy will give an **elevated BUN-to-creatinine ratio of > 15:1**, similar to that seen in prerenal azotemia.

Clues to obstructive uropathy are the following:

- **Distended bladder** on exam
- **Large volume diuresis** after passing a urinary catheter
- **Bilateral hydronephrosis on ultrasound**

Intrarenal Causes of Renal Failure

Intrarenal causes of renal failure result in the following:

- **BUN-to-creatinine ratio closer to 10:1**
- **Urinary sodium > 40**
- **Urine osmolality < 350**

Acute tubular necrosis (ATN) can be caused by either **hypoperfusion** to the point of death of the tubular cells or by various **toxic injuries to the kidney.** It is often caused by a combination of both.

Toxin-Induced Renal Insufficiency

In these cases, there is *no* single test to prove that a particular toxin caused the renal failure. Common causes are these:

- **Aminoglycosides,** such as gentamicin, tobramycin, or amikacin: Hypomagnesemia is suggestive of aminoglycoside-induced renal failure, but it is *not* conclusive. It usually takes 4–5 days of use to effect damage.
- **Amphotericin**
- **Contrast agents:** Urine sodium low (< 20); can happen 12 hours later
- **Chemotherapy,** such as cisplatin

Contrast is extremely rapid in onset.

Basic Science Correlate

Mechanism of Rapid Onset of Renal Failure with Contrast Agent

Contrast agents are directly toxic to kidney tubules, as are aminoglycosides. Contrast also causes an intense vasoconstriction of the afferent arteriole. This combination of direct toxicity and decreased perfusion is why there is such a rapid rise in creatinine during contrast-induced renal failure. It is also why contrast-induced renal failure causes a low urine sodium, as in prerenal azotemia.

The urinalysis may show **"muddy brown" or granular casts.** There is *no* specific therapy to reverse toxin-induced renal failure.

A man is admitted for pneumonia from a nursing home. He is placed on piperacillin-tazobactam, and he becomes afebrile. Two days later, his BUN and creatinine start to rise. He develops a new fever and a rash. What is the most likely diagnosis, and what is the most accurate diagnostic test?

Answer: **Allergic interstitial nephritis** is a hypersensitivity reaction to medications such as penicillin or sulfa drugs. Other common culprits are phenytoin, allopurinol, cyclosporine, quinidine, quinolones, or rifampin. The clue to the diagnosis is the **fever and rash.** The best initial test is a **urinalysis (UA) that shows white cells.** However, the UA is not capable of distinguishing between neutrophils and eosinophils. The most accurate test is a **Wright stain** or **Hansel's stain of the urine** that will show eosinophils. This is more sensitive than either the blood eosinophil level or an elevated IgE level. There is no specific therapy generally given for allergic interstitial nephritis; it resolves on its own.

Cyclophosphamide causes hemorrhagic cystitis, *not* renal failure.

Rhabdomyolysis

In cases of rhabdomyolysis, large-volume **muscular necrosis** is associated with renal failure from the direct **toxic effect of myoglobin on the kidney tubule.** Look for the following in presentation:

- Crush injury
- Seizure or cocaine toxicity
- Prolonged immobility in an intoxicated patient
- Hypokalemia resulting in muscle necrosis
- A patient recently started on a "statin" medication for hyperlipidemia

Diagnostic Testing

- Best initial test: **Urinalysis** showing dipstick positive for large amounts of blood with no cells seen on the microscopic examination
- **CPK level:** Will be elevated.
- Most accurate test: **Urine myoglobin** is probably the single most accurate test.
- On a CCS, also order the following:
  - **Potassium level (hyperkalemia):** Potassium goes up from any cellular destruction, such as from a tumor lysis, hemolysis, or rhabdomyolysis.
  - **Calcium level (hypocalcemia):** Damaged muscle binds increased amounts of calcium. Hyperphosphatemia may lead to binding of calcium with the phosphate.
  - **Chemistries especially for detecting a decreased serum bicarbonate**

Basic Science Correlate

Mechanism of Low Calcium in Rhabdomyolysis

Damaged muscle binds calcium. Each skeletal muscle cell contains sarcoplasmic endoplasmic reticulum for calcium (SERCA). SERCA is the normal mechanism for ending contraction, which it achieves by pulling all the cell calcium out of the cytosol. When the outside covering, or sarcolemma, is damaged, the SERCA can suck up calcium and lower the blood level.

Treatment

- **Bolus of normal saline**
- **Mannitol and diuresis** to decrease the contact time of myoglobin with the tubule
- **Alkalinization of the urine** may decrease precipitation of myoglobin at the tubule

A patient is brought to the emergency department after a seizure leading to prolonged immobility on a sidewalk. He has dark urine and myalgias. What is the most urgent step in the management of this patient?

a. Urinalysis
b. Urine myoglobin level
c. EKG
d. CPK level
e. Phosphate level
f. Creatinine

Answer: **C.** EKG is the most urgent step in an acute case of rhabdomyolysis. This case tests your knowledge of how people die with rhabdomyolysis. Severe muscle necrosis leads to **hyperkalemia,** which leads to **arrhythmia.** If this is a CCS case, then all of the tests should be done simultaneously. A specific diagnosis with urinalysis or urine myoglobin is not as important as detecting and treating potentially life-threatening conditions, such as hyperkalemia with peaked T waves. This condition would be treated with immediate intravenous calcium gluconate, insulin, and glucose.

Crystal-Induced Renal Failure

This condition can result from oxalate crystals or uric acid crystals.

- Oxalate crystals: Look for **suicide by antifreeze ingestion** (ethylene glycol). The patient will be intoxicated with metabolic acidosis with an elevated anion gap.
  - Best initial test: **Urinalysis** showing **envelope-shaped oxalate crystals**
  - Best initial treatment: **Ethanol** or **fomepizole** with **immediate dialysis**

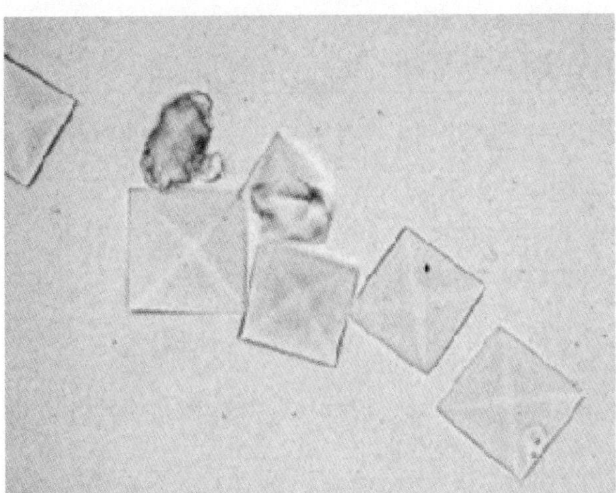

Oxalate crystals

- **Uric acid crystals:** Look for **tumor lysis syndrome,** most often after chemotherapy for lymphoma.
  - Treat with hydration, allopurinol, and rasburicase.

Rasburicase breaks down uric acid.

Prevention of Contrast-Induced Renal Failure

To test your knowledge of this situation, the case will describe a patient who *must* have a radiologic procedure with contrast *and* common reasons for renal insufficiency, such as an elderly patient with hypertension and diabetes. There will be no attempt to hide the etiology. Mild renal insufficiency with a creatinine just above the normal range at 1.5 to 2.5 will be shown.

What is the best method to prevent contrast induced renal failure?

Answer: Give hydration with **normal saline** and possibly **bicarbonate, N-acetyl cysteine,** or **both.**

Step 3 wants you to know that even a very slight elevation in creatinine means the *loss of 60–70 percent of renal function* at a minimum. Preserve what is left!

Kidney Damage Caused by NSAIDs

NSAIDS can cause the following:

- **Direct toxicity and papillary necrosis**
- **Allergic interstitial nephritis** with eosinophils in the urine
- **Nephrotic syndrome**
- **Afferent arteriolar vasoconstriction and decreased perfusion of the glomerulus,** worsening renal function

Glomerulonephritis

All forms of glomerulonephritis (GN) can have the following characteristics:

- **Red blood cells** in the urine
- **Red cell casts** in the urine
- Mild degrees of **proteinuria** (< 2 g per 24 hours)
- **Edema**
- May lead to **nephrotic syndrome**
- Are most accurately diagnosed with **kidney biopsy,** although this is not always necessary

Think: What are the few extra words to remember about each disease in order to answer the diagnostic and treatment questions? Step 3 does *not* generally emphasize the "most likely diagnosis" question.

Goodpasture's Syndrome

Cough, hemoptysis, shortness of breath, and lung findings will be present in the case.

Diagnostic Testing

- Best initial test: **Anti–basement membrane antibodies**
- Most accurate test: **Renal biopsy showing "linear deposits"**

Treatment

Treatment is with **plasmapheresis** and **steroids.**

Churg-Strauss Syndrome

Asthma, cough, and eosinophilia are present in addition to the **renal abnormalities.**

Diagnostic Testing

- Best initial test: **CBC for eosinophil count**
- Most accurate test: **Biopsy**

Treatment

- Best initial therapy: **Glucocorticoids** (e.g., prednisone)
- If there is no response to prednisone, add **cyclophosphamide.**

Wegener's Granulomatosis

Upper respiratory problems such as **sinusitis and otitis** are the key to diagnosis. **Lung problems** (cough, hemoptysis, abnormal chest x-ray) are present as well.

Wegener's is a **systemic vasculitis,** so joint, skin, eye, brain, and GI problems are also present, but the key is both upper and lower respiratory involvement *in addition* to renal involvement. Often the case will be misdiagnosed as pneumonia.

Diagnostic Testing

- Best initial test: **c-ANCA** (antineutrophil cytoplasmic antibodies)
- Most accurate test: **Biopsy of kidney**

Treatment

The best initial therapy is **cyclophosphamide and steroids.**

Polyarteritis Nodosa (PAN)

Polyarteritis nodosa is a **systemic vasculitis** with involvement of every organ *except* the lung.

Presentations include the following:

- Renal
- Myalgias
- GI bleeding and abdominal pain
- Purpuric skin lesion
- Stroke
- Uveitis
- Neuropathy

The very nonspecific findings of fever, weight loss, and fatigue will also be present. **Multiple motor and sensory neuropathy with pain** are key to diagnosis.

Diagnostic Testing

- Best initial test: **ESR and markers of inflammation**
- Most accurate test: **Biopsy of sural nerve or the kidney**
- Test for **hepatitis B and C,** which can be associated with 30 percent of PAN.
- **Angiography showing "beading"** can spare the need for biopsy.

Treatment

The best initial therapy is **cyclophosphamide and steroids.**

IgA Nephropathy (Berger's Disease)

This condition presents with **painless recurrent hematuria,** particularly in an **Asian patient** after a very **recent viral respiratory tract infection.** Proteinuria and red cells and red cell casts can be present in all forms of glomerular disease. There is *no* specific physical finding that clearly defines the disease.

Diagnostic Testing

- Best initial test: There is *no* specific blood test. IgA levels are sometimes elevated.
- Most accurate test: **Renal biopsy is essential,** because there is no blood test or specific physical findings to use in diagnosis. Complement levels are normal.

Treatment

There is *no* proven effective therapy to reverse IgA nephropathy.

- **Steroids** are used in boluses when there is a sudden worsening of proteinuria.
- **ACE inhibitors** are used as they are for all patients with proteinuria.
- **Fish oil** *may* have some effect in delaying progression.

Henoch-Schönlein Purpura

This presents in an **adolescent or child** with the following symptoms:

- **Raised, nontender, purpuric skin lesions,** particularly on the buttocks
- **Abdominal pain**
- Possible **bleeding**
- **Joint pain**
- **Renal involvement**

Diagnostic Testing

- Best initial test: The presentation of GI, joint, skin, and renal involvement is the best indicator of Henoch-Schönlein purpura.
- Most accurate test: Although a biopsy is the most accurate test, showing deposition of IgA, it is *not* necessary.

Treatment

No specific therapy is necessary because Henoch-Schönlein purpura **resolves spontaneously** over time.

Post-Streptococcal Glomerulonephritis (PSGN)

PSGN results in dark urine, described as "tea colored" or "cola colored." **Periorbital edema** and **hypertension** also occur. Many other infections can lead to glomerulonephritis; both throat and skin infections can lead to PSGN.

Diagnostic Testing

- **Best initial test:** Antistreptolysin O (ASLO), anti-DNase, antihyaluronidase in blood. Complement levels are low.
- **Most accurate test:** Although **biopsy** is the most accurate test, it should *not* be done routinely, because the blood tests are most often sufficient. Biopsy shows subepithelial deposits of IgG and C3.

Treatment

- **Penicillin and other antibiotics** for the infection should be given, although they do *not* clearly reverse the disease.
- Control the hypertension and fluid overload with **diuretics.**

Cryoglobulinemia

This presents in a patient with a history of **hepatitis C with renal involvement.** The patient may have **joint pain and purpuric skin lesions.**

New oral drugs for hepatitis C:

- boceprevir
- telaprevir
- simeprevir
- sofosbuvir

Diagnostic Testing

- Best initial test: **Serum cryoglobulin component levels** (immunoglobulins and light chains, IgM). Complement levels (especially C4) are low.
- Most accurate test: **Biopsy**

Treatment

Ledipasvir and sofosbuvir are used for type 1. Ribavirin is added for treatment-experienced patients. Use sofosbuvir and ribavirin for other genotypes.

Lupus (SLE) Nephritis

The patient presents with a history of SLE. Note that drug-induced lupus spares the kidney and brain.

Diagnostic Testing

- Best initial test: **ANA and anti-double-stranded DNA**
- Most accurate test: **Renal biopsy.** The biopsy in the case of lupus nephritis is very important. It is not to diagnose the presence of renal involvement but to **determine the extent of disease to guide therapy.**

Treatment

- **Sclerosis only:** *No* treatment. This is a "scar" of the kidney.
- **Mild disease, early stage, nonproliferative: Steroids**
- **Severe disease, advanced, proliferative: Mycophenolate mofetil and steroids.** Mycophenolate is superior to cyclophosphamide.

Alport Syndrome

Alport's syndrome is a congenital problem with **eye and ear problems,** such as **deafness.** Renal failure occurs in the second or third decade of life.

There is *no* specific therapy.

Thrombotic Thrombocytopenic Purpura (TTP) and Hemolytic Uremic Syndrome (HUS)

Look for a history of **E. coli 0157:H7 for HUS.** There is no specific diagnostic test for these conditions.

HUS is a triad:

- **Intravascular hemolysis** (fragmented cells on smear)
- **Elevated creatinine**
- **Thrombocytopenia**

TTP has the same 3 findings *plus* the following:

- **Fever**
- **Neurological abnormalities**

Treatment is with plasmapheresis in severe cases.

> Do *not* give platelets for hemolytic uremic syndrome or thrombotic thrombocytopenic purpura. They can make HUS and TTP worse. Also, do *not* give antibiotics for the infection; doing so may worsen the disease.

Nephrotic Syndrome

Any of the glomerular diseases just described can lead to nephrotic syndrome if they are severe. Nephrotic syndrome is often a term of **severity of renal disease.** Hypertension is common.

- When the damage becomes severe enough, the condition leads to the **loss of more than 3.5 g per day of protein in the urine.** When this happens, **albumin levels in the blood fall,** and there is also **edema.**
- **Hyperlipidemia** is a part of nephrotic syndrome.

> **Basic Science Correlate**
>
> LDL and VLDL are removed from serum by lipoprotein signals. If the lipoprotein is lost in the urine with nephrotic syndrome, then the lipid levels in the blood rise.

- **Thrombosis** can occur because of the loss of antithrombin III, protein C, and protein S in the urine.

Nephrotic syndrome is defined as follows:

- **Hyperproteinuria**
- **Hypoproteinemia**
- **Hyperlipidemia**
- **Edema**

Diagnostic Testing

- Best initial test: **Urinalysis showing a markedly elevated protein level**
- The next best test is one of these:
  - **Spot urine for a protein-to-creatinine ratio > 3.5:1.** The spot urine protein creatinine level is equal in accuracy to a 24-hour urine collection.
  - **24-hour urine protein collection showing > 3.5 g of protein**
- Most accurate test: **Renal biopsy**

> Urine protein:creatinine ratio is same as 24-hour urine.

Other Primary Renal Disorders

In addition to the glomerular diseases previously described with systemic manifestations and specific blood tests, there are several primary renal disorders with *no* specific physical findings to make a precise diagnosis. There are features in the history that are suggestive. The following table summarizes specific types of nephrotic syndromes and their associations.

Children	Adults, Cancer Such as Lymphoma	Hepatitis C	HIV, Heroin Use	Unclear
Minimal change disease	Membranous	Membranoproliferative	Focal segmental	Mesangial

Diagnostic Testing

In all of these cases, testing is as follows:

- Best initial tests: **Urinalysis,** followed by **spot protein-to-creatinine ratio** or **24-hour urine**
- Most accurate test: Renal biopsy

Treatment

Treatment for all of these cases is as follows:

- Best initial therapy: **Steroids**
- If there is no response, such as a decrease in urine protein excretion after 12 weeks, **cyclophosphamide** is used.

Proteinuria

At any given time, 2–10 percent of the population has mild proteinuria. The first step when this presents is always to **repeat the urinalysis.** Very often, the proteinuria disappears on repeat testing. These patients need no further follow-up.

If proteinuria persists, you should see if the patient has a reason for transient mild proteinuria, such as the following:

- **CHF**
- **Fever**
- **Exercise**
- **Infection**

If these reasons are not present, the next possibility is **orthostatic proteinuria.** Look for a history of **a job in which people must stand all day,** such as waiters, teachers, security, and so on.

Diagnostic Testing

The first step to confirm orthostatic proteinuria is to **split the urine.** Do a morning urine for protein and then one in the afternoon. If protein is present in the afternoon and not in the morning, then the patient likely has orthostatic proteinuria. Orthostatic proteinuria does *not* need to be treated.

If proteinuria is persistent and not orthostatic, a **24-hour urine** or **spot protein/creatinine ratio** is necessary. If this is elevated, a renal biopsy should be performed.

Steps for proteinuria evaluation:

1. Repeat the UA.
2. Evaluate for orthostatic proteinuria.
3. Get a protein/creatinine ratio.
4. Perform a renal biopsy.

End-Stage Renal Disease

When is dialysis indicated?

Answer: **Dialysis is essential with renal failure in the following circumstances:**

- **Hyperkalemia**
- **Metabolic acidosis**
- **Uremia with encephalopathy**
- **Fluid overload**
- **Uremia with pericarditis**
- **No renal failure, but patient has toxicity with dialyzable drug, such as lithium, ethylene glycol, or aspirin.**
- **Uremia-induced malnutrition**

Phosphate binders:

- sevelamer
- lanthanum
- calcium acetate
- calcium carbonate

The following table summarizes other manifestations of uremia and their treatment.

Hyperphosphatemia	Calcium acetate, calcium carbonate phosphate binders
Hypermagnesemia	Dietary magnesium restriction
Anemia	Erythropoietin replacement
Hypocalcemia	Vitamin D replacement

Hypernatremia

Elevated serum sodium always implies a free water deficit. Dehydration is treated with **normal saline replacement** at first. Step 3 does *not* require knowledge of specific dosing. However, fluids should be first ordered as a bolus, then given continuously.

Besides **simple dehydration,** which can occur from poor oral intake, fever, pneumonia, or other types of increased insensible losses, the other main cause is **diabetes insipidus (DI).** Diabetes insipidus can be caused by either:

- **failure to produce antidiuretic hormone (ADH) in the brain (central);** or
- **insensitivity of the kidney (nephrogenic).** Nephrogenic DI can result from hypokalemia, hypercalcemia, or lithium toxicity.

Hypernatremia leads to **neurological abnormalities,** such as confusion, disorientation, or seizures. The worst manifestation is a **coma.** Sodium disorders do not cause cardiac rhythm disturbance.

Both central and nephrogenic DI give the following results:

- **Low urine osmolality**
- **Low urine sodium**
- **Increased urine volume**
- *No* change in urine osmolality with water deprivation

The following table summarizes specific diagnostic tests and treatment for central DI and nephrogenic DI.

	Central DI	Nephrogenic DI
Urine volume	Prompt **decrease** in urine volume with administration of vasopressin (DDAVP)	**No change** in urine volume with DDAVP
Urine osmolality	Prompt **increase** in urine osmolality with DDAVP	**No change** in urine osmolality with DDAVP
Treatment	Treat with **DDAVP** or **vasopressin**	**Correct underlying cause,** such as hypokalemia or hypercalcemia. **Thiazide diuretics** are used in other cases.

Hyponatremia

Hyponatremia presents with **neurological abnormalities, such as confusion, disorientation, seizures, or coma.** There will be *neither* edema *nor* signs of dehydration.

The first step in the management of hyponatremia is to **assess volume status** to determine the cause and, therefore, the treatment.

Hypervolemic Hyponatremia

Hypervolemic causes of hyponatremia are the following:

- **Congestive heart failure (CHF)**
- **Nephrotic syndrome**
- **Cirrhosis**

These are managed by correcting/managing the underlying cause.

Hypovolemic Hyponatremia

Hypovolemic causes of hyponatremia are the following:

- **Diuretics** (urine sodium elevated)
- **GI loss of fluids (vomiting, diarrhea)** (urine sodium low)
- **Skin loss of fluids (burns, sweating)** (urine sodium low)

The diuretic, sweating, or other cause makes the patient lose water and a little salt, but the patient replaces free water only. Over time the sodium level drops. **Correct the underlying cause and replace with normal (isotonic) saline.** Remember to check serum sodium frequently.

Euvolemic (Normal) Volume Status

This can be caused by the following:

- **Syndrome of inappropriate ADH release (SIADH)**
- **Hypothyroidism**
- **Psychogenic polydipsia**
- **Hyperglycemia:** Glucose above normal drops sodium by 1.6 points for each 100 mg above normal glucose

Addison's Disease

Addison's disease also causes hyponatremia from **insufficient aldosterone production.** The key to this diagnosis is the presence of hyponatremia with **hyperkalemia and mild metabolic acidosis.** Treat with **aldosterone replacement, such as fludrocortisone.**

SIADH

SIADH can be caused by the following:

- Any **CNS abnormalities**
- Any **lung disease**
- Medications such as **sulfonylureas, SSRIs, carbamazepine**
- **Cancer**

SIADH is associated with the following:

- Inappropriately **high urine sodium** (> 20 mEq/L)
- Inappropriately **high urine osmolality** (> 100 mOsm/kg)
- **Low serum osmolality** (< 290 mOsm/kg)
- **Low serum uric acid**
- Normal BUN, creatinine, and bicarbonate

Hyperglycemia causes an artificial drop in sodium by 1.6 points of sodium for each 100 points of glucose.

Treatment

Mild Hyponatremia (no symptoms)

Treat by restricting fluids.

Moderate to Severe Hyponatremia (confused, seizures)

Treat as follows:

- **Saline infusion** with loop diuretics
- **Hypertonic (3 percent) saline**
- **Check serum sodium frequently**
- **ADH blockers (conivaptan, tolvaptan)**

Conivaptan raises sodium as an ADH blocker.

Do not correct serum sodium more than 10–12 mEq/L in the first 24 hours or more than 18 mEq/L in the first 48 hours. Otherwise, you run the risk of **central pontine myelinosis.**

Chronic SIADH (as from malignancy)

Demeclocycline blocks the effect of ADH at the kidney. Conivaptan and tolvaptan are inhibitors of ADH at the V2 receptor of the collecting duct.

Hyperkalemia

Hyperkalemia is predominantly caused by **increased potassium release from tissues, such as muscles, or red blood cells, such as in rhabdomyolysis or hemolysis.** Increased dietary potassium can *only* cause hyperkalemia if it is associated with renal insufficiency. If kidney function is normal, it is almost impossible to ingest potassium faster than the kidney can excrete it. Also, the GI tract is not able to absorb potassium faster than the kidney can excrete it. Aldosterone normally functions to excrete potassium from the body. If there is a **deficiency or blockade of aldosterone,** potassium levels will rise.

Other causes of hyperkalemia are the following:

- **Metabolic acidosis** from transcellular shift out of the cells
- **Adrenal aldosterone deficiency,** such as from Addison's disease
- **Beta blockers**
- **Digoxin toxicity**

- **Insulin deficiency,** such as from diabetic ketoacidosis (DKA)
- **Diuretics,** such as spironolactone
- **ACE inhibitors and angiotensin receptor blockers,** which inhibit aldosterone
- **Prolonged immobility, seizures, rhabdomyolysis, or crush injury**
- **Type IV renal tubular acidosis,** resulting from decreased aldosterone effect
- **Renal failure,** preventing potassium excretion

Basic Science Correlate

Mechanism of Hyperkalemia with Beta Blocker Use

Normal Na/K ATPase activity lowers blood potassium. Beta blockers decrease the activity of the sodium/potassium ATPase. When you inhibit Na/K ATPase with a beta blocker, potassium levels can go up.

Pseudohyperkalemia is an artifact caused by the hemolysis of red cells in the laboratory or prolonged tourniquet placement during phlebotomy. Pseudohyperkalemia does not need therapy; you need only repeat the test.

Hyperkalemia can lead to **cardiac arrhythmia.** Potassium disorders are not associated with seizures or neurological disorders.

Remember: First peaked T-waves occur, then loss of the P-wave, and then the widened QRS complex occurs.

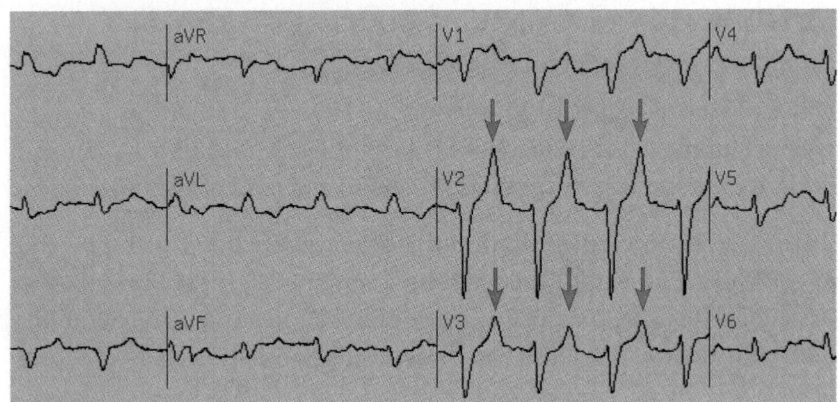

Hyperkalemia Peaked T-Waves

Treatment

Severe Hyperkalemia (EKG abnormalities, such as peaked T-waves)

- Administer **calcium gluconate intravenously** to protect the heart.
- Follow with **insulin and glucose intravenously.**
- Conclude with **kayexalate.**

Moderate Hyperkalemia (no EKG abnormalities)

- Administer **insulin and glucose intravenously.**
- Use **bicarbonate** to shift potassium into the cell when acidosis is the cause of the hyperkalemia or there is rhabdomyolysis, hemolysis, or another reason to alkalinize the urine.
- **Kayexalate** (potassium-binding resin) is administered **orally** to remove potassium from the body. This takes several hours.

Basic Science Correlate

Mechanism of How Bicarbonate Lowers Potassium

When alkalosis pulls hydrogen cations out of cells, another cation must go in to maintain electrical neutrality. As hydrogen ions come out of cells, potassium goes in.

Hypokalemia

Dietary insufficiency can lead to hypokalemia. Other causes are:

- Increased urinary loss caused by **diuretics**
- **High-aldosterone states, such as Conn syndrome**
- **Vomiting** leads to metabolic alkalosis, which shifts potassium intracellularly, and volume depletion, which leads to increased aldosterone.
- **Proximal and distal renal tubular acidosis (RTA)**
- **Amphotericin** from the RTA it causes
- **Bartter syndrome** is the inability of the loop of Henle to absorb sodium and chloride. It causes secondary hyperaldosteronism and renal potassium wasting.

Hypokalemia leads to **cardiac rhythm disturbance.** The EKG will show **"U-waves,"** which have an extra wave after the T-wave indicative of Purkinje fiber repolarization. Hypokalemia can also cause muscular weakness from its **ability to inhibit contraction;** this effect can be so severe that rhabdomyolysis occurs.

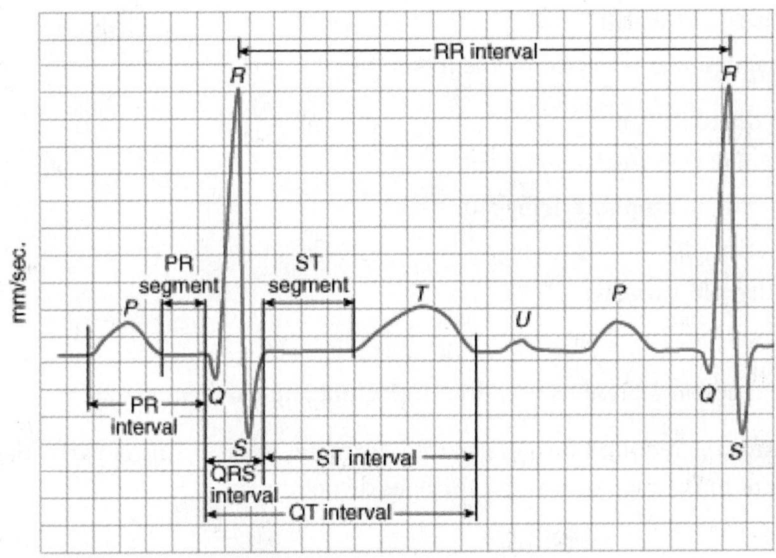

EKG-Normal Intervals

Treatment

Therapy is to **replace potassium.** There is no maximum rate on oral potassium replacement; the bowel will regulate the rate of absorption.

Avoid glucose-containing fluids in cases of hypokalemia. They will increase insulin release and worsen the hypokalemia.

> In hypokalemia cases, IV potassium replacement must be *slow* so as not to cause an arrhythmia with overly rapid administration.

Magnesium Disorders

Hypermagnesemia

Hypermagnesemia is caused by the **overuse of magnesium-containing laxatives** or from **iatrogenic administration,** such as during premature labor when it is administered as a tocolytic. It is rare to have hypermagnesemia without renal insufficiency. Hypermagnesemia leads to **muscular weakness and loss of deep tendon reflexes.**

Treat hypermagnesemia as follows:

- **Restricting intake**
- **Saline administration** to provoke diuresis
- Occasionally **dialysis**

Hypomagnesemia

Hypomagnesemia is caused by the following:

- **Loop diuretics**
- **Alcohol withdrawal, starvation**
- **Gentamicin, amphotericin, diuretics**
- **Cisplatin**
- **Parathyroid surgery**
- **Pancreatitis**

Hypomagnesemia presents with **hypocalcemia and cardiac arrhythmias.**

Magnesium is required for parathyroid hormone release. This is particularly important in the management of torsades de pointes.

Metabolic Acidosis

Metabolic Acidosis with an Increased Anion Gap

This condition is caused by the following:

Lactic Acidosis

This is caused by any form of **hypoperfusion,** such as hypotension, resulting in **anaerobic metabolism.** Anaerobic metabolism leads to glycolysis, which results in the accumulation of lactic acid.

Treat the underlying cause of hypoperfusion.

Aspirin Overdose

Aspirin overdose originally gives **respiratory alkalosis from hyperventilation.** Over a short period, **metabolic acidosis** develops from poisoning of mitochondria and the loss of aerobic metabolism. This gives lactic acidosis.

Treat with **bicarbonate,** which corrects the acidosis and increases urinary excretion of aspirin.

Methanol Intoxication

This toxic alcohol leads to **formic acid and formaldehyde production.** Look for an **intoxicated patient with visual disturbance.**

After **getting a methanol level,** order **fomepizole** or **ethanol** administration. These substances block the production of formic acid and allow time for **dialysis** to remove the methanol.

Uremia

Renal failure prevents the excretion of the 1 mEq/kg of organic acid that is formed each day.

This is an indication for dialysis.

Diabetic Ketoacidosis

Acetone, acetoacetate, and beta hydroxybutyric acid lead to an increased anion gap.

A **low serum bicarbonate** is the fastest single test to tell if a patient's hyperglycemia is life threatening. Treat with normal **saline hydration and insulin.** Place the patient in the **ICU.**

Isoniazid Toxicity

Just **stop the medication** and move the clock forward on CCS.

Ethylene Glycol

Look for an **intoxicated patient with a renal abnormality,** such as oxalate crystals in the urine. There is also renal failure and hypocalcemia, because the oxalate binds with calcium to form crystals. **Suicide attempt with ethylene glycol is key.**

Treat the same as methanol intoxication with **fomepizole** or **ethanol,** which blocks the production of oxalic acid and allows time for dialysis to remove the ethylene glycol.

Metabolic Acidosis with a Normal Anion Gap

This results from either **diarrhea** or **renal tubular acidosis (RTA).**

Diarrhea

Diarrhea causes metabolic acidosis via **increased bicarbonate loss from the colon.** The colon secretes both bicarbonate and potassium, so the potassium level will be low (**hypokalemia**) as well. Because there is increased chloride reabsorption, there is **hyperchloremia,** and that is why there is a normal anion gap.

Renal Tubular Acidosis (RTA)

- **Distal RTA (Type I):** There is an **inability to excrete acid of hydrogen ions in the distal tubule.** This results in the accumulation of acid in the body. The urine pH rises because the body cannot excrete acid. In an alkaline environment, stones will form. **Serum potassium is low** (body excretes + ions in the form of K^+ since it can't excrete H^+) and **serum bicarbonate is low.**
  - Test by **intravenously administering acid** (ammonium chloride—which should lower urine pH secondary to increased H^+ formation). In distal RTA the person cannot excrete the acid, and the urine pH stays abnormally basic.

- Treat by administering **bicarbonate**. The proximal tubule is still working; therefore the patient will still absorb the bicarbonate.

- **Proximal RTA (Type II):** There is an **inability to reabsorb bicarbonate in the proximal renal tubule**. Initially there is an elevated urine pH, but when the body loses substantial amounts of bicarbonate, the **urine pH drops**. Because urine pH is often low, kidney stones do *not* develop. A low serum bicarbonate leaches calcium out of the bones, and there is also **osteomalacia**.
  - Test by giving **bicarbonate**. A normal person with metabolic acidosis will absorb all of the bicarbonate, and there should still be a low urine pH in a normal patient. In proximal RTA, the patient cannot absorb the bicarbonate and the urine pH rises from the bicarbonate malabsorption.
  - Treat by giving a **thiazide diuretic**, which results in a volume contraction. The contracted blood volume raises the concentration of serum bicarbonate. Large quantities of serum bicarbonate are also given (bicarbonate is generally ineffective and that is why they must be used in such high amounts).
- **Hyporeninemic hypoaldosteronism (Type IV):** There is **decreased aldosterone production or effect.** Look for a **diabetic patient with a normal anion gap metabolic acidosis.** This is the *only* RTA with an **elevated potassium level.**
  - Treat with **aldosterone** administration in the form of **fludrocortisone,** which is the steroid with the highest mineralocorticoid content.

The following table compares Types I, II, and IV RTA.

	Distal RTA (Type I)	Proximal RTA (Type II)	Type IV (Diabetes)
Urine pH	High	Low	Low
Serum Potassium	Low	Low	High
Stones	Yes	No	No
Test	Give acid	Give bicarbonate	Urine sodium loss
Treatment	Bicarbonate	Thiazide diuretic **High dose** bicarbonate	Fludrocortisone

Urine Anion Gap (UAG)

The UAG is the way to **distinguish between diarrhea and RTA** as the cause of the normal anion gap metabolic acidosis:

- **UAG = Urine Na^+ – Urine Cl^-**

When acid is excreted from the kidney, it goes out as NH_4Cl. Acid excretion from the kidney goes out with chloride.

If you *can* excrete acid from the kidney, the urine chloride goes up. If the urine chloride is up, then the number (UAG) is negative. **Diarrhea causes a negative UAG**, because the kidney can excrete acid and the net UAG is negative. In metabolic acidosis, a **negative UAG means the kidney works.**

If you *cannot* excrete acid from the kidney, the urine chloride goes down. This gives a positive number (UAG). **In RTA, you cannot excrete acid from the kidney.** The urine chloride will be low, and the **UAG will be positive.**

Metabolic Alkalosis

Volume Contraction

Volume contraction leads to metabolic alkalosis because there is a **secondary hyperaldosteronism,** which causes increased urinary loss of acid.

Treat the underlying cause.

Conn Syndrome or Cushing Syndrome

Hyperaldosteronism resulting from primary hyperaldosteronism (Conn syndrome) or Cushing syndrome causes urinary acid loss.

Surgically remove the adenoma. Also look for **hypokalemia,** which often accompanies the increased urinary acid loss.

Hypokalemia

Hypokalemia causes metabolic alkalosis, because **potassium ions shift out of the cell** to correct the hypokalemia. This shifts hydrogen ions into the cell in exchange for the potassium ions leaving.

Milk-Alkali Syndrome

Metabolic alkalosis occurs from the administration of **too much liquid antacid.**

Vomiting

Vomiting causes a **loss of acid from the stomach.** In addition, the loss of fluids leads to **volume contraction** and secondary hyperaldosteronism.

Cystic Disease

Cystic disease presents with **recurrent hematuria, stones, and infections.** There are **cysts throughout the body,** such as in the liver, ovaries, and circle of Willis; **mitral valve prolapse; and diverticulosis.** The most common site of extrarenal cysts is the **liver.** The most common cause of death is **end-stage renal disease.**

> Subarachnoid hemorrhage is *not* the most common cause of death in cystic disease.

There is *no* specific therapy.

Incontinence

The following table summarizes the presentation, diagnosis, and treatment of incontinence.

	Urge Incontinence	Stress Incontinence
Presentation	Pain followed by urge to urinate	*No* pain
	No relationship to coughing, laughing, or straining	Brought on by coughing and laughing
Testing	Urodynamic pressure monitoring	Observe leakage with coughing
Treatment	• Behavior modification • Anticholinergic medications - Tolterodine - Trospium - Darifenacin - Solifenacin - Oxybutynin	• Kegel exercises • Estrogen cream

Hypertension

A man comes to the office for a routine visit. He is found to have a blood pressure of 145/95. What is the next best step in management?

Answer: Repeat the blood pressure measurement in 1–2 weeks.

Diagnostic Testing

The first step when a case of hypertension presents is to **repeat the blood pressure measurement.** It may take 3–6 measurements to get an accurate assessment of blood pressure.

CCS Tip: Routine tests for hypertension cases on CCS are:

- **Urinalysis**
- **EKG**
- **Eye exam** for retinopathy
- **Cardiac exam** for murmur and S4 gallop

Treatment

If the blood pressure is repeatedly abnormal, initiate lifestyle modifications such as these:

- **Sodium restriction**
- **Weight loss**
- **Dietary modification**
- **Exercise**
- **Relaxation techniques**

What is the most effective lifestyle modification for hypertension?

Answer: **Weight loss**

If lifestyle modifications have no effect over 3–6 months, initiate medical therapy:

- Use a **thiazide diuretic,** such as **hydrochlorothiazide** or **chlorthalidone,** and a calcium blocker or ACE inhibitor.
- In **diabetics,** however, use **ACEI/ARB** as the first-line therapy.

About 60–70 percent of patients will be controlled with one drug. If pressure control is not achieved with the first drug, add a second and possibly a third drug:

- **Beta blocker** (metoprolol, carvelodil)
- **ACE inhibitor**
- **Angiotensin receptor blocker (ARB)**
- **Calcium channel blocker (CCB)**

About 90–95 percent of patients should achieve control with the use of 3 medications. If 2 drugs do not work, **add a third drug. Investigate for causes of secondary hypertension if 3 drugs do not work.**

Compelling Indications for Specific Medications

If any of the conditions in the following table are present, do not start with a diuretic. Go straight to the specific medication.

Thiazides are not better than CCBs, ACEIs, or ARBs as a first drug.

Condition	Medication
Coronary artery disease	Beta blocker
Congestive heart failure	Beta blocker, ACEI, or ARB
Migraine	Beta blocker, CCB
Hyperthyroidism	Beta blocker
Osteoporosis	Thiazide
Depression	*No* beta blockers
Asthma	*No* beta blockers
Pregnancy	Alpha methyldopa
BPH	Alpha blockers
Diabetes	ACEI/ARB

BP target for those age >60 is 150/90.

Thiazides are not better as a first choice than ACE inhibitors, ARBs, or calcium channel blockers. Diabetes alone can be controlled to 140/90. Start with 2 medications if baseline blood pressure is > 160/100. In those over age 60, blood pressure need only be controlled to <150/90.

Secondary Hypertension

Investigate for secondary hypertension if you see the following:

- Young (< 30) or old (> 60) patient
- Failure to control pressure with 3 medications
- Specific findings in the history or physical (see table below)

Specific Findings in the History or Physical

Condition	Finding
Closure of renal artery (stenosis)	Bruit
Pheochromocytoma	Episodic hypertension
Conn syndrome	Hypokalemia
Cushing syndrome	Buffalo hump, truncal obesity, striae
Coarctation of the aorta	Upper extremity > lower extremity pressure
Congenital adrenal hyperplasia	Hirsutism

Renal Artery Stenosis

Look for an **abnormal sound (bruit)** auscultated in the flanks or abdomen. **Hypokalemia** may be present.

Diagnostic Testing

- Best initial test: **Renal ultrasound with Doppler**
- If a **small kidney** is seen, any of the following tests can be done next:
  - **Magnetic resonance angiography (MRA)**
  - **Duplex ultrasonogram**
  - **Nuclear renogram**
- Most accurate test: **Renal angiogram**

Treatment

- Best initial therapy: **Renal artery angioplasty and stenting**

Basic Science Correlate

Diameter and Flow

Flow markedly increases as radius of a tube increases. The flow increases to the fourth power of the radius. For example, if the radius or diameter doubles in size, flow will go up 16 times, or 2 × 2 × 2 × 2.

Oncology

11

For Step 3 in oncology, the most important thing to know *by far* is the **screening tests.**

Which of the following screening tests lowers mortality *the most*?

a. Mammography above age 50
b. Mammography above age 40
c. Colonoscopy
d. Pap smear
e. Prostate-specific antigen (PSA)

Answer: **A.** Mammography above age 50 lowers mortality the most. Although **screening should start at the age of 50,** the mortality benefit is also greatest above the age of 50, because the number of cases of cancer detected will be greater above the age of 50. The age cutoff for mammography is somewhat controversial. Step 3 will likely avoid the issue.

Breast Cancer

Diagnostic Testing

Screening mammography should be done as follows:

- Age 50: Begins
- Age 75: Not routinely indicated above age 75

When a mammogram shows an abnormality, it should be followed up by a **biopsy.** The biopsy will both show the cancer, if present, and allow testing for the presence of **estrogen and progesterone receptors.**

Sentinel node biopsy follows an abnormal mammogram: A dye or tracer is placed into the operative field. The *first* node it goes to is biopsied. This is the "sentinel node."

- If this node is free of cancer, then an axillary node dissection is *not* necessary.
- If the node *does* have cancer, then an axillary lymph node dissection is performed.

BRCA

BRCA genetic testing is *not* a routine screening test. All that can be said for sure about BRCA is:

> Use tamoxifen if 2 or more first-degree relatives have breast cancer.

- BRCA is associated with an **increased risk of familial breast cancer.**
- BRCA is associated with an **increased risk of ovarian cancer.**

Treatment

- Best initial therapy: **Lumpectomy with radiation treatment** of the site at the breast is equal to modified radical mastectomy.
- Primary preventive therapy: **Tamoxifen** should be used in any patient with **multiple first-degree relatives** (mother, sister) with breast cancer. Tamoxifen decreases risk by 50 percent. Start at age 40.

A 42-year-old woman has a 2-cm breast cancer tumor removed by lumpectomy, and the breast is irradiated. The cancer is negative for estrogen receptors and positive for progesterone receptors. Three of 14 nodes removed from the axilla are positive for cancer. What is the next best step in management?

a. Adjuvant chemotherapy and radiation of the axilla
b. Tamoxifen for 5 years
c. Anastrozole (aromatase inhibitor) for 5 years
d. Tamoxifen and adjuvant chemotherapy
e. Oophorectomy and chemotherapy

Answer: **D.** Tamoxifen is used whenever there are either estrogen receptors or progesterone receptors positive. If both receptors are positive, tamoxifen will be of greater benefit. Adjuvant chemotherapy is used whenever the axillary nodes are positive or the cancer is > 1 cm in size.

Hormonal Inhibition Therapy

Tamoxifen or **raloxifene** is used if *either* the estrogen or progesterone receptors are positive. The response is greater if both are positive. Following are the adverse effects of tamoxifen:

- **Deep venous thrombosis (DVT)**
- **Hot flashes**
- **Endometrial cancer**

Aromatase inhibitors are pure estrogen antagonists. They do *not* have the selective estrogen receptor agonist (stimulatory) activity that tamoxifen does. Aromatase inhibitors (anastrozole, letrozole, exemestane) do *not* lead to DVT, but they can lead to **osteoporosis,** because they are antagonistic to estrogen receptors in the bone.

Adjuvant Chemotherapy

Adjuvant chemotherapy is appropriate under the following circumstances:

- Cancer is in the **axilla.**
- Cancer is **larger than 1 cm.**
- It is *more* efficacious when the **patient is still menstruating.** Breast cancer in menstruating women will not likely be controlled with estrogen antagonists, such as tamoxifen or aromatase inhibitors.

Tamoxifen decreases risk of breast cancer. BRCA does not.

Trastuzumab

- A monoclonal antibody against the breast cancer antigen **HER-2/NEU**
- Useful in metastatic disease
- Modest efficacy with few adverse effects

Colon Cancer

The most important knowledge to have for Step 3 is the **screening** schedule and indicators. Colon cancer is treated with **surgical resection of the colon** and **chemotherapy** centered around a **5-fluorouracil** regimen if high-risk stage 2 cancer or stage 3 or more.

The table below shows the recommended screening for colon cancer.

Routine	Single Family Member with Colon Cancer	HNPCC Three Family Members, Two Generations, One Premature (< 50)	Familial Adenomatous Polyposis	Juvenile Polyposis, Peutz-Jeghers, Turcot's Syndrome, Gardner's Syndrome
• Colonoscopy starting at age 50, then every 10 years • Occult blood testing starting at age 50, then yearly	Colonoscopy at age 40 or 10 years earlier than the age at which the family member contracted cancer, whichever is earlier, then every 10 years	Colonoscopy at age 25, then every 1–2 years	Screening sigmoidoscopy at age 12, then every 1–2 years	No additional screening

Screening test for lung cancer: CT scanning has been shown to lower mortality.

Lung Cancer

A 52-year-old smoker has a 1.5-cm calcified nodule found on chest x-ray done for other reasons. He has no symptoms. What should you do?

Answer: **Excisional biopsy** should be done on solitary lung nodules > 1 cm in size in patients who are smokers. Age > 50 lends additional urgency to the need for biopsy. Even though calcification goes against malignancy, the age of the patient, size of the nodule, and history of smoking are more important.

Diagnostic Testing

Lung cancer screening should be performed in all smokers with more than 30 pack-years of smoking history between the ages of 55–75. A chest CT should be performed. Screen long-term smokers with chest CT at age 55.

Treatment

The most important issue in the treatment of lung cancer is whether the **disease is localized enough to be surgically resectable.** Surgery *cannot* be performed if any of the following are present:

- Bilateral disease
- Metastases
- Malignant pleural effusion
- Involvement of the aorta, vena cava, or heart
- Lesions within 1–2 cm of the carina

Small-cell cancer is nonresectable because one of these features is present in > 95 percent of cases.

The size of the lesion alone is *not* the reason a cancer may be unresectable. If the lesion is large but is peripheral, without metastases, it can be resected.

Cervical Cancer

Start Pap at age 21. Repeat every 3 years until age 29. Then do Pap combined with HPV testing every 5 years.

Follow up abnormal Pap smears as follows:

1. Abnormal Pap smears with low-grade or high-grade dysplasia should be followed by colposcopy and biopsy.

2a. If the Pap smear shows atypical squamous cells of undetermined significance (ASCUS), the patient should undergo HPV testing.

2b. If the patient is HPV-positive, then proceed to colposcopy; otherwise, repeat the Pap smear in 6–12 months.

The bottom line on cervical cancer screening is:

- Age 21–65
- Sexual activity is irrelevant.
- For age 30–65, it can be performed every 5 years if combined with HPV testing.

> - Start Pap smears at age 21 regardless of the onset of sexual activity.
> - Frequency should be every 2–3 years until age 65. Or go every 5 years with Pap and HPV test from age 30.
> - Administer HPV quadrivalent vaccine (Gardasil) to all women ages 13–26.

Prostate Cancer

A 65-year-old man comes to you requesting screening for prostate cancer. What should you do?

Answer: Patients requesting screening for prostate cancer should undergo **PSA and digital rectal exam.** Though seemingly self-contradictory, the recommendation is that the physician should not "routinely offer" screening but, if requested, should perform it if the age < 75.

> No PSA testing.

Diagnostic Testing

Prostate-specific antigen (PSA) and digital rectal exam are not proven to lower mortality from prostate cancer. The area of prostate cancer screening is controversial.

> There is *no* proven screening method that lowers mortality for prostate cancer.

Besides the **spread of the disease,** the most important prognostic factor for prostate cancer is the **Gleason score.** The Gleason score is a measure of the level of differentiation of the histology. The higher the score, the more aggressive the cancer.

Treatment

- **Localized prostate cancer: Surgery** and either **external radiation** or **implanted radioactive pellets** are nearly *equal* in efficacy.
- **Metastatic prostate cancer: Androgen blockade** is the standard of care: use **flutamide (testosterone receptor blocker) and leuprolide** *or* **goserelin (gonadotropin-releasing hormone [GnRH] agonists).** There is no particularly good chemotherapy for metastatic prostate cancer. The treatments are hormonal in nature.

Do *not* confuse therapies for prostate cancer with the 5 alpha-reductase inhibitor finasteride. Finasteride treats benign prostatic hypertrophy and male pattern hair loss—not prostate cancer.

What is the fastest way to lower androgen/testosterone levels?

Answer: **Orchiectomy.** We did not say to do it, but this is the fastest way.

A man with prostate cancer presents with severe, sudden back pain. His MRI shows cord compression, and he is started on steroids. What is the next best step in management?

a. Flutamide
b. Flutamide and leuprolide simultaneously
c. Leuprolide followed by flutamide
d. Ketoconazole

Answer: **A.** Flutamide should be started first to block the temporary flare up in androgen levels that accompanies GnRH agonist treatments. When cord compression is described, GnRH agonists, if used too soon, can worsen the compression. Ketoconazole, at a high dose, blocks the production of androgens, but it is not as effective as the other therapies.

Ovarian Cancer

Look for a woman > 50 with **increasing abdominal girth** at the same time as **weight loss.**

Diagnostic Testing

There is *no* routine screening test for ovarian cancer. **CA125** is a marker of progression and response to therapy for ovarian cancer, *not* a diagnostic test.

Treatment

Treatment is **surgical debulking** followed by **chemotherapy,** even in cases of extensive local metastatic disease. Ovarian cancer is unique in that surgical resection is beneficial even when **there is a large volume of tumor spread through the pelvis and abdomen.** Removing all visible tumor still helps.

Testicular Cancer

Presents with a painless **scrotal lump** in a man under 35.

> Testicular cancer is **extremely curable** with a 90–95 percent 5-year survival rate. It is *not* diagnosed by biopsy of the testicle: This is the wrong answer.

Diagnostic Testing

Do *not* do a needle biopsy of the testicle. Simply perform **inguinal orchiectomy** of the affected testicle.

Of all testicular cancers, 95 percent are **germ cell tumors (seminoma** and **nonseminoma).** Alpha fetoprotein (AFP) is secreted *only* by nonseminomas. Measure **AFP, LDH, and beta-hCG.** Stage with a **CT scan of the abdomen and pelvis.**

Treatment

- **Local disease: Radiation**
- **Widespread disease: Chemotherapy.** Chemotherapy can cure even metastatic disease.

Section 2
Preventive Medicine

Cancer Prevention

The single most important oncology question on Step 3 is about prevention. While what you need to know in terms of volume is extremely small, it is very highly tested.

Breast Cancer Screening

The cancer screening test that lowers mortality the most is the **mammogram.** The mortality benefit is greatest in patients > 50 years old. The test should be started in all women > 50.

Routine breast self-examination has *no* proven benefit.

> Mammography guidelines are controversial at this time. Benefit is greatest above age 50.

Cervical Cancer Screening

Cervical cancer screening with Pap smear also lowers mortality. The Pap smear should start at **age 21. This is regardless of the onset of sexual activity,** whichever comes first. Pap smears should be done at least **every 3 years** until age 65, when they can be stopped.

> HPV testing is right for ASCUS. If ASCUS is HPV-positive, do colposcopy.

Summary of Cancer Screening Guidelines	
Breast cancer	Mammography at age 50, then every 1–2 years
Colon cancer	Colonoscopy at age 50, then every 10 years
Cervical cancer	Pap smear at age 21, then every 2–3 years; stop at age 65 unless no previous screening

Colon Cancer Screening

Colon cancer screening is started with a **colonoscopy at age 50** and is performed **every 10 years.**

Other forms of colon cancer screening, such as sigmoidoscopy, barium enema, or stool for fecal occult blood testing, are not as effective in detecting cancer as colonoscopy. Virtual colonoscopy with CT scanning is not accurate.

If a **close family member has had the disease** then screening should begin at 40 or 10 years earlier than the family member was diagnosed, whichever is earlier. **Hereditary nonpolyposis colon cancer syndrome (HNPCC),** known formerly as Lynch syndrome, is defined as colon cancer in 3 family members in 2 generations having the disease, with 1 having it prematurely (defined as occurring before the age of 50). In this case, screening should begin at age 25 and be done every 1–2 years.

Prostate Cancer Screening

There is *no* recommendation to screen patients routinely for prostate cancer with either a prostate-specific antigen (PSA) or a digital rectal examination. There is specific evidence to recommend *against* the PSA for men > 75 on the basis that they will accrue the disadvantages of treatment, such as erectile dysfunction or incontinence, without any benefit.

Lung Cancer Screening

Perform lung cancer screening using CT scan once, at age 55, in long-term smokers with 30 pack-years.

Vaccinations

Influenza and Pneumococcal Vaccine

The indications for influenza vaccination and pneumococcal pneumonia vaccination have a lot of overlap:

- Patients with chronic lung, heart, liver, kidney, and cancer conditions
- HIV-positive patients
- Patients on steroids
- Patients with diabetes

Influenza vaccine is recommended yearly in the general population. It has the **greatest benefit** in the following persons:

- Everyone > 50
- Pregnant women
- Health care workers

Flu vaccine is **acceptable** for everyone yearly.

Pneumococcal vaccine is *different* from influenza vaccine in that:

- It is indicated for all patients > 65
- It is administered as a single injection.

Influenza vaccine is acceptable in everyone in the general population yearly.

Meningococcal Vaccination

Meningococcal vaccination is now routine at **age 11.** Children at especially high risk, who should be vaccinated even earlier, are those with **functional or anatomic asplenia** or those with **terminal complement deficiency.**

HPV Vaccination

This is a quadrivalent vaccine that should be administered to **all females between 13 and 26.** Studies are looking at the benefits of administering the vaccine to women outside this age range, but currently the guideline is ages 13–26. HPV vaccine is acceptable in boys.

Varicella-Zoster Vaccine

Vaccination against the reactivation of varicella-zoster (shingles) should be performed in everyone above age 60. The vaccine is a higher-dose form of the varicella vaccine given to children.

Smoking Cessation

All patients should be screened for tobacco use and advised against it. The most effective method of achieving smoking cessation is the use of **oral medication, such as bupropion and varenicline.** Less effective therapies that can be tried first are **nicotine patches and gums.**

Osteoporosis

All women should be screened with bone densitometry at age 65.

Abdominal Aortic Aneurysm

All men about **age 65** who were **ever smokers** should be screened once with an ultrasound.

Diabetes

Diabetes screening is routine only in those with hypertension

Hypertension

All patients above age 18 should have their blood pressure checked at every office visit.

Hyperlipidemia

Men > 35 and women > 45 should be screened for hyperlipidemia.

Section 3
Dermatology

Bullous and Blistering Diseases

Pemphigus Vulgaris

This is an **autoimmune disease** of unclear etiology in which the body becomes, essentially, allergic to its own skin. Antibodies are produced against antigens **in the intercellular spaces of the epidermal cells.** Its causes are as follows:

- Idiopathic
- ACE inhibitors
- Penicillamine

Pemphigus vulgaris acts like a burn, because the bullae occur from destruction *within* the epidermis and so are **relatively thin and fragile.**

Nikolsky's sign is present: Nikolsky's sign is the easy removal of skin by just a little pressure, with the examiner's finger pulling it off like a sheet. Note that Nikolsky's sign is present in pemphigus vulgaris, staphylococcal scalded skin syndrome, and toxic epidermal necrolysis.

The lesions of pemphigus vulgaris are **painful,** not pruritic.

Diagnostic Testing

The most accurate diagnostic test is a biopsy of the skin.

Treatment

Treatment is as follows:

- Use **glucocorticoids,** such as prednisone.
- When steroids are ineffective, use the following:
  - **Azathioprine**

- **Mycophenolate**
- **Cyclophosphamide**

Bullous Pemphigoid

Pemphigoid can be drug induced by sulfa drugs and others.

The fracture of the skin causing the blisters is **relatively deep,** and the **bullae are thicker walled and much less likely to rupture** than the bullae of pemphigus vulgaris. Oral lesions are rare. Because the bullae are tense and intact, the skin is better protected. There is no dressing for skin as good as the skin. Hence, there is much less fluid loss and infection is much less likely as compared with pemphigus vulgaris. Mortality is much less likely in bullous pemphigoid.

Diagnostic Testing

Test for bullous pemphigoid by performing a **biopsy with immunofluorescent antibodies.**

Treatment

Treatment is as follows:

- Use **systemic steroids,** such as prednisone.
- Alternatives to steroids:
  - **Tetracycline**
  - **Erythromycin with nicotinamide**

The following table compares pemphigus vulgaris and bullous pemphigoid.

	Pemphigus Vulgaris	Bullous Pemphigoid
Age range	30s and 40s	70s and 80s
Severity	Life-threatening	Resolves
Bullae	Thin and fragile	Thick and intact
Mouth involved	Yes	No
Other features	Nikolsky's sign	

Pemphigus Foliaceus

This blistering disease is associated with **other autoimmune diseases,** or it can be **drug induced by ACE inhibitors or NSAIDs.** Foliaceus is much more superficial than pemphigus vulgaris and bullous pemphigoid, and intact bullae are not seen because they break so easily. There are no oral lesions.

Foliaceus is **diagnosed by biopsy** and **treated with steroids** in the same fashion as pemphigus vulgaris.

Porphyria Cutanea Tarda (PCT)

This is a disorder of porphyrin metabolism resulting in a **photosensitivity reaction** to an **abnormally high accumulation of porphyrins.**

The following are associated with PCT:

- Alcoholism
- Liver disease
- Chronic hepatitis C
- Oral contraceptives
- Liver disease, such as chronic hepatitis or hemochromatosis PCT, is associated with increased liver iron stores.
- Diabetes is found in 25 percent of patients.

PCT presents with the following:

- **Nonhealing blisters on the sun-exposed parts of the body,** such as the backs of the hands and the face
- **Hyperpigmentation of the skin**
- **Hypertrichosis of the face**

Diagnostic Testing

Test for **urinary uroporphyrins.** Uroporphyrins are elevated 2–5 times above the coproporphyrins in this disease.

Treatment

Manage this disease as follows:

- **Stop drinking alcohol.**
- **Stop all estrogen use.**
- **Use barrier sun protection.**
- **Use phlebotomy** to remove iron. **Deferoxamine** is used to remove iron if phlebotomy is not possible.
- **Chloroquine** increases the excretion of porphyrins.

Drug Eruptions/Hypersensitivity

Urticaria

Acute urticaria is a **hypersensitivity reaction,** most often **mediated by IgE and mast cell activation,** which results in **evanescent wheals and hives.** It is a type of localized, cutaneous anaphylaxis but without hypotension and hemodynamic instability. The onset of the wheals and hives is usually within 30 minutes and lasts for < 24 hours. **Itching** is prominent.

The most common causes are:

- **Medications** (aspirin, NSAIDs, morphine, codeine, penicillins, phenytoin, and quinolones)
- **Insect bites**
- **Foods** (peanuts, shellfish, tomatoes, and strawberries)
- **Emotions** (occasionally)
- **Contact with latex** (in any form)

Chronic urticaria is associated with:

- **Pressure on the skin:** Pressure on the skin resulting in localized urticaria is also known as **dermatographism.**
- **Cold**
- **Vibration**

Treat urticaria with the following:

- **H1 antihistamines:** Severe, acute urticaria is treated with older medications, such as **diphenhydramine** (Benadryl), **hydroxyzine** (Atarax), or **cyproheptadine.**
- For **life-threatening** reactions, add **systemic steroids.**
- **Chronic therapy:** Treat with newer, nonsedating antihistamines, such as **loratadine, desloratadine, fexofenadine,** or **cetirizine.**
- **Desensitization** is the answer when the **trigger cannot be avoided.** An example of this is a bee sting in a person who is a farmer. Beta blocker medications *must* be stopped prior to desensitization, because they inhibit the epinephrine that may be used if there is an anaphylactic *re*action.

Morbilliform Rash

Morbilliform rash is a milder version of a hypersensitivity reaction than urticaria. This is the **"typical" type of drug reaction** and is usually secondary to medications to which the patient is allergic, such as penicillin, sulfa, allopurinol, or phenytoin. The rash **resembles measles;** it is a **generalized maculopapular eruption that blanches with pressure.** The reaction can appear a few days after the exposure and may begin even after the medication has been stopped.

Morbilliform rash is lymphocyte mediated and is treated with **antihistamines.** Steroids are rarely necessary.

Erythema Multiforme (EM)

Erythema multiforme is caused by the following:

- **Penicillins**
- **Phenytoin**
- **NSAIDs**
- **Sulfa drugs**
- **Infection with herpes simplex or mycoplasma**

This condition presents with **targetlike lesions** that especially occur on the **palms and soles.** These lesions can also be described as "irislike." Bullae are not uniformly found. EM of this type usually does not involve mucous membranes.

Treatment is with **antihistamines** and **treatment of the underlying infection.**

Stevens-Johnson Syndrome (SJS)

It is sometimes difficult to distinguish SJS from toxic epidermal necrolysis (TEN), and, in fact, the 2 diseases may be considered as being on a spectrum of severity of the same disorder.

Disorders along this spectrum may arise as a **hypersensitivity response** to the same set of medications, such as **penicillins, sulfa drugs, NSAIDs, phenytoin, and phenobarbital.** SJS usually involves < 10–15 percent of the total body surface area, and the overall mortality is < 5–10 percent. There is **mucous membrane involvement,** most often of the oral cavity and the conjunctivae, although there may be extensive involvement of the respiratory tract. **Respiratory tract involvement may be so severe as to require mechanical ventilation.** These patients should be managed **in a burn unit.** Death occurs from a combination of infection, dehydration, and malnutrition.

Steroids have *no* proven benefit. Therapies of possible value are intravenous immunoglobulins, cyclophosphamide, cyclosporine, and thalidomide.

Toxic Epidermal Necrolysis (TEN)

TEN is the **most serious version** of cutaneous hypersensitivity reaction.

- Much more of the body surface area (BSA) is involved, up to 30–100 percent.
- Mortality may be as high as 40–50 percent.

Nikolsky's sign is present, and the **skin easily sloughs off.** TEN has certain similar features to staphylococcal scalded skin syndrome. However, TEN is drug induced as opposed to being caused by a toxin coming from an organism. Sepsis is the most common cause of death, but prophylactic systemic antibiotics are *not* indicated.

Diagnosis is with a **skin biopsy.** Systemic steroids are *not* an effective treatment and may, in fact, decrease chances of survival.

Fixed Drug Reaction

This is a **localized allergic drug reaction** that recurs at precisely the same anatomic site on the skin with repeated drug exposure. Fixed drug reactions are generally **round, sharply demarcated lesions that leave a hyperpigmented spot at the site** after they resolve.

Fixed drug reactions can be treated with **topical steroids.**

Erythema Nodosum

This condition presents as follows:

- Painful, red, raised nodules appear on the anterior surface of the lower extremities.
- Nodules are tender to palpation.
- Nodules do not ulcerate.
- Nodules last about 6 weeks.

Erythema nodosum is **secondary to recent infections or inflammatory conditions,** including the following:

- **Pregnancy**
- **Recent streptococcal infection**
- **Coccidioidomycosis**
- **Histoplasmosis**
- **Sarcoidosis**
- **Inflammatory bowel disease**
- **Syphilis**
- **Hepatitis**
- **Enteric infections,** such as *Yersinia*

Treatment is with **analgesics and NSAIDs** and by **treating the underlying disease.**

Infections

Fungal Infections

These are the following:

- **Tinea pedis**
- **Tinea cruris**
- **Tinea corporis**
- **Tinea versicolor**
- **Tinea capitis**
- **Onychomycosis**

Diagnostic Testing

- Best initial test: **Potassium hydroxide (KOH) test of the skin.** The leading edge of the lesion on the skin or nails is scraped with a scalpel to remove some of the epithelial cells or some of the nail and hair. KOH has the ability to dissolve the epithelial cells and collagen of the nail but not the fungus.
- Most accurate test: **Culture the fungus.** Molds that grow on the skin (dermatophytes) take up to 6 weeks to grow, even on specialized fungal media. A specific species usually does not need to be isolated in most cases, unless the infection is of the hair or nails.

Treatment

For onychomycosis (nail infection) or **hair infection** (tinea capitis), the medications with the greatest efficacy are **oral terbinafine or itraconazole.** These medications are used for 6 weeks for fingernails and 12 weeks for toenails.

- **Terbinafine is potentially hepatotoxic,** and it is important to check liver function tests periodically.
- Griseofulvin must be used for 6–12 months and has much less antifungal efficacy than terbinafine.

All of the other fungal infections of the skin that don't involve the hair or nails may be treated with any of the following topical medications:

- **Ketoconazole**
- **Clotrimazole**
- **Econazole**
- **Terbinafine**
- **Miconazole**
- **Sertaconazole**
- **Sulconazole**
- **Tolnaftate**
- **Naftifine**

There is no clear difference in efficacy or adverse effects among them when they are used topically.

When used systemically, **ketoconazole** has the following adverse effects: **hepatotoxicity and gynecomastia.** This is why ketoconazole is not a good choice for onychomycosis.

There is no topical form of fluconazole. Fluconazole also has less efficacy for dermatophytes of the nails when used systemically.

Bacterial Infections

These include the following:

- **Impetigo**
- **Erysipelas**
- **Cellulitis**
- **Folliculitis**
- **Furuncles**
- **Carbuncles**
- **Necrotizing fasciitis**
- **Paronychia**

Treatment

Bacterial skin infections in general (including impetigo, erysipelas, cellulitis, folliculitis, furuncles, and carbuncles) are treated as follows:

- **Dicloxacillin, cephalexin (Keflex), or cefadroxil (Duricef)**
- The intravenous equivalent of dicloxacillin is **oxacillin or nafcillin.** The intravenous equivalent of cefadroxil is **cefazolin.**
- If a patient is allergic to penicillin but the reaction is **only a rash,** then **cephalosporins** can be safely used. There is far less than 1 percent cross-reaction between penicillins and cephalosporins. (The cross-reactivity is actually estimated to be 0.1 percent.)
- If the penicillin reaction is **anaphylaxis,** cephalosporins *cannot* be used. The alternative antibiotics that will treat the skin are **macrolides,** such as **erythromycin, azithromycin, and clarithromycin,** or the **newer fluoroquinolones levofloxacin, gatifloxacin,** or **moxifloxacin.**
  - Ciprofloxacin will *not* adequately cover the skin.
  - Vancomycin is *only* for intravenous use for skin infections. Oral vancomycin is not absorbed and is used only for *Clostridium difficile* intestinal infection.
- Consider using **IV vancomycin** if you suspect methicillin-resistant *Staphylococcus aureus* (MRSA), such as in a nursing home patient or a patient who has been in the hospital for a long time. The oral alternative would be **linezolid or Bactrim.**

Impetigo

This is a **superficial bacterial infection** of the skin limited largely to the epidermis and not spreading below the dermal-epidermal junction. The infection is described as **"weeping," "oozing," "honey-colored," or "draining."** It occurs more often in **warm, humid conditions,** particularly when there is poverty and crowding of children. It is both contagious and autoinoculable. Impetigo can cause glomerulonephritis, but it will not cause rheumatic fever.

Impetigo is more often caused by **Staphylococcus** but is sometimes caused by **Streptococcus pyogenes,** also known as group A *Streptococcus.*

Impetigo is treated as follows:

- Apply **topical antibiotics,** such as **mupirocin.**
- If topical antibiotics are not effective, then **antistaphylococcal oral antibiotics** should be used.

Erysipelas

Erysipelas involves both the dermis and epidermis and is most commonly caused by **group A Streptococcus (pyogenes).** Erysipelas is more likely than other bacterial infections to result in the following:

- Fever, chills, and bacteremia
- Bright red, angry, swollen appearance to the face

Treatment is as follows:

- **Use the systemic oral or intravenous antibiotics previously described.**
- If there is culture confirmation of the organism as *Streptococcus,* then **penicillin G** or ampicillin can be used.

Cellulitis

This is a bacterial infection of the dermis and subcutaneous tissues with *Staph* and *Strep.*

Cellulitis is treated with **the antibiotics previously described,** based on the severity of the disease. If there is **fever, hypotension, or signs of sepsis** or if **oral therapy has not been effective,** then the patient should receive intravenous therapy. **Oxacillin, nafcillin,** or **cefazolin** is the best therapy. Treatment is generally empiric, because injecting and aspirating sterile saline for a specific microbiological diagnosis has only a 20 percent sensitivity. For minor skin infections with MRSA, use TMP/SMZ, doxycycline, or clindamycin.

Folliculitis, Furuncles, and Carbuncles

These 3 disorders represent 3 different degrees of severity of **staphylococcal infection occurring around a hair follicle.** Occasionally, folliculitis can occur from **Pseudomonas** in those who contract it in a **whirlpool or hot tub.** As folliculitis worsens from a simple infection superficially around the hair follicle, it becomes a small collection of infected material known as a **furuncle.** When several furuncles become confluent into a single lesion, it becomes known as a **carbuncle,** essentially a localized skin abscess that must be drained. Folliculitis is rarely tender, while furuncles and carbuncles are often extremely tender.

Treatment is as follows:

- Folliculitis can be treated with **topical mupirocin.**
- Furuncles and carbuncles must be treated with **systemic antistaphylococcal antibiotics,** such as **dicloxacillin** or **cefadroxil.**

Necrotizing Fasciitis

This is an **extremely severe, life-threatening infection** of the skin. It starts as a **cellulitis that dissects into the fascial planes of the skin. Streptococcus and Clostridia** are the most common organisms involved, because they produce a toxin that worsens the damage to the fascia. **Diabetes** increases the risk of developing fasciitis.

Necrotizing fasciitis presents as follows:

- **Very high fever**
- **Portal of entry into the skin**
- **Pain out of proportion to the superficial appearance**
- **Bullae**
- **Palpable crepitus**

Diagnostic Testing

The following diagnostic tests can be used:

- Elevated CPK
- X-ray, CT scan, or MRI that shows air in the tissue or necrosis

All of these laboratory methods of establishing a diagnosis *lack both sensitivity and specificity.* **Surgical debridement** is both the best way to confirm the diagnosis, as well as being the mainstay of therapy.

> If presented with an obvious clinical case with **crepitus,** pain, high fever, and a portal of entry, answer surgery, *not* a test, such as x-ray, as the best initial step.

Treatment

Treat with **beta lactam/beta lactamase combination medications:**

- **Ampicillin/sulbactam (Unasyn)**
- **Ticarcillin/clavulanate (Timentin)**
- **Piperacillin/tazobactam (Zosyn)**

If there is a definite diagnosis of **group A Streptococcus (pyogenes),** then the treatment is with **clindamycin and penicillin.**

Without adequate therapy, necrotizing fasciitis has an **80 percent mortality.**

Paronychia

This is an infection **loculated under the skin surrounding a nail.**

It is generally treated with a **small incision** to allow drainage and **antistaphylococcal antibiotics** as previously described.

Viral Infections

Herpes Simplex

Herpes simplex infections of the **genitals** are characterized by **multiple, painful vesicles.** They are usually obvious by examination, and you should proceed directly to therapy with **acyclovir, famciclovir,** or **valacyclovir.**

Diagnostic Testing

- Best initial test: In the event that the diagnosis is not clear or the lesions have become confluent into an ulcer, then the best initial test is a **Tzanck smear.** The Tzanck smear is somewhat nonspecific in that it will only determine that the infection is in the herpes virus family. Tzanck smears detect multinucleated giant cells and are similar in technique to a Pap smear. A scraping of the lesion is immediately placed on a slide and sprayed with fixative.
- Most accurate test: **Viral culture.** This grows in 24–48 hours.

> The most common wrong answer is serology. Serology is *not* a useful test for diagnosing acute herpes infections.

Treatment

- **Oral acyclovir, famciclovir, or valacyclovir**
- Topical acyclovir has extremely little efficacy.
- Topical penciclovir has some utility for oral herpetic lesions, but it must be used every 2 hours.
- The treatment of acyclovir-resistant herpes is with **foscarnet.**

Herpes Zoster/Varicella

Chickenpox is primarily a disease of children. It is generally *not* treated with antivirals. *If* the child is immunocompromised or the primary infection occurs in an adult, then **acyclovir, valacyclovir, or famciclovir** should be given.

Complications of varicella are the following:

- **Pneumonia**
- **Hepatitis**
- **Dissemination**

Outbreaks of **shingles,** also known as **dermatomal herpes zoster,** occur more frequently in the elderly and those with defects of the lymphocytic portion of the immune system, such as leukemia, lymphoma, or HIV, or those on steroids.

The vesicles are 2–3 mm in size at all stages of development and are on an erythematous base.

Diagnostic Testing

Although Tzanck prep and PCR are the best initial and most accurate diagnostic tests, they are generally *not* necessary, because little else will produce a band of vesicles in a dermatomal distribution besides herpes zoster. PCR is more accurate than viral culture.

Treatment

Treat with the following:

- **Steroid** use is still not clearly beneficial, although the best evidence for its efficacy is in **elderly patients with severe pain.**
- The **rapid administration of acyclovir** still has the best efficacy for decreasing the risk of postherpetic neuralgia.
- Other treatments for managing the pain:
  - **Gabapentin:** The most effective analgesic specifically for postherpetic neuralgia
  - **Tricyclic antidepressants**
  - **Topical capsaicin**
- **Nonimmune adults exposed to chickenpox** should receive **varicella zoster immune globulin within 96 hours** of the exposure for it to be effective.

Sexually Transmitted Diseases (STDs)

Human Papillomavirus (HPV)

Warts caused by HPV, or condylomata acuminata, present as heaped up, translucent, white or flesh-colored lesions on mucous surfaces.

Diagnostic Testing

No form of testing is routinely necessary. Biopsy, scraping, smears, and serology are of *no* definite benefit. There is *no* benefit to routine subtyping of the specific strain of papillomavirus.

Treatment

- **Mechanical removal:** This can involve **cryotherapy** with liquid nitrogen, **laser removal,** or **trichloroacetic acid** or **podophyllin** to melt them away.
- **Imiquimod** is a local immunostimulant that takes several weeks to result in sloughing off of the wart. Resolution is slower; however, there is *never* any damage to the surround normal tissue and *no* pain.
- Podophyllin is potentially teratogenic and should be scrupulously avoided in pregnancy.

Syphilis

Both primary and secondary syphilis present mainly with **cutaneous disorders.**

Primary Syphilis

The chancre of primary syphilis is an **ulceration with heaped-up indurated edges** that is painless the majority of the time.

The best initial test is a **darkfield examination.** This is because there is a false negative rate of 25 percent for both the VDRL and RPR. In other words, these serologic tests need several weeks to become positive, and they are only 75 percent sensitive in primary syphilis.

Both primary and secondary syphilis are treated with a **single intramuscular dose of penicillin.** In those patients allergic to penicillin, **doxycycline orally for 2 weeks** is the alternative therapy.

Secondary Syphilis

Secondary syphilis presents with a generalized copper-colored, maculopapular rash that is particularly intense on the palms and soles of the feet. The other manifestations of secondary syphilis are predominantly dermatologic as well: the **mucous patch, alopecia areata, and condylomata lata.**

The **VDRL and RPR tests** have nearly 100 percent sensitivity in secondary syphilis.

As above, both primary and secondary syphilis are treated with a **single intramuscular dose of penicillin.** In those patients allergic to penicillin, **doxycycline orally for 2 weeks** is the alternative therapy.

Scabies and Pediculosis

Scabies

Scabies involves primarily the **web spaces of the hands and feet** but can also cause **pruritic lesions around the penis and breast. Itching** can be extreme in both cases. Because *Sarcoptes scabiei* is quite small, all that can be seen with the naked eye are the **burrows and excoriations around small pruritic vesicles.** Scabies often *spares* the head.

Immunocompromised patients, such as those with HIV, are particularly vulnerable to an extremely exuberant form of scabies with severe crusting known as "Norwegian scabies."

Diagnostic Testing

Scabies is confirmed by **scraping out the organism after mineral oil is applied to a burrow.**

Treatment

Treatment is with **permethrin.** Lindane has equal efficacy but greater toxicity; thus, it is *not* the best initial therapy. Scabies, particularly Norwegian scabies, can be treated with **ivermectin orally.**

Pediculosis (Lice and Crabs)

Pediculosis **tends to include the head** and is **easily transmitted** by sharing hats and hairbrushes. Both organisms have an enormously high rate of transmission through sexual contact, with 90 percent transmission from a single contact. They are sometimes rust colored from their ingestion of blood.

Diagnostic Testing

Because pediculosis is caused by a much larger organism, scraping is *not* necessary. The organisms can readily be **seen attached to hair-bearing areas,** particularly under magnification.

Treatment

As with scabies, treatment is with **permethrin.** Lindane has equal efficacy but greater toxicity; thus, it is *not* the best initial therapy. Pediculosis can be treated with **over-the-counter pyrethrins.**

Lyme Disease

More than 85 percent of patients who have Lyme disease develop a rash. The **rash must be erythematous with central clearing and be at least 5 cm in diameter.** It usually occurs 7–10 days after the tick bite.

This rash is so characteristic of Lyme that it is more important than serological testing in terms of confirming a diagnosis. If the rash is described, then go straight to therapy with **oral doxycycline, amoxicillin,** or **cefuroxime.** Without therapy,

- two-thirds of these patients will develop **joint disease.**
- a smaller number will develop **neurological or cardiac disorders.**

Toxin-Mediated Diseases

Toxic Shock Syndrome (TSS)

TSS is caused by **Staphylococcus attached to a foreign body.** Nasal packing, retained sutures, or any other form of surgical material retained in the body can promote the growth of the type of *Staph* that produces the toxin.

Diagnostic Testing

Because there is no single specific test, cases are matters of definition. The definition of a case of toxic shock syndrome is as follows:

- **Fever > 102°F**
- **Systolic blood pressure < 90**
- **Desquamative rash**
- **Vomiting**
- **Involvement of the mucous membranes of the eye, mouth, and genitals**

In addition, toxic shock is a systemic disease that

- **raises the creatinine, CPK, and liver function tests;**
- **lowers the platelet count;** and
- can cause **central nervous system dysfunction,** such as confusion.

Treatment

- **Vigorous fluid resuscitation**
- **Pressors,** such as **dopamine**
- **Antistaphylococcal medications,** such as **oxacillin, nafcillin,** or **cefazolin**
- For methicillin- (oxacillin-) resistant strains, **vancomycin** or **linezolid** can be used.

Staphylococcal Scalded Skin Syndrome (SSSS)

SSSS is mediated by a **toxin from Staphylococcus.** It presents with **loss of the superficial layers of the epidermis in sheets** and **Nikolsky's sign.** SSSS differs from other conditions as follows:

- Unlike TSS, SSSS presents with normal blood pressure and no involvement of the liver, kidney, bone marrow, or central nervous system.
- Unlike TEN, which results from drug toxicity, SSSS is caused by an infection. In addition, SSSS only splits off the superficial granular layer of skin and is not a full thickness split, such as in TEN.

This condition should be managed in a **burn unit.** Give **oxacillin/nafcillin** or other antistaphylococcal antibiotics.

Anthrax

Bacillus anthracis is usually a **cutaneous infection** acquired from **contact with infected livestock.** It is an occupational hazard of wool sorters. **Bioterrorism** is also a potential source. A papule appears that later becomes inflamed and develops **central necrosis that is black in color;** hence the name *anthrax,* which is the Greek word for "coal." Of untreated cases, 20 percent are fatal.

The diagnosis is confirmed with **gram stain and culture of the lesion. Ciprofloxacin** or **doxycycline** is the treatment.

Malignant and Premalignant Diseases

Benign Lesions

The predominant method of distinguishing between benign and malignant lesions is by the **shape and color of the lesion. Benign lesions,** such as the junctional or intradermal nevus, have the following characteristics:

- They do not grow in size.
- They have smooth, regular borders.
- Their diameter is usually < 1 cm.
- They are homogenous in color, and the color remains constant.

Biopsy is the most accurate method of making a diagnosis. Benign lesions only need to be removed for cosmetic purposes.

Melanoma

These **malignant** lesions **grow in size, have irregular borders, are uneven in shape, and have inconsistent coloring.**

Biopsy diagnosis is best performed with a full thickness sample, because **tumor thickness** is by far the most important prognostic factor. Treatment of melanoma is by **excision. Interferon** seems to reduce the recurrence rates of melanoma.

Seborrheic Keratosis

This is a **benign** condition with **hyperpigmented lesions occurring in the elderly with a "stuck on" appearance.** They are most common on the face, shoulders, chest, and back.

They are removed with **liquid nitrogen** or **curettage** *only* for cosmetic purposes and have *no* malignant potential. There is *no* relationship to either actinic keratosis or seborrheic dermatitis.

Actinic Keratosis

Actinic keratoses are **precancerous** lesions occurring on **sun-exposed areas of the body in older persons.** They occur more often in those with light skin color. Although they are usually asymptomatic, they can be tender to the touch.

Therapy is universally with **sunscreen** to prevent their progression and recurrence. Lesions should be removed with **cryotherapy, topical 5 fluorouracil (5FU), imiquimod, topical retinoic acid derivatives,** or **even curettage.**

Squamous Cell Carcinoma

Of all skin cancers, 10–25 percent are squamous cell. Squamous cell carcinoma develops on **sun-exposed skin surfaces in elderly patients.** It is particularly common on the lip, where the carcinogenic potential of tobacco is multiplicative. **Ulceration** of the lesion is common. Metastases are rare, with only 3–7 percent of patients developing them.

Diagnosis is with a **biopsy,** and the treatment is **surgical removal.**

Basal Cell Carcinoma

Of all skin cancers, 65–80 percent are basal cell. Basal cell carcinoma has a shiny or "pearly" appearance. The rate of metastases is < 0.1 percent.

The diagnosis is confirmed by **shave or punch biopsy.** Treatment is with **surgical removal. Mohs microsurgery** has the greatest cure rate. In this technique, instant frozen sections are done to determine when enough tissue has been removed to give a clean margin.

Kaposi's Sarcoma

These are **purplish lesions found on the skin predominantly of patients with HIV and CD4 counts < 100.** Human herpes virus 8 is the causative organism.

The best therapy is to **start antiretroviral therapy and raise the CD4 count.** In those in whom this does not occur, the specific chemotherapy for Kaposi's sarcoma is **liposomal Adriamycin and vinblastine.**

Scaling Disorders (Eczema)/Papulosquamous Dermatitis

Psoriasis

Silvery scales develop on the extensor surfaces. Psoriasis can be local or enormously extensive. **Nail pitting** is a common accompaniment. A **Koebner phenomenon** is the development of lesions to the site of an epidermal injury.

Treatment

All patients should use **emollients,** such as Eucerin, Lubriderm, Aquaphor, and Vaseline or mineral oil. **Salicylic acid** is used to remove heaped up collections of scaly material so the other therapies can make contact.

- If the disease is relatively localized, **topical steroids** are used.
- Severe disease also needs **coal tar** or **anthralin derivatives.**
- To avoid the long-term use of steroids, which can cause skin atrophy, and to avoid coal tars, which are messy, one can substitute **topical vitamin D and vitamin A derivatives.** The vitamin D derivative most frequently used is **calcipotriene. Tazarotene** is a topical vitamin A.

When > 30 percent of the body surface area is involved, it is difficult to use topical therapy routinely to control disease. Such patients can be treated with **ultraviolet light.** This is the most rapid way to control extensive disease.

The most severe, widespread, and progressive forms of the disease can be controlled with **methotrexate.** However, this therapy has the highest toxicity and may cause **liver fibrosis.**

The newest therapies are **immunomodulatory biological agents,** such as **alefacept, efalizumab, etanercept, and infliximab.**

Xerosis/Asteatotic Dermatitis

Xerosis and dry skin are managed with **humidifiers and emollients,** such as Lubriderm, Eucerin, Vaseline, Dermasil, mineral oil, or Lac-Hydrin. In those whose skin is especially inflamed, **topical steroids** can be used briefly.

Atopic Dermatitis

This extraordinarily pruritic disorder presents with the following:

- **High IgE levels**
- **Red, itchy plaques of the flexor surfaces**

Treatment

- **Preventive therapy:** Keep the skin moist with emollients, avoid hot water and drying soaps, and use only cotton clothes, because these patients are extremely sensitive to drying.
- **Active disease** is managed with the following:
  - **Topical steroids**
  - **Antihistamines**
  - **Coal tars**
  - **Phototherapy**
  - **Antistaphylococcal antibiotics,** if there is impetiginization of the skin
  - **Topical immunosuppressants,** such as tacrolimus and pimecrolimus, can be used to decrease dependence on steroid use.
  - **Every effort has to be made to avoid scratching.** The topical tricyclic **doxepin** can be used to help stop pruritus.

Seborrheic Dermatitis

An **oversecretion of sebaceous material,** as well as a **hypersensitivity reaction to a superficial fungal organism, Pityrosporum ovale,** underlies seborrheic dermatitis. These patients present with **"dandruff," which may also occur on the face.** Scaly, greasy, flaky skin is found on a red base on the scalp, around the eyebrows, and in the nasolabial fold.

Treatment

- **Low-potency topical steroids,** such as **hydrocortisone**
- **Topical antifungal,** such as **ketoconazole** or **selenium sulfide**
- **Zinc pyrithione** used as a shampoo

Stasis Dermatitis

This is a **hyperpigmentation** that is built up from hemosiderin in the tissue. It occurs over a long period from **venous incompetence of the lower extremities** leading to the microscopic extravasation of blood in the dermis. There is *no* way to reverse this problem.

Prevention of progression is with **elevation of the legs and lower extremity support hose.**

Contact Dermatitis

This is a **hypersensitivity reaction to soaps, detergents, latex, sunscreens, or neomycin** over the area of contact. Jewelry is a frequent cause, as is contact with the metal nickel from belt buckle and wristwatches. It can present as **linear streaked vesicles,** particularly when it is caused by **poison ivy.**

Diagnostic Testing

A definitive diagnosis can be determined with **patch testing.**

Treatment

Treatment is by properly **identifying the causative agent** and with **antihistamines and topical steroids.**

Pityriasis Rosea

This is a **pruritic eruption** that begins with a **"herald patch"** 70–80 percent of the time. It is **erythematous and salmon colored** and looks like secondary syphilis, except that it spares the palms and soles, has a herald patch, and the VDRL/RPR is negative. The lesions on the back appear in a pattern like a Christmas tree (if the observer is especially imaginative).

It is **mild and self-limited** and usually resolves in 8 weeks without scarring. Lesions that are very itchy may be treated with topical steroids.

Acne

Pustules and cysts occur and rupture, releasing free fatty acids that cause further irritation. The contributing organism is *Propionibacterium acnes.* The discharge, although purulent, is odorless.

Treatment

Mild disease is treated with the following:

- **Topical antibiotics,** such as **clindamycin, erythromycin,** or **sulfacetamide.** In addition, the bacteriostatic agent **benzoyl peroxide** is used.
- **Topical retinoids** are used if these attempts to control the load of bacteria locally are ineffective.

Moderate disease is treated with the following:

- **Benzoyl peroxide,** combined with the retinoids **tazarotene, tretinoin, and adapalene.**

Severe cystic acne is treated with the following:

- **Oral antibiotics, such as minocycline, tetracycline, clindamycin, and isotretinoin:** Oral retinoic acid derivatives are **strong teratogens.** Check urine pregnancy test and make sure patients are on oral contraceptives if they are females of childbearing age.

Section 4
Surgery

contributing author Niket Sonpal, MD

Trauma

Airway

Establishing and securing the airway is always the first step in management in any patient with acute trauma or change in mental status. **Altered mental status** is the most common indication for intubation in the trauma patient (unconscious patients can't maintain their airways). The exam will want you to know the *best* step in securing an airway.

- **Orotracheal intubation** is the preferred method of securing an airway.
- If the case describes **trauma with cervical spine injury,** orotracheal intubation can still be performed with manual cervical immobilization. The best answer is **the use of a flexible bronchoscope.**
- If the case describes **extensive facial trauma and bleeding into the airway** (listen for gurgling sounds), **cricothyroidotomy** is the best answer. **Percutaneous tracheostomy** is also acceptable.

Breathing

Always check the oxygen saturation. If the saturation is < 90 percent, do the following:

- Obtain an **arterial blood gas (ABG).**
- **Determine likely causes of hypoxia** based on the history.

Basic Science Correlate

Normal PCO2 = 40
Normal bicarb = 24

Circulation

Chest Trauma

Circulatory disturbances in the setting of trauma may have 1 of 3 major causes. In the exam, you will need to determine quickly the likely cause to institute prompt therapy.

Do *not* be distracted by head trauma or dilated pupils in a hypotensive trauma patient. Intracranial bleeds are *never* the cause of hypotensive shock. The first step in management is to identify and control the site of bleeding.

1. **Hypovolemic shock** is the most common type of shock.
   - Look for a source of bleeding. (The patient may lose a large volume of blood in the abdomen or thigh following diaphyseal fracture of the femur.)

Basic Science Correlate

In hypovolemic shock:

- Right atrial pressure is decreased.
- Pulmonary capillary wedge pressure is decreased.
- Cardiac index is decreased.
- Systemic vascular resistance is increased.
- Mixed venous saturation is decreased.

2. **Pericardial tamponade** and **tension pneumothorax** can both result from thoracic trauma.
   - Both result in **distended neck veins,** or a high central venous pressure (CVP).

Pericardial tamponade involves the following:

- An **enlarged heart** on chest x-ray.
- Immediately perform pericardiocentesis. If unsuccessful, proceed with pericardial window.
- **Electrical alternans** on EKG.
- **Pulsus paradoxus** on vital signs.

3. **Tension pneumothorax:**
   - Look for **respiratory distress, tracheal deviation, absent breath sounds, and hyperresonance to percussion.**
   - Immediately place a **large-bore needle or IV catheter** into the pleural space at the second intercostal space. *Then* place a **chest tube.**
   - *Never* wait for a chest x-ray for diagnosis.

Abdominal Trauma

A 24-year-old male with a history of gang violence presents to the emergency room with 3 stab wounds to the abdomen. He was intubated in the field for airway protection and is barely conscious. Blood pressure is 70/30 mm Hg and pulse is 140/min. On exam, 3 penetrating wounds covered by abdominal pressure pads are noted. Which of the following is the best next step in management of this patient?

a. Direct pressure to the abdomen
b. Abdominal x-ray
c. IV fluids
d. IV antibiotics
e. Obtain consent for surgery

Answer: **C.** This patient is in hemorrhagic shock and requires immediate resuscitation. Of the choices listed, the best next step in management is IV fluids after obtaining venous access. The best form of venous access is 2 large-bore IVs in the periphery and/or central venous access. Applying direct pressure to the abdomen (a) does not treat the underlying cause. Getting an abdominal x-ray (b) will take too long for a patient with this rate of blood loss. IV antibiotics (c) may be needed later in the care of this patient, but stabilizing blood pressure is now the more urgent need. Surgical consent (e) is implied in a life-threatening emergency in which a patient cannot communicate his wishes.

Management of circulatory disturbances in cases of abdominal trauma involves the following:

- While doing your initial survey of the patient, it is imperative to simultaneously **control the site of bleeding**.
  - Apply **direct local pressure** when the site is visible (e.g., extremity).
  - Blind clamping and the use of a tourniquet is *never* the answer.
- **Fluid resuscitation** is always the best next step in management in a patient who is hemodynamically unstable.
- Do several things at once in **preparation for immediate exploratory laparotomy:**
  - Set up 2 large-gauge IV lines
  - Give fluids and blood
  - Type and screen
  - Insert Foley catheter
  - Administer IV antibiotics.
- **If surgery isn't needed** (e.g., blunt trauma), **fluid resuscitation is the first step in management and is also diagnostic.** (If the patient responds promptly, then he's probably no longer bleeding.)

> Intraosseous cannulation in the proximal tibia is used in children (generally < 6 years old). Give an initial bolus of Ringer's lactate at 20 mL/kg of body weight.

Vasomotor Shock

Vasomotor shock is the cause of hypotension and tachycardia in patients who are **warm and flushed** (rather than pale and cold). Look for a history of **medication use** (e.g., penicillin that may have triggered a penicillin allergy), **spinal anesthesia,** or **exposure to allergen** (e.g., bee sting).

> **Basic Science Correlate**
>
> On exposure to an foreign substance, IgE binds to the antigen, forming an antigen-antibody complex. This complex activates the high-affinity receptor for the Fc region of immunoglobulin E (FcεRI), leading to mast cell and basophil degranulation and the release of inflammatory mediators such as histamine. These mediators cause vasodilation, bronchoconstriction, tachycardia, and swelling.

The first step in management is to administer **vasoconstrictors and fluids.**

Trauma to Localized Sites

All penetrating wounds with damage to internal organs will need to go to the OR. If the case describes an object embedded in the patient, *never* remove it in the ER or at the scene of the accident.

> All impaled objects are to be removed in the OR under a controlled setting.

Head Trauma

Management Steps for the Exam

A man was hit over the head with a baseball bat during a mugging. He has a scalp laceration and a linear skull fracture on CT scan. He denies loss of consciousness. There are no neurological signs on exam. Is surgery indicated?

Answer: No surgical intervention is needed for an **asymptomatic head injury with a closed skull fracture** (no overlying wound) alone. The next step in management is to **clean any lacerations.**

A woman was hit over the head with a baseball bat during a mugging. She has a scalp laceration, and a comminuted, depressed fracture is seen on CT scan. She denies loss of consciousness. There are no neurological signs on exam. Is surgery indicated?

Answer: **Surgery** (repair or craniotomy) is always done for **comminuted** or **depressed skull fracture,** even if the patient is asymptomatic. Send the patient to the OR.

A man is hit over the head with a baseball bat during a mugging. He reports "being out of it for a few seconds," but then he came to without any symptoms. There are no neurological signs on exam. What is the next step in management? He wants to go home—what will you tell him?

Answer: For **head trauma and loss of consciousness,** the first step in management is to order a **CT of the head and neck without contrast.** If the head CT and neurological exam are normal, he can go home if someone can closely observe him over the next 24 hours (i.e., wake him up frequently and watch for changes in mentation).

Give **tetanus toxoid and prophylactic antibiotics** to *all* patients with open skull fractures.

Basal Skull Fracture

Look for ecchymosis around both eyes **(raccoon eyes)** or behind the ear **(Battle's sign)** or **clear fluid dripping from the ear or nose** (cerebrospinal fluid [CSF] leak).

Management of this injury involves:

- **CT scan of the head and neck** (which will show a basal skull fracture). X-ray is *not* the correct answer.
- A CSF leak will stop by itself and requires no specific management. Prophylactic antibiotics are *not* indicated.
- **Facial palsy** may occur 2–3 days later due to neurapraxia.

Epidural Hematoma

A 14-year-old boy is hit over the side of the head with a baseball bat. He loses consciousness for a few minutes, but he recovers promptly and wishes to continue playing. He is brought to the ER; the CT is shown in image below. The patient has no complaints and has no neurologic dysfunction on exam.

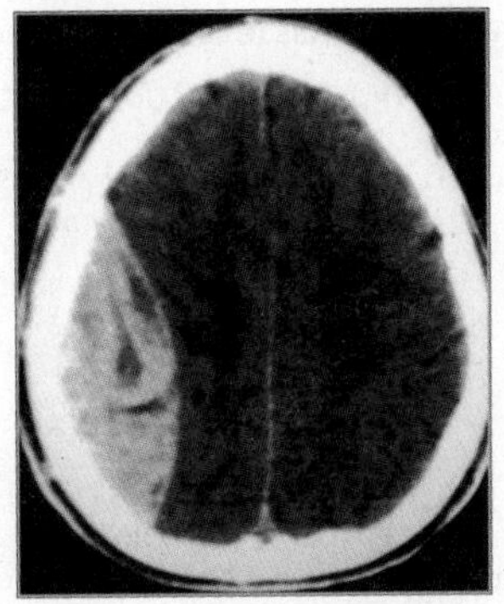

What is the next step in management?

a. Admit and observe for 24 hours.
b. Perform emergency craniotomy.
c. Give mannitol.
d. Send the patient home with frequent neurological checks.

Answer: **B.** The patient is at risk of sudden deterioration. Emergency craniotomy is needed for all epidural hematomas.

> Epidural → biconvex → middle meningeal artery → lucid interval

Epidural hematomas present with **trauma** and **sudden loss of consciousness.** The period when the patient immediately awakes and appears normal is referred to as the lucid interval, but then the patient quickly deteriorates. It is important to move quickly.

- **Diagnosis: CT scan** shows a **lens-shaped hematoma** with or without midline deviation.
- **Management:** Perform an **emergency craniotomy.** If the patient is treated, the prognosis is good; if not, epidural hematoma is fatal within hours.

> Subdural → crescent shaped → bridging veins → gradual loss of consciousness

Basic Science Correlate

The middle meningeal artery is the third branch of the maxillary artery, which is a branch of the external carotid artery.

Chronic Subdural Hematoma

Bleeding is low pressure from the venous system. Suspect chronic subdural hematoma in cases of **head trauma with fluctuating consciousness** (gradual headaches, memory loss, personality changes, dementia, confusion, and drowsiness).

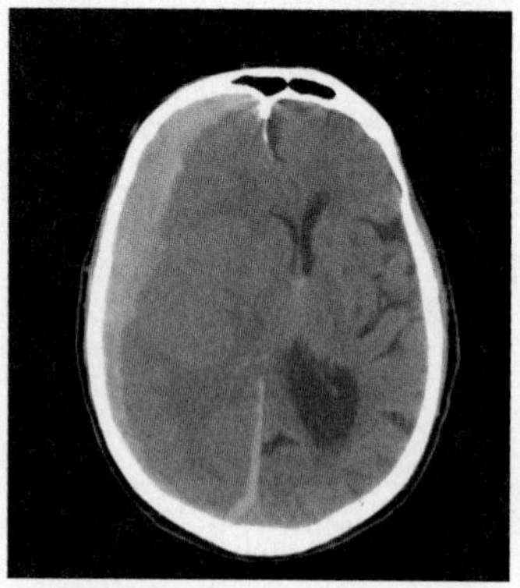

Subdural Hematoma

- **Diagnosis: CT scan** shows **semilunar, crescent-shaped hematoma** with or without midline deviation.
- **Management:** Emergency craniotomy is done only if there are lateralizing signs and midline displacement.

> **Basic Science Correlate**
>
> Bridging veins drain the neural tissue and puncture through the dura mater to empty into the dural sinuses.

> To rule out bleeds in the brain, order CT scans **without contrast**. Blood and contrast look the same on CTs, giving a false positive.

Diffuse Axonal Injury

Diffuse axonal injury results from **acceleration-deceleration injuries to the head.** The patient will be deeply unconscious.

- **Prognosis is terrible,** and surgery *cannot* help.
- Therapy is directed at **preventing further injury** from increased intracranial pressure (ICP).

Elevated Intracranial Pressure (ICP)

The classic history proceeds as follows:

1. **Briefly depressed consciousness after head trauma**
2. **Improvement**
3. **Progressive drowsiness**

Elevated intracranial pressure is a **medical emergency.**

Diagnostic Testing

- **Gradual dilatation of one pupil and a decreasing responsiveness to light** is an important sign, as it indicates clot expansion on the ipsilateral hemisphere.
- Get a head CT and look for midline shift or dilated ventricles.
- Do *not* think about performing a lumbar tap in anyone *without* first getting a head CT. If you perform a lumbar puncture on a person with increased intracranial pressure, you will herniate the brain, kill the patient, and fail the exam.

> **Basic Science Correlate**
>
> Hyperventilation causes vasoconstriction and decreased blood volume in the brain, lowering ICP.

Steroids are good for cerebral edema secondary to tumors and abscesses, but they have *no* role in head trauma patients.

Management

- **First-line measures** are the following:
  - **Head elevation**
  - **Hyperventilation**
  - **Avoid fluid overload**
- **Second-line measures** are the following:
  - **Mannitol:** Use *very* cautiously; it can reduce cerebral perfusion.
  - **Sedation and/or hypothermia:** These lower oxygen demand.

Basic Science Correlate

Mannitol is filtered by the glomeruli but not reabsorbed from the renal tubule. The result is decreased water and Na+ reabsorption, which subsequently leads to decreased extracellular fluid volume.

Caution! Do *not* overdo the treatment for elevated intracranial pressure. Lowering ICP is *not* the ultimate goal; **preserving brain perfusion** is. Systemic hypotension or excessive cerebral vasoconstriction may be counterproductive.

General Surgery

Acute Abdomen

The 4 main causes of an acute abdomen are these:

1. Perforation
2. Obstruction
3. Inflammatory/infection
4. Ischemia

The most important question to ask yourself when presented a case of an acute abdomen is **when to operate and when to treat medically.**

Primary peritonitis is spontaneous inflammation in children with nephrosis or an adult with ascites and mild abdominal pain (even if there is fever and leukocytosis).

When is **surgery** the answer?

- **Peritonitis** (excluding primary peritonitis)
- **Abdominal pain/tenderness plus signs of sepsis**
- **Acute intestinal ischemia**
- **Pneumoperitoneum**

In all of the above cases, make sure pancreatitis is first ruled out.

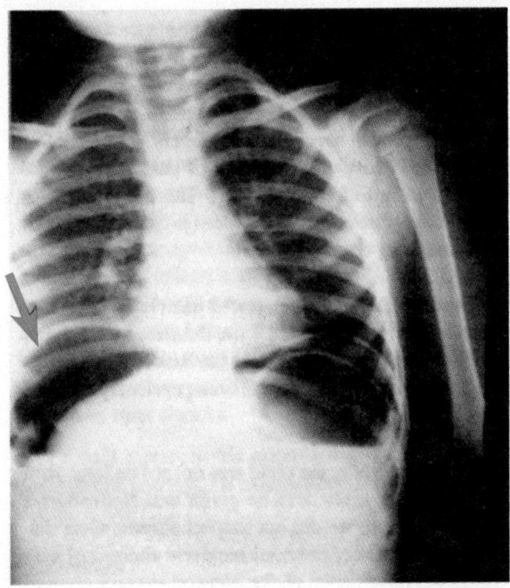

Pneumoperitoneum in a child with perforated small bowel

Cholangitis is a gastrointestinal **medical emergency**, and intervention with an emergency ERCP is the treatment of choice.

When is **"treat medically"** the answer?

- **Primary peritonitis**
- **Pancreatitis**
- **Cholangitis**
- **Urinary stones**
- Things that can mimic an acute abdomen:
  - **Lower lobe pneumonia:** Look for infiltrate on chest x-ray.
  - **Myocardial ischemia:** Look for EKG changes.
  - **Pulmonary embolism:** Always suspect this in any immobilized patient.
- **Ruptured ovarian cysts**

Nonsurgical causes of an acute abdomen are the following:

- Myocardial infarction, acute pericarditis
- Lower lobe pneumonia, pulmonary infarction
- Hepatitis, GERD
- DKA, adrenal insufficiency
- Pyelonephritis, acute salpingitis
- Sickle cell crisis
- Acute porphyria

Be careful to differentiate GERD from peptic ulcer perforation, which *is* a surgical emergency.

Perforation

Gastrointestinal Perforation

The question will describe **acute abdominal pain that is sudden, severe, constant, and generalized.** Pain is excruciating with any movement (it may be blunted in elderly patients). The most common causes of gastrointestinal perforation are these:

- **Diverticulitis:** Elderly patient with lower abdominal pain and fever
- **Perforated peptic ulcer:** Epigastric pain that classically wakes patient at night and, possibly, referred pain to the scapula
- **Crohn's disease**

Diagnostic Testing

Diagnose with an **erect chest x-ray** (free air under diaphragm, or falciform ligament) or **left lateral decubitus x-ray** if patient is too sick to stand up.

Treatment

Management is as follows:

- Order **nothing by mouth (NPO) and IV fluid hydration.**
- IV antibiotics such as:
  - metronidazole and Cipro
  - second-generation cephalosporins (cefotetan or cefoxitin)
  - ampicillin-sulbactam
  - piperacillin-tazobactam

Basic Science Correlate

Metronidazole covalently binds to DNA. This disrupts its helical structure, inhibits bacterial nucleic acid synthesis, and results in bacterial death.

- Perform **emergency surgery.**

Esophageal Perforation

Classic presentation for perforation is after endoscopy.

The most common cause of esophageal perforation is **iatrogenic.** The case will describe the following:

- Pain in chest or upper abdomen
- Dysphagia or odynophagia
- Subcutaneous emphysema shortly after endoscopy

Esophageal perforation is a **surgical emergency. Gastrografin contrast esophagram** is the first study of choice (do *not* use barium).

Obstruction

Suspect obstruction in patients with the following symptoms:

- **Severe colicky pain**
- **Absence of flatus or feces**
- **High-pitched bowel sounds**
- **Nausea and vomiting** in patients with these **risk factors:**
  - Prior surgery (think adhesions)
  - Elderly patient with weight loss and anemia or melanotic stools (think tumor)
  - History of recurrent lower abdominal pain (think diverticulitis)
  - History of hernia (incarcerated hernia)
  - Sudden abdominal pain in elderly patient (don't forget about volvulus)
- **Constant movement,** as the patient tries to find a position of comfort

Diagnostic Testing

- **CBC and lactate level (elevated)**
- **Supine and erect abdominal x-ray:** Look for dilated loops of bowel, absence of gas in rectum, bird's beak sign for volvulus.
- **CT scan of the abdomen and pelvis with contrast** is the most accurate test, and can at times show a transition point. The transition point is the location at which the obstruction has occurred.

In a patient with a hernia, immediate surgery is the answer *if* the case describes fever, leukocytosis, constant pain, and signs of peritoneal irritation (think strangulated obstruction).

Treatment

- **NPO, nasogastric (NG) suction, and IV fluid hydration**
- Consider **gastrografin contrast study** (until perforation has been ruled out).

Basic Science Correlate

Gastrografin is water soluble, unlike barium, which is caustic if it extravasates.

- **Volvulus:** Perform **proctosigmoidoscopy** with rigid instrument. Leave the rectal tube in place. Perform **sigmoid resection** for recurrent cases.
- **Abdominal hernias:** Perform **elective repair** for all abdominal hernias, *except* umbilical hernia in patients < 2 years old and esophageal sliding hiatal hernia.
- **All other obstructions:** Perform **emergency surgery.**

Inflammation

Inflammatory causes of acute abdomen include the following:

- **Acute diverticulitis**
- **Acute pancreatitis**
- **Acute appendicitis**

The question will describe the following:

- Gradual onset of constant abdominal pain that slowly builds up over several hours
- Initially ill-defined pain that eventually becomes localized to the site of inflammation
- Note that signs of peritoneal irritation are absent in pancreatitis.

When diagnosing acute diverticulitis, don't forget to order a **urine pregnancy test** on *all* women of childbearing age.

Acute Diverticulitis

Acute diverticulitis is one of the very few inflammatory processes presenting with acute abdominal pain in the **left lower quadrant.** Look for a patient in **middle age or older with fever, leukocytosis, and peritoneal irritation in the left lower quadrant with a palpable tender mass.** In women, think about fallopian tube and ovaries as potential sources.

Basic Science Correlate

The common location for diverticulosis is the sigmoid colon. This is because it has the smallest diameter and therefore the highest intraluminal pressure. Concurrently, the sigmoid has the highest degree of diverticulitis.

Colonoscopy is **absolutely contraindicated** in acute diverticulitis, as it raises the risk of perforation.

Diagnostic Testing

The most accurate diagnostic test is CT with contrast to look for abscess or free air. Fat stranding is common around the inflamed bowel.

Look out for the risk factors for acute pancreatitis:

- Alcoholism
- Gallstones
- Medications (didanosine, pentamidine, Flagyl, tetracycline, thiazides, furosemide)
- Hypertriglyceridemia
- Trauma
- Post-ERCP

Treatment

- **No peritoneal signs:** Manage as outpatient with antibiotics.
- **Localized peritoneal signs and abscess:** Admit the patient. Order NPO, IV fluids, IV antibiotics, and CT-guided percutaneous drainage of the abcess.
- **Generalized peritonitis or perforation:** Perform *emergency* surgery.
- **Recurrent attacks of diverticulitis:** Perform *elective* surgery.

Acute Pancreatitis

Suspect this in the **alcoholic** who develops an **acute (over several hours) upper abdominal pain, radiating to the back, with nausea and vomiting.** Acute pancreatitis may be

- **edematous,**
- **hemorrhagic,** or
- **suppurative** (pancreatic abscess).

Late complications include **pancreatic pseudocyst and chronic pancreatitis.**

Diagnostic Testing

Diagnose with a **serum or urinary amylase or lipase** (serum from 12 to 48 hours, urinary from 3rd to 6th days). Perform a **CT** if diagnosis is uncertain.

Warning signs for **hemorrhagic pancreatitis** are the following:

- Lower hematocrit that continues to fall the day after presentation
- Very high WBC (> 18,000), glucose, BUN
- Very low calcium

Basic Science Correlate

Pancreatitis can lead to low calcium levels due to the presence of insoluble calcium salts in the pancreas. The free fatty acids avidly chelate the salts, resulting in calcium deposition in the retroperitoneum.

Treatment

Treat with **NPO, NG suction, and IV fluids.**

Complications can include the following:

- **Abscess:** Often appears 10 days after onset with persistent fevers and high WBC count. **Surgical drainage** is the treatment.
- **Pseudocyst:** Appears 5 weeks after initial symptoms, when a collection of pancreatic juice causes anorexia, pain, and a palpable mass.
  - If **painless**: Do not drain.
  - If **painful** *and* > 6 cm *and* > 6 weeks: Perform **surgical internal drainage** or **endoscopic drainage**. If infected, **percutaneous external drainage** is performed.
- **Chronic damage:** Causes diabetes and steatorrhea. Treat with **insulin and pancreatic enzyme supplements.**

Amylase = highest sensitivity
Lipase = highest specificity

Acute Appendicitis

Acute appendicitis presents as follows:

- It classically begins with **anorexia**
- This is followed by vague **periumbilical pain,** which several hours later becomes sharp, severe, constant, and localized to the **right lower quadrant of the abdomen.**
- **Tenderness, guarding, and rebound are found to the right and below the umbilicus** (but not elsewhere in the belly).

Rovsing's sign: palpation of LLQ increases the pain felt in RLQ

Diagnostic Testing

- Look for **fever and leukocytosis in the 10,000–15,000 range,** with neutrophilia and immature forms.
- If diagnosis is unclear by clinical history and exam, the best imaging study is **CT scan**; less optimal is **ultrasound** of the abdomen.

Treatment

- Administer **IV antibiotics before appendectomy**:
  - Cipro *and* metronidazole
  - Ampicillin/sulbactam
  - Levofloxacin *and* clindamycin
  - Cefoxitin *or* cefotetan
- If appendix is **perforated, continue IV** until fever and WBC count have normalized.

Chronic Ulcerative Colitis (CUC)

CUC is managed medically. *Elective* surgery is the answer under the following conditions:

- Disease has been **present more than 20 years** (high incidence of malignant degeneration).
- There have been **multiple hospitalizations.**
- The patient needs chronic **high-dose steroids** or **immunosuppressant.**
- There is **toxic megacolon** (abdominal pain, fever, leukocytosis, epigastric tenderness, massively distended transverse colon on x-rays with gas within the wall of the colon).

Basic Science Correlate

Ulcerative colitis extends from the anal verge in an uninterrupted pattern to the entire colon.

Ischemia

Always consider the following:

- Acute mesenteric ischemia in older patients
- History of arrhythmia (atrial fibrillation)
- Coronary artery disease
- Recent MI

> **Basic Science Correlate**
>
> The intestine is supplied by 3 major gastrointestinal arteries that arise from the abdominal aorta: the celiac axis, the superior mesenteric artery (SMA), and the inferior mesenteric artery (IMA).

Classically, **pain is out of proportion to the exam.** Diagnosis is clinical but look for acidosis and signs of sepsis. If ischemia is suspected, do *not* wait for lab findings (acidosis, elevated lactate); go straight to **surgery** or **order angiography.**

- If diagnosis is during surgery: **Perform embolectomy and revascularization or resection.**
- If diagnosis is during angiography: **Give vasodilators** or **thrombolysis.**

CCS Tip: When you think a patient has an acute abdomen or one that may become acute, make sure to get a *surgical consultation* on the CCS. The consultation will not offer useful information; the test is checking if you know to get surgery involved.

> **Basic Science Correlate**
>
> The most common vessel affected is the superior mesenteric artery, due to the acuity of its angle and because it is a direct branch off the aorta.

Abscess

Intra-Abdominal Abscess

Consider the possibility of an abscess in any patient with a **history of a previous operation, trauma, or intra-abdominal infection/inflammation.** Abscesses can occur anywhere in the abdomen or retroperitoneum.

Diagnostic Testing

Diagnose with a **CBC and a contrast CT of the abdomen/pelvis.**

Treatment

- Always **drain an intra-abdominal abscess** (either surgically or percutaneously).
- Give **antibiotics** to prevent spread of infection (does not cure abscess).

Surgical Jaundice

Obstructive Jaundice Caused by Stones

The question will describe an **obese, fecund woman in her 40s** with the following signs:

- **Recurrent episodes of abdominal pain**
- **High alkaline phosphatase**
- **Dilated ducts on sonogram**
- **Nondilated gallbladder full of stones**
- **Direct hyperbilirubinemia**

Basic Science Correlate

The common hepatic duct and cystic duct merge to form the common bile duct, which merges with the pancreatic duct and allows enzyme and bile exit through the sphincter of Oddi.

ERCP and EUS are never the first step in diagnosis. ERCP is most often a management step on the exam.

Diagnostic Testing

1. Order a **sonogram.**
2. Confirm with **endoscopic ultrasound** (**EUS**) or **magnetic resonance cholangiopancreatography** (**MRCP**).

Treatment

1. Perform **endoscopic retrograde cholangiopancreatography** (**ERCP**) with sphincterotomy.
2. **Cholecystectomy** should follow.

Obstructive Jaundice Caused by Tumor

In patients with progressive symptoms in the preceding weeks and weight loss, suspect a **tumor:**

- Adenocarcinoma at the head of the pancreas
- Adenocarcinoma of the ampulla of Vater
- Cholangiocarcinoma arising in the common duct itself

Diagnostic Testing

- Sonogram
- CT scan
  - For lesions seen on CT scan, obtain a tissue diagnosis via EUS.
  - If no lesion is seen on CT scan, order an MRCP (shows ampullary or common bile duct tumors not seen on CT scan) and obtain tissue diagnosis via ERCP.

Treatment

Management is with **surgical resection.**

Gallstones

Biliary Colic

Temporary occlusion of the cystic duct causes **colicky pain in the right upper quadrant, radiating to the right shoulder and back,** often triggered by **fatty food.** Episodes are **brief** (20 minutes), and there are *no* signs of peritoneal irritation or systemic signs.

Diagnosis is with a **sonogram.**

Treatment is with *elective* **cholecystectomy.**

Acute Cholecystitis

Persistent occlusion of the cystic duct from a stone causes **constant pain,** as well as **fever, leukocytosis, and peritoneal irritation in the right upper quadrant.**

Murphy's sign: pain on palpation of RUQ during inhalation

Diagnosis is with a **sonogram,** which will show gallstones, a thick-walled gallbladder, and pericholecystic fluid.

Treatment is as follows:

1. **NG suction, NPO, IV fluids, and antibiotics**
2. These are followed by **cholecystectomy** (after 6–12 weeks).

Emergency cholecystectomy is needed if there is **generalized peritonitis** or **emphysematous cholecystitis** (suggestive of perforation or gangrene).

Acute Ascending Cholangitis

Reynolds's pentad: jaundice, fever, abdominal pain, altered mental status, and shock

Obstruction of the common duct causes **obstruction and ascending infection.** There is **high fever and very high white blood cell count.** Key findings are **high levels of alkaline phosphatase** and high levels of total bilirubin and direct bilirubin with mild elevation of transaminases.

Treatment is with the following:

- **IV antibiotics**
- **Emergency decompression of the common duct** is lifesaving:
  - Ideally by ERCP
  - Alternatively through the liver by **percutaneous transhepatic cholangiogram (PTC)**
  - Rarely by surgery
- Eventually **cholecystectomy** must follow

Fecal Incontinence

Fecal incontinence is involuntary passage of bowel contents for at least one month in a patient age > 3.

The diagnosis is made through a combination of clinical history and flexible sigmoidoscopy or anoscopy (best initial test). The most accurate test is anorectal manometry. Patients with a history of anatomic injury should undergo endorectal manometry.

Treatment

Best initial treatment: Combine bulking agents (e.g., fiber) with biofeedback techniques (e.g., control exercises and muscle strengthening exercises). The best next step is endoscopic injection of dextranomer/hyaluronic acid in an effort to create a pseudo-sphincter. This technique has reduced incontinence episodes by 50 percent. If this fails, colorectal surgery is needed.

Preoperative and Postoperative Care

Preoperative Assessment

The most important aspect of preoperative assessment is being able to **identify comorbidities that preclude surgery.** Other aspects of preoperative assessment include understanding the modifications that may need to be instituted to **prepare patients for surgery.**

A 42-year-old man with hepatitis C cirrhosis presents with a large umbilical hernia with intermittent pain. On examination he has large amounts of ascites. Surgical intervention is being considered. His bilirubin is 3.0, his prothrombin time is 32 seconds, INR 2.2, and his serum albumin is 1.9. Which of the following is the best next step in management?

a. Proceed to emergency surgery.
b. Proceed with surgery after first giving vitamin K.
c. Proceed with surgery after total parenteral nutrition (TPN).
d. Proceed with surgery after albumin infusion.
e. Do not perform surgery.

Answer: **E.** Do not do surgery in any patients with multiple derangements in hepatic risk factors. Any 1 of the hepatic risks alone—bilirubin above 2, albumin below 3, prothrombin above 16, and encephalopathy (as suggested by altered mental status)—predicts a mortality of over 40 percent. If 3 of them are present, the risk is 85 percent; all 4 risks constitute almost 100 percent risk of mortality.

A 59-year-old man is scheduled for prostatectomy. He has a history of HTN, COPD, and diabetes mellitus. He takes atenolol for blood pressure, tiotropium and albuterol for COPD, and glipizide for diabetes. BP is 145/89 mm Hg, and HgbA1c is 7.1. Recent pulmonary tests document FEV_1 1.3. Blood CO_2 is 47. Which of the following is this patient most at risk of developing?

a. Intraoperative myocardial infarction
b. Pneumothorax
c. Postoperative pneumonia
d. Hypercapnic failure

Answer: **C.** Severe COPD ($FEV_1 < 1.5$ L) increases surgical risk, mainly because patients have an ineffective cough and cannot clear secretions. They are subsequently at risk for postoperative pneumonia.

The table below summarizes important principles in preoperative assessment.

Organ System	Risk Factor	Modifications/Interventions
Cardiac risk	Ejection fraction < 35%	Prohibits noncardiac surgery.
	Jugular venous distention (sign of CHF)	Optimize medications with ACE inhibitors, beta blockers, digitalis, and diuretics prior to surgery.
	Recent myocardial infarction	Defer surgery for 6 months after MI.
	Severe progressive angina	Perform cardiac catheterization to evaluate for possible coronary revascularization.
Pulmonary risk	Smoking (compromised ventilation: high pCO_2, FEV_1 < 1.5	Order PFTs to evaluate FEV_1. If FEV_1 is abnormal, obtain blood gas. Cessation of smoking for **8 weeks** prior to surgery.
Hepatic risk	Bilirubin > 2.0 Prothrombin time > 16 Serum albumin < 3.0 Encephalopathy	~ 40% mortality with any single risk factor. ~ 80–85% mortality is predictable if 3 or more risk factors are present.
Nutritional risk	Loss of 20% of body weight over several months Serum albumin < 3.0 Anergy to skin antigens Serum transferrin < 200 mg/dL Diabetic coma	Provide 5–10 days of nutritional supplements (preferably via gut) before surgery. Absolute contraindication to surgery. First stabilize diabetes. Rehydrate and normalize acidosis prior to surgery.

The following table shows the calculation of the cardiac risk index in noncardiac surgery.

Cardiac Risk Index in Noncardiac Surgery		
Criterion	**Finding**	**Points***
Age	> 70	5
Cardiac status	MI within 6 months	10
	Ventricular gallop or jugular venous distention (signs of heart failure)	11
	Significant aortic stenosis	3
	Arrhythmia other than sinus or premature atrial contractions	7
	≥ 5 premature ventricular contractions/minute	7
General medical condition	$pO_2 < 60$ mm Hg, $pCO_2 > 50$ mm Hg, $K < 3$ mmol/L, $HCO_3 < 20$ mmol/L, BUN > 50 mg/dL, serum creatinine > 3 mg/dL, elevated AST, a chronic liver disorder, or bedbound	3
Type of surgery needed	Emergency surgery	4
	Intraperitoneal, intrathoracic, or aortic surgery	3

*Risk is based on the total number of points:

Level I: 0–5

Level II: 6–12

Level III: 13–25

Level IV: > 25

Adapted from Goldman L, Caldera DL, Nussbaum SR, et al. Multifactorial index of cardiac risk in noncardiac surgical procedures. *New England Journal of Medicine.* 1997; 297 (lb):845–850.

Postoperative Complications

In each of the following cases, which diagnostic tests will likely show the cause of the patient's postoperative fever?

1. **A patient who had major abdominal surgery is afebrile during the first 2 postoperative days but on Day 3 has a fever to 103°F.**
2. **A patient who had major abdominal surgery is afebrile during the first 4 postoperative days but on Day 5 has a fever to 103°F.**
3. **A patient who had major abdominal surgery is afebrile during the first 6 postoperative days but on Day 7 has a fever to 103°F.**

a. **Chest x-ray**
b. **CT of the abdomen**
c. **CT of the chest**
d. **Doppler of the lower extremities**
e. **Urinalysis**

Answers:
1. **E.** Urinalysis
2. **D.** Doppler of the lower extremities
3. **B.** CT of the abdomen

Every potential source of post-op fever must be investigated, but the timing of the first febrile episode gives a clue as to the most likely source. While not a hard-and-fast rule, the "four Ws" mnemonic gives a clue to the likely cause of the fever:

- **"Wind"** for atelectasis, common post-op Day 1: Order a **chest x-ray.**
- **"Water"** for urinary tract infections, common post-op Day 3: Order **urinalysis and urine culture.**
- **"Walking"** for thrombophlebitis, common post-op Day 5: Order a **Doppler.**
- **"Wound"** for wound infections, common post-op Day 7: Conduct a **complete physical exam** and consider **CT scan** to evaluate for deep infections.

A 46-year-old woman with medical history significant for large fibroids and anemia becomes disoriented 18 hours after an uncomplicated hysterectomy. What is the next step in management?

a. Obtain arterial blood gas.
b. Obtain CT scan of the pelvis.
c. Give intravenous fluids.
d. Give lorazepam.
e. Give blood transfusion.

Answer: **A.** There is a long list of causes for post-op disorientation; however, the most lethal one if not recognized and treated early is **hypoxia.** Unless the vignette clearly identifies other possible metabolic causes of disorientation—uremia, hyponatremia, hypernatremia, ammonium, hyperglycemia, delirium tremens (DTs), or iatrogenic medications—the safest thing is to obtain a blood gas first.

A 52-year-old woman is found to have brown feculent fluid draining from her wound drain 9 days after a sigmoid resection for colorectal cancer. The patient is afebrile, has stable vital signs, and is without complaints. What is the next step in management?

a. Administer intravenous antibiotics.
b. Order a CT of the abdomen.
c. Flush the drain with normal saline.
d. Perform an urgent laparotomy.
e. Observation only.

Answer: **E.** Observation is all that is needed. A fecal fistula, if draining to the outside, is not serious. It will close eventually with little or no therapy. If feces were accumulating on the inside, the patient would be febrile and would have other systemic signs. This would require drainage and probably a diverting colostomy.

The leakage of fecal, gastric, or duodenal contents to the outside postoperatively is *not* an indication for emergency surgery. Observe stable patients. Dehydration and electrolyte derangements must be corrected.

Nutritional support should always first be given via the gut whenever possible. Total parenteral nutrition is almost *never* the right answer on the exam due to the high risk of infection, but it is needed if there is upper GI fistula.

The following table summarizes the features and management of postoperative complications.

Postoperative Complication	Features	Management
Fever		
Malignant hyperthermia exceeding 104°F	Shortly after the onset of the anesthetic (halothane or succinylcholine) Treat with IV dantrolene, 100 percent oxygen, correction of the acidosis, and cooling blankets	Watch for development of myoglobinuria
Bacteremia exceeding 104°F	Within 30–45 minutes of invasive procedures (instrumentation of the urinary tract is a classic example)	Blood cultures times 3 Start empiric antibiotics
Postoperative fever in the usual range (101°–103°F)	Atelectasis (Day 1)	Incentive spirometry
	Pneumonia (Day 3)	CXR: Infiltrate Sputum culture Antibiotics (hospital-acquired pneumonia)
	Urinary tract infection (Day 3)	Urinalysis and urinary culture Antibiotics
	Deep venous thrombophlebitis (Day 5)	Doppler ultrasound of deep veins of legs and pelvis Anticoagulation
	Wound infection (Day 7)	Antibiotics if only cellulitis Incision and drainage if abscess is present
	Deep abscesses (subphrenic, pelvic, or subhepatic) (Days 10–15)	CT scan of the appropriate body cavity is diagnostic Percutaneous radiologically guided drainage is therapeutic
Perioperative myocardial infarction	Precipitated by hypotension when intraoperative Post-op MI seldom presents with chest pain	Thrombolytics are contraindicated, even in post-op setting Mortality rate is higher than for nonsurgery-related MI

(continued next page)

Postoperative Complication	Features	Management
Fever		
Pulmonary embolus (PE) (Day 7)	Tachycardia, shortness of breath, hypoxia, increased A-a gradient	CTA (CT angiogram) Anticoagulate with heparin IVC filter if recurrent PE
Aspiration	Shortness of breath, hypoxia, infiltrate on x-ray	Lavage and remove gastric contents Bronchodilators and respiratory support Steroids do *not* help
Intraoperative tension pneumothorax	Positive-pressure breathing; patient becomes progressively more difficult to "bag" BP steadily declines, and CVP steadily rises	Insert needle to decompress and place chest tube later
Postoperative confusion	Suspect hypoxia first Consider sepsis	Check blood gases Get blood cultures and CBC
Acute respiratory distress syndrome (ARDS)	Bilateral pulmonary infiltrates and hypoxia, with no evidence of CHF	Positive end-expiratory pressure (PEEP)
Delirium tremens (Days 2–3)	Tachycardia, hyperthermia, hypertension, altered mental status	Give benzodiazepines (barbiturates are second-line agents because of lower therapeutic range); watch for seizures and rhabdomyolysis

Pediatric Surgery

Conditions That Need Surgery at Birth

Congenital anomalies constitute the conditions that need surgery at birth. On the Step 3 exam, the most important first step before surgery is to rule out other associated congenital conditions. In any of the following presentations, look for other associated elements of the VACTER (vertebral, anal, cardiac, tracheal, esophageal, renal, and radial) constellation:

- Look at anus for imperforation.
- Check the x-ray for vertebral and radial anomalies.
- Do echocardiogram looking for cardiac anomalies.
- Do sonogram looking for renal anomalies.

Esophageal Atresia

Excessive salivation is noted shortly after birth, or **choking spells** are noticed when first feeding is attempted.

Basic Science Correlate

Ventrally displaced location of the notochord in an embryo can lead to a failure of apoptosis in the developing foregut and cause esophageal atresia.

Confirm the diagnosis with an **NG tube,** which becomes coiled in the upper chest on x-ray.

Treat as follows:

- Primary **surgical repair** is indicated.
- If surgery needs to be delayed for further workup, perform **gastrostomy** to protect the lungs from acid reflux.

Anal Atresia

This is indicated by an **absence of flatus or stool.** The anal canal is absent on exam.

Treat as follows:

- Look for a **fistula nearby** (to vagina or perineum).
  - If **present,** delay repair until further growth (but before toilet training time).
  - If **not present,** a **colostomy** needs to be done for high rectal pouches.

VACTERL syndrome = association of:
V: Vertebral anomalies
A: Anal atresia
C: Cardiovascular anomalies
TE: TracheoEsophageal fistula
R: Renal (kidney) and/or radial anomalies
L: Limb defects

Congenital Diaphragmatic Hernia

Dyspnea is noted at birth, and **loops of bowel in left chest are seen on x-ray.** The primary abnormality is the **hypoplastic lung with fetal-type circulation.**

Basic Science Correlate

Left-sided hernias allow herniation of intra-abdominal organs into the thoracic cavity, while right-sided hernias allow the liver to herniate.

Treat by performing **endotracheal intubation, low-pressure ventilation, sedation, and NG suction.** Delay repair 3–4 days to allow lung maturation.

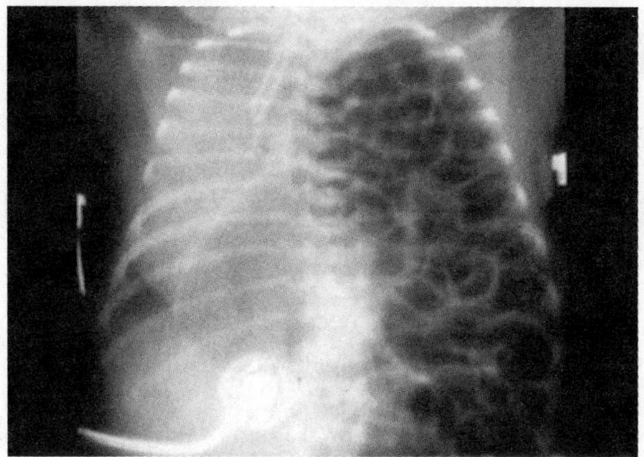

Congenital Diaphragmatic Hernia

Gastroschisis and Omphalocele

- **Gastroschisis:** The umbilical cord is normal (it reaches the baby); the defect is to the right of the cord, where there is no protective membrane and the bowel looks angry and matted.

> **Basic Science Correlate**
>
> Gastroschisis occurs when the neural crest fails to migrate, resulting in the absence of enteric neurons within the myenteric plexus and submucosal plexus.

- **Omphalocele:** The umbilical cord goes to the defect, which has a thin membrane under which one can see normal-looking bowel and a little slice of liver.

> **Basic Science Correlate**
>
> **Embryology and Omphalocele**
>
> Incomplete fusion during the fourth week of development results in a defect that allows abdominal viscera to protrude through the anterior body wall, which is made when the lateral body folds move ventrally and fuse in the midline.

Basic Science Correlate

Edward's syndrome (Trisomy 18) and Patau syndrome (Trisomy 13) are associated with omphalocele.

Treat as follows:

- **Small defects:** Close small defects primarily.
- **Large defects:** These require a silastic "silo" to protect the bowel and **manual replacement of the bowel daily** until complete closure (in about 1 week). In the meantime, give parenteral nutrition (the bowel will not work in gastroschisis) and IV antibiotics.

Exstrophy of the Urinary Bladder

This is an abdominal wall defect over the pubis.

Transfer the patient to a specialized center that offers surgical repair in first 1–2 days of life. Do *not* delay surgery.

A newborn is vomiting greenish liquid material. A "double-bubble" is seen on x-ray. What is the diagnosis?

a. Annular pancreas
b. Congenital diaphragmatic hernia
c. Gastroschisis
d. Imperforated anus
e. Intestinal atresia

Answer: **A.** Don't be fooled into thinking that only duodenal atresia presents with double-bubble sign. Annular pancreas and malrotation also present with double-bubble sign. All of these anomalies require surgical correction, but malrotation is the most dangerous because the bowel can twist on itself, cut off its blood supply, and become necrotic.

Intestinal Atresia

Like annular pancreas, this condition also presents with green vomiting. But instead of a double-bubble, there are **multiple air-fluid levels throughout the abdomen.** There is no need to suspect other congenital anomalies, because this condition results from a vascular accident in utero.

Surgical Conditions in the First 2 Months of Life

Necrotizing Enterocolitis

This shows up as **feeding intolerance in premature infants** when they are first fed. There is **abdominal distention** and a **rapidly dropping platelet count** (in babies, this is a sign of sepsis).

> **Basic Science Correlate**
>
> The most common pathogens in necrotizing enterocolitis are *Escherichia coli* and *Klebsiella pneumonia.*

Treatment is as follows:

- **Stop all feedings.**
- Prescribe **broad-spectrum antibiotics.**
- Deliver **IV fluids and nutrition.**
- Do **surgery** if there are signs of necrosis or perforation (abdominal wall erythema, portal vein gas, or gas in the bowel wall).

Meconium Ileus

Symptoms are **feeding intolerance and bilious vomiting** in a baby with **cystic fibrosis** (look for cystic fibrosis in family history).

> **Basic Science Correlate**
>
> Cystic fibrosis, an autosomal recessive disease, results from a point mutation at position 508 of the CFTR gene that causes the mistranslation of phenylalanine.

Diagnose by **x-rays,** which show **multiple dilated loops of small bowel** and a **ground-glass appearance** in the lower abdomen.

Gastrografin enema is both

- **diagnostic** (microcolon and inspissated pellets of meconium in the terminal ileum); and
- **therapeutic** (gastrografin draws fluid in and dissolves the pellets).

Hypertrophic Pyloric Stenosis

This shows up as **nonbilious projectile vomiting after each feeding** at approximately 3 weeks of age. Look for **gastric peristaltic waves** and a **palpable "olive-size" mass** in the right upper quadrant.

Diagnose with a **sonogram.**

Treat as follows:

- **First correct dehydration and associated hypochloremic, hypokalemic metabolic alkalosis.**
- Follow this with **pyloromyotomy.**

Biliary Atresia

This appears in 6- to 8-week-old babies who have **persistent, progressively increasing jaundice** (conjugated bilirubin).

Diagnose in the following ways:

- Conduct **serologies and sweat test** to rule out other problems.
- Order **HIDA scan** after 1 week of phenobarbital (a powerful choleretic).
- If no bile reaches the duodenum even with phenobarbital stimulation, **surgical exploration** is needed.

Hirschsprung Disease (Aganglionic Megacolon)

The most important clue to diagnosis is **chronic constipation.** A **rectal exam** may lead to explosive expulsion of stool and flatus with relief of abdominal distention.

Diagnose by getting a **full-thickness biopsy of rectal mucosa.**

Surgical Conditions Later in Infancy

Intussusception

This presents in 6- to 12-month-old **chubby, healthy-looking kids** with **brief episodes of colicky abdominal pain** that makes them "double up and squat." There is also the following:

- A vague mass on the right side of the abdomen
- An "empty" right lower quadrant
- "Currant jelly" stools

A barium or air enema is both diagnostic and therapeutic. Perform **surgery** if enema fails to achieve reduction.

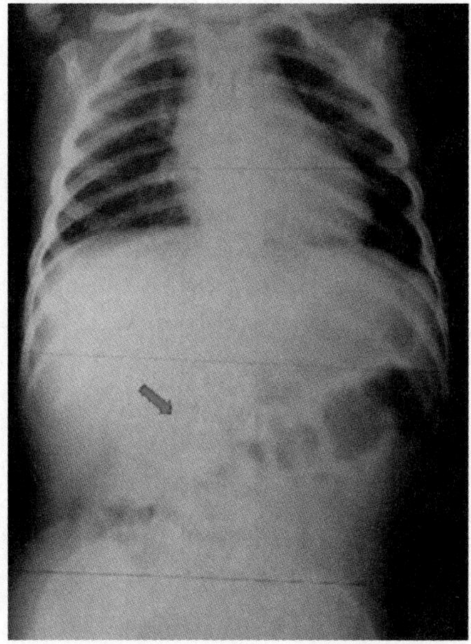

Intussusception

Meckel Diverticulum

This presents as **lower GI bleeding** in a child of pediatric age.

> **Basic Science Correlate**
>
> Meckel diverticulum is a true diverticulum consisting of all 3 layers of the bowel wall: mucosa, submucosa, and muscularis propria.

Diagnosis is with a **radioisotope scan,** which looks for gastric mucosa in the lower abdomen. **Surgical resection** is the best therapy.

Orthopedics

Common Adult Orthopedic Injuries

General Rules about Fractures

- When you suspect a fracture, order **2 views at 90° to one another** and *always* include the joints above and below the broken bone.
- *Always* x-ray other sites **"in the line of force"** (e.g., lumbar spine for someone who falls and lands on the feet, hips in a patient who has been in a motor vehicle accident with force of knees against the dashboard).

> Always worry about **gas gangrene** in any deep-penetrating or dirty wounds. Three days later, the patient will be septic with a tender, swollen injury site with gas crepitus. Treatment is large doses of **IV penicillin and hyperbaric oxygen.**

- **Closed reduction** is the answer for fractures that are not badly displaced or angulated.
- **Open reduction and internal fixation** is the answer when the fracture is severely displaced or angulated or cannot be aligned.
- **Open fractures** (the broken bone sticking out through a wound) require cleaning in the OR and reduction within 6 hours from the time of the injury.
- *Always* perform **cervical spine films** in any patient with **facial injuries.**

Fracture Management

A 27-year-old woman with a known seizure disorder has a grand mal seizure. She complains of left shoulder pain. PA and lateral x-rays are obtained and fail to reveal fracture or dislocation. She is given ibuprofen for pain. She returns 3 days later with persistent pain with her arm held close to her side. She reports that she is unable to move the left arm. What is the next step in management?

a. Axillary radiograph of the left shoulder
b. Change analgesic to Percocet
c. CT of the left shoulder
d. MRI of the left shoulder
e. Ultrasound of tendon insertion sites

Answer: **A.** Although **anterior shoulder dislocations** are easily seen on erect posteroanterior (PA) and lateral films—look for adducted arm and externally rotated forearm with numbness over deltoid (axillary nerve is stretched)—posterior shoulder dislocations are commonly missed on these views. **Posterior shoulder dislocations** should be suspected in a patient with a recent seizure or electrical burn and shoulder injury or pain. Order axillary or scapular views of the affected shoulder.

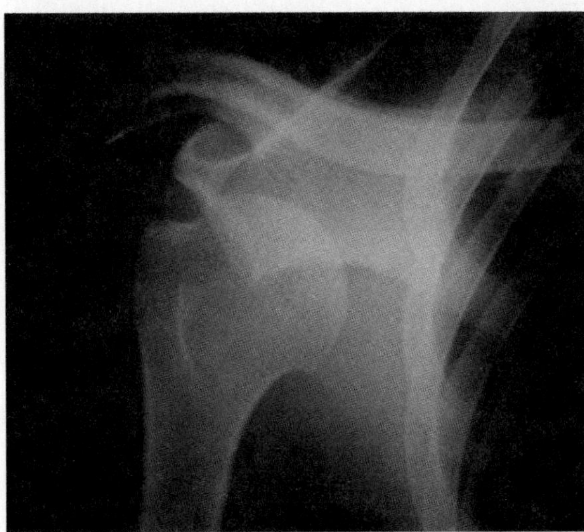

Anterior Dislocation of the Shoulder

- **Anterior dislocation:** This is the most common shoulder dislocation. Look for an arm held close to the body but an externally rotated forearm and associated numbness over the deltoid muscle (axillary nerve is stretched).
- **Posterior dislocation:** The arm is held close to the body, and the forearm is internally rotated.

Following are the best choices for the management of fractures:

> Open femoral shaft fractures are an orthopedic emergency and can result in massive blood loss and a high rate of infection. Immediate surgery and cleaning within 6 hours is needed.

- **Clavicular fractures: Figure-eight sling**
- **Colles' fracture: Closed reduction and casting** (Presents often in an elderly woman who falls on an outstretched hand. Look for a painful wrist with a "dinner-fork" deformity.")
- **Direct blow to the ulna (Monteggia fracture) or radius (Galeazzi fracture)** results in a combination of diaphyseal fracture and displaced dislocation of the nearby joint. **Open reduction and internal fixation** is needed for the diaphyseal fracture, and **closed reduction** for the dislocated joint.
- Fall on an outstretched hand with persistent pain in the anatomical snuffbox is a **scaphoid fracture** until proven otherwise (takes > 3 weeks to be seen on x-ray). Place **thumb spica cast** to help prevent nonunion.
- Consider the possibility of a **hip fracture** in *any* elderly patient who sustains a fall. Look for externally rotated and shortened leg.
  - **Femoral neck fractures** are at high risk of avascular necrosis (tenuous blood supply) and are best treated with **femoral head replacement.**
  - **Intertrochanteric fractures** are treated with **open reduction and pinning.**
  - **Femoral shaft fractures** are treated with **intramedullary rod fixation.** Be aware of a high risk for fat emboli.

> Femoral shaft fractures cause fat emboli.

- **Trigger finger** (woman who awakens at night with an acutely flexed finger that "snaps" when forcibly extended) and **De Quervain tenosynovitis** (young mother carrying baby with flexed wrist and extended thumb to stabilize the baby's head): Steroid injection is the best initial therapy.
- **Dupuytren contracture** (contracture of the palm with palmar fascial nodules): **Surgery** is the treatment if collagenase fails.
- **Posterior dislocation of the hip** (history of head-on car collision where the knees hit the dashboard) is an orthopedic emergency. Differentiate it from hip fracture by an *internally* rotated leg (the leg is also shortened). **Emergency reduction** is needed to avoid avascular necrosis.
- **Knee injuries:**
  - **Medial/lateral collateral ligament injury** (caused by a direct blow to the opposite side of the joint): **Casting** if isolated ligament injury; **surgical repair** if multiple ligaments injured.
  - **Anterior/posterior cruciate ligament injuries** (swelling pain and anterior/posterior drawer sign): Young athletes need **arthroscopic repair.** Older patients may be treated with **immobilization and rehabilitation.**
  - **Meniscal injury** (prolonged pain and swelling with "catching" and "locking" during ambulation). Treat with arthroscopic repair.
- **Tibial stress injury** (e.g., history of military or cadet marches): x-ray may be negative initially. Treat with **cast,** order the patient **not to bear weight,** and **repeat films in 2 weeks.**

> Tinel's sign has greater specificity than Phalen's sign.

- **Rupture of the Achilles tendon** (middle-aged man "overdoes it" at tennis or basketball, or patient with history of fluoroquinolone use, complaining of sudden "popping" and limping): Treat with **casting in equinus position** or **surgical repair.**

Wrist Injuries

Carpal tunnel syndrome (CTS) is entrapment of the median nerve that causes pain and paresthesias. The most common causes are idiopathic: **rheumatoid arthritis, acromegaly, and hypothyroidism** are conditions that predispose one to CTS.

Diagnostic Testing

The best initial test is the history and physical. **Phalen's test** causes symptoms by flexing the wrist gently and holding the position. **Tinel's sign** causes symptoms by tapping the nerve over the flexor retinaculum and awaiting paresthesias.

Treatment

The best initial therapy is **NSAIDs and splinting**. If this does not alleviate symptoms, local steroid injections have been shown to help in some cases. Surgical release is recommended when splinting no longer controls the patient's symptoms.

Compartment Syndrome

This is most frequent in the forearm or lower leg. Look for a history of **prolonged ischemia followed by reperfusion, crushing injuries, or other types of trauma.** There is pain, and the affected area feels tight and tender to palpation. The classic sign is **excruciating pain with passive extension.** Pulses may be *normal.*

When a patient complains of pain at the site of a cast, *always* remove the cast and examine for compartment syndrome.

The first step in management is **emergency fasciotomy.**

Neurovascular Injuries

The table below summarizes injuries that involve neurovascular complications.

Primary Injury	Neurovascular Complication	Signs/Symptoms	Next Step in Management
Oblique distal humerus	Radial nerve	Unable to dorsiflex (extend) the wrist Function regained after reduction	Surgery is indicated if paralysis persists after reduction
Posterior dislocation of the knee	Popliteal artery injuries	Decreased distal pulses	Doppler studies or arteriogram Prophylactic fasciotomy if reduction is delayed

Back Pain

Disc Herniation

A 45-year-old man with a history of back pain for several months presents with sudden-onset severe back pain that came on when he was moving a television. He describes an "electrical shock" that shoots down his leg, which is worse when he coughs or strains and is partially relieved by flexing his legs. The pain has prevented him from ambulating. Straight leg raising gives excruciating pain. What is the next step in management?

a. CT of the spine
b. Dexamethasone
c. Immediate surgery
d. Ibuprofen and brief bed rest
e. MRI of the spine

Answer: **D.** This is the classic presentation of **lumbar disc herniation.** It occurs almost exclusively at L4–L5 or L5–S1. Peak age is 43–46. Anti-inflammatories and a brief period of bed rest is all that is needed at this stage. Immediate surgical compression is needed if the history suggests **cauda equina syndrome** (look for bowel/bladder incontinence, flaccid anal sphincter, and saddle anesthesia). MRI can confirm both disc herniation and cauda equina, but do not answer MRI in classic cases of disc herniation. Trial of anti-inflammatories is also the first step in management.

Basic Science Correlate

A sluggish ankle jerk reflex is suggestive of pathology at S1/S2. A sluggish patellar reflex is suggestive of pathology at L4/L5.

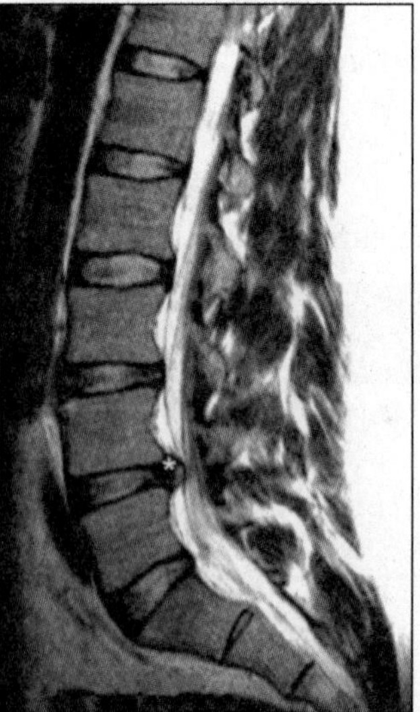

Lumbar Disc Herniation

Ankylosing Spondylitis

This presents in men in their 30s or early 40s with **chronic back pain and morning stiffness that improve with activity.** X-rays eventually show a **"bamboo spine."**

It is associated with the HLA B-27 antigen; **screen for uveitis and inflammatory bowel disease,** which are also associated with HLA-B27.

Management involves **anti-inflammatory agents and physical therapy.**

> In cases of ankylosing spondylitis, do *not* answer HLA-B27 antigen testing in first-degree relatives. Risk of developing ankylosing spondylitis based on HLA-B27 positivity is low, and it is not indicated for screening.

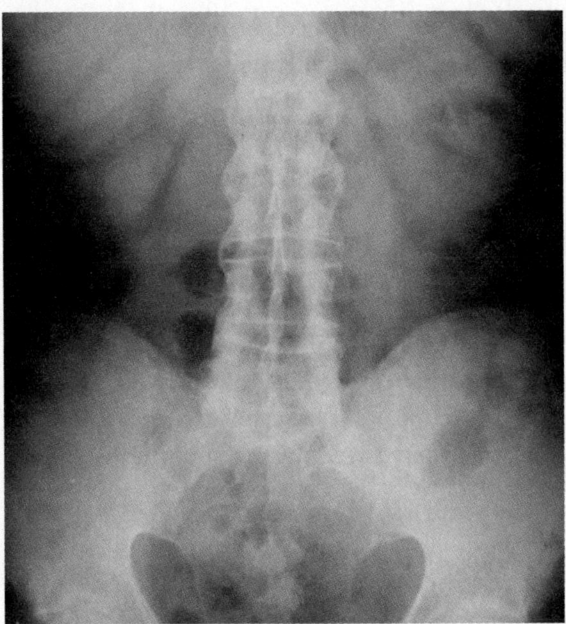

Ankylosing spondylitis: Note fused sacroiliac joints and spicules bridging the vertebral bodies, giving characteristic "bamboo spine" appearance.

Metastatic Malignancy

Suspect metastatic malignancy in an **elderly patient** with **progressive and constant back pain that is worse at night and unrelieved by rest.** There will be a history of **weight loss. X-rays** will show the lytic (also look for hypercalcemia and/or elevated alkaline phosphatase) or blastic lesions. Always include a workup for the most likely malignancy based on history and type of bone lesion.

> - Blastic metastatic lesions: Prostate cancer and breast cancer
> - Lytic metastatic lesions: Lung, renal, breast, thyroid, multiple myeloma

Perform the following imaging:

- First order plain **radiographs** (especially important in multiple myeloma).
- **Bone scan** is most sensitive in early disease.
- **MRI** shows the greatest amount of detail and is the diagnostic test of choice if there are any neurologic symptoms (to rule out cord compression).

> Bone scans will not be helpful in purely lytic lesions (e.g., multiple myeloma). Instead order plain radiographs or MRI.

Basic Science Correlate

Lytic lesions can be caused by multiple myeloma and kidney and thyroid metastasis, while blastic lesions are caused by metastatic prostate cancer.

Foot Pain

Plantar Fasciitis

The pain in plantar fasciitis feels like a tack in the bottom of the foot and resolves quickly after walking.

Plantar fasciitis commonly presents in **older, overweight patients with sharp heel pain every time their foot strikes the ground.** Pain is worse in the mornings. X-rays may show a bony spur matching the location of the pain, and there is exquisite tenderness to palpation over the spur. However, surgical resection of the **bony spur** is not indicated, so x-ray makes no difference.

Give **symptomatic treatment;** resolution occurs spontaneously in 12–18 months.

Morton Neuroma

Morton neuroma is **inflammation of the common digital nerve at the 3rd interspace,** between the 3rd and 4th toes, caused by wearing pointy-toed shows. The **neuroma is palpable,** and there is very tender spot there.

Management is **analgesics and appropriate footwear.** If this does not work, follow with surgical excision.

Urology

Urologic Emergencies

A 24-year-old man presents in the emergency room with very severe pain. His temperature on presentation is 102.3°F. His testes appear swollen and are tender to palpation. Urinalysis reveals 50 white blood cells, 0 red blood cells. Which of the following is the next step in management?

a. Antibiotics
b. Culture and sensitivity
c. Inguinal lymph node biopsy
d. Testicular ultrasound
e. Prostate biopsy

Answer: **A.** The most likely diagnosis is orchitis/epididymitis, so starting antibiotics is the best next step in management.

Testicular Torsion

Testicular torsion classically presents as **severe, sudden-onset testicular pain without fever or pyuria.** The testis is swollen, exquisitely tender, "high riding," and with a "horizontal lie."

Basic Science Correlate

The sensory and motor components of the cremasteric reflex are at L1/L2. Their absence is suggestive of testicular torsion.

Diagnose with **ultrasound**, but do not wait for results to do surgery. Treat with **immediate surgical intervention with bilateral orchiopexy.**

Acute Epididymitis

The patient presents with **acute scrotal pain** (sometimes referred to the abdomen), **fever, and urinary symptoms.**

To diagnose, get a **urinalysis** and **urine cultures** and obtain a **culture of discharge** if present.

Treatment is as follows:

- **Males < 35:** Treat for gonorrhea/chlamydia with **ceftriaxone and doxycycline.**
- **Older males:** Treat as a urinary tract infection (*E. coli*) with **levofloxacin.**

Basic Science Correlate

Serotypes D–K of *Chlamydia trachomatis* (obligate intracellular) are responsible for urethritis and other STD-related sequelae.

A 72-year-old man is being observed; he has a ureteral stone that is expected to pass spontaneously. He develops chills, a temperature of 102.9°F, flank pain, and elevated creatinine. Which of the following is the next step in management?

a. Prescribe oral antibiotics
b. Prescribe loop diuretics
c. Perform lithotripsy
d. Place Foley catheter
e. Place percutaneous stent

Answer: **E.** Place a percutaneous stent to relieve the obstruction.

Urologic Obstructions

The combination of **obstruction and infection** of the urinary tract is a urologic emergency. It can lead to destruction of the kidney in a few hours and, potentially, to death from sepsis.

Treat urologic obstructions in the following way:

- **Immediate decompression of the urinary tract** above the obstruction is required.
- **IV antibiotics** are given to treat the infection.
- A **ureteral stent** or **percutaneous nephrostomy** is the most important intervention; defer more elaborate instrumentations for a later, safer date.

Congenital Urologic Diseases

Following are the urologic diseases that possibly require surgery:

- The most common reason for a newborn boy not to urinate during the first day of life is **posterior urethral valves.**
  - **Catheterize** to empty the bladder.
  - Diagnose with **voiding cystourethrogram.**
- **Hypospadias** (urethral opening on ventral side of penis) is easily seen on routine newborn physical exam.
  - *Never* perform circumcision on this child. The prepuce will be needed for the **plastic reconstruction.**
- A child who has **hematuria from trivial trauma** has an **undiagnosed congenital anomaly** until proven otherwise.
- A child with a **urinary tract infection** has an **undiagnosed congenital anomaly** until proven otherwise (e.g., vesicoureteral reflux).
  - Order a voiding cystogram to look for the reflux.
  - If found, give long-term antibiotics until the child "grows out of the problem."
- Suspect **low implantation of a ureter** in girls who void appropriately but are also found to be constantly wet from **urinating into the vagina.**
- **Ureteropelvic junction (UPJ) obstruction** is only symptomatic when diuresis occurs. UPJ presents classically in a teenager who drinks large volumes of beer and develops **colicky flank pain.**

Vascular Surgery

A 48-year-old laborer complains of coldness and tingling in his left hand as well as pain in the forearm when he does strenuous work. Recently he's complained of dizziness, with blurred vision and trouble keeping steady during these episodes. Which of the following is the most important management?

a. Aspirin
b. Clopidogrel
c. Warfarin
d. Bypass surgery
e. Carotid endarterectomy

Answer: **D.** Bypass surgery is needed for **subclavian steal syndrome.**

Subclavian Steal Syndrome

Although this condition is rare in practice, it is a classic board vignette. An arteriosclerotic stenotic plaque at the origin of the subclavian allows enough blood supply to reach the arm for normal activity but not enough to meet the increased demands of an exercised arm, resulting in **blood being "stolen" from the vertebral artery.** When the arm is raised, increasing oxygen demand, the vessels in the arm dilate to increase perfusion. This dilation acts as a vacuum to blood in the head, neck, and shoulder, leading to syncopal episodes. Classic symptoms are the following:

- **Posterior neurological signs:** Visual symptoms, equilibrium problems
- **Claudication** in the arm during arm exercises

Don't confuse this condition with thoracic outlet syndrome, which causes vascular symptoms only, with *no* neurologic signs.

Diagnose with an **angiography.**

Treatment is with **bypass surgery.**

Aortic Aneurysm

A 66-year-old man has vague, poorly described epigastric and upper back discomfort. He is found on physical examination to have a pulsatile mass, which is very tender to palpation. Ultrasound reveals a 6-cm abdominal aneurysm. What is the next step in management?

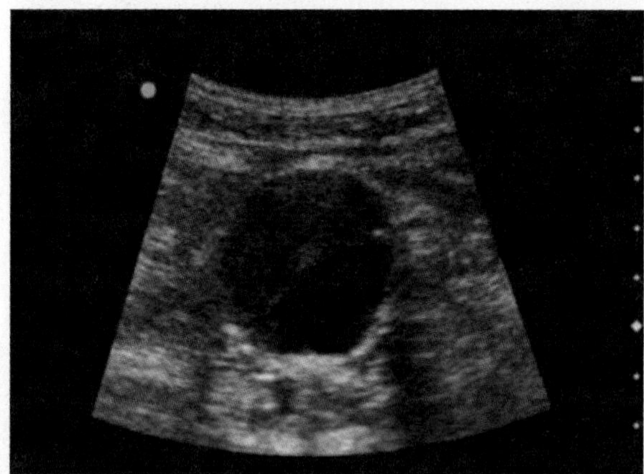

Abdominal Aortic Aneurysm with Mural Thrombus

> **Abdominal aortic aneurysm (AAA):** one-time screening by ultrasonography in men age 65–75 who have **ever** smoked

a. ACE inhibitors
b. Urgent surgery
c. Elective repair
d. Repeat abdominal ultrasound in 6 months
e. Order CT angiogram of the chest

Answer: **B.** Urgent surgery within the next day is the most appropriate management in a patient with asymptomatic abdominal aortic aneurysm. Signs (hypotension) and symptoms (excruciating abdominal pain radiating to the back) suggest leaking or ruptured aneurysm and necessitate emergency surgery.

Size and symptoms are key to management of abdominal aortic aneurysm.

- Aneurysms < 5 cm can be observed with **serial annual imaging.**
- Aneurysms ≥ 5 cm should have **elective repair.**

More urgent surgery is needed in the following cases:

- A **tender abdominal aortic aneurysm** will rupture within a day or two and, thus, requires **urgent repair.**
- **Excruciating back pain in a patient with a large abdominal aortic aneurysm** means that the aneurysm is already leaking, necessitating **emergency surgery.**

Basic Science Correlate

The abdominal aorta has 3 layers: intima, media, and adventitia.

A 65-year-old man presents with severe sharp chest and back pain down the spine that started 1 hour ago. His blood pressure is 219/115 mm Hg. Chest x-ray is shown. EKG and cardiac enzymes are nonrevealing. Which of the following is the most important intervention that would have prevented this presentation?

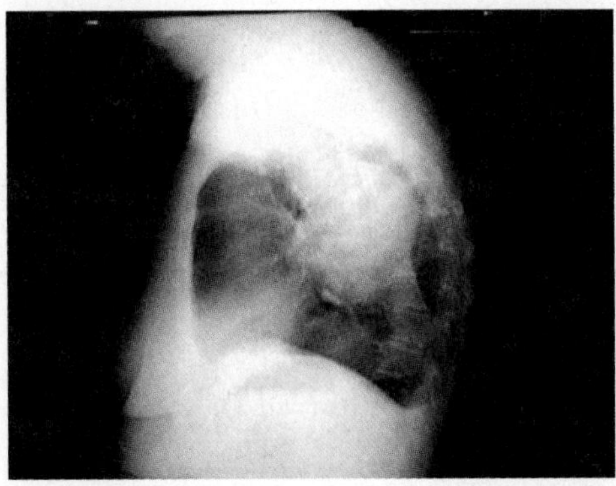

a. Aspirin prophylaxis
b. Blood pressure control
c. Cessation of smoking
d. Low fat diet
e. Serial CT scans

Answer: **B.** Blood pressure control is the most important strategy to prevent progression of thoracic aortic aneurysms.

Risk Factors

The following contribute to the *development* of thoracic aortic aneurysms:

- **Chronic hypertension**
- **Hyperlipidemia**
- **Smoking**
- **Marfan syndrome**
- **Untreated tertiary syphilis**

The most important modifiable risk to prevent *worsening* of existing aneurysms is **uncontrolled hypertension.**

- **Asymptomatic lesions: Blood pressure management** is the most important factor in controlling asymptomatic lesions.
- **Symptomatic lesions,** including active dissection (look for chest pain and sudden-onset "tearing" pain in the back): These require **surgical intervention.**

Arteriosclerotic Occlusive Disease of the Lower Extremities

The classic presentation of this condition is **pain in the legs on exercise that is relieved by rest** (intermittent claudication).

If the claudication does *not* interfere significantly with the patient's lifestyle, *no* workup is indicated. The only management indicated is

- **cessation of smoking** and
- the use of **cilostazol and aspirin.**

> **Basic Science Correlate**
>
> Cilostazol is a selective inhibitor of phosphodiesterase 3 (PDE3).

If the pain is more severe, diagnosis is with the following:

- Doppler studies looking for a pressure gradient (ankle-brachial index [ABI] <0.90)
- Arteriogram to identify stenosis

If the case describes **disabling symptoms** (affects work or activities of daily living) or if there is **impending ischemia to the extremity,** then **surgery** is indicated. This involves the following:

- Angioplasty and stenting for stenotic segments
- More extensive disease requires bypass grafts or sequential stents.

Pain at rest indicates **end-stage disease** (the patient complains of calf pain at night with disturbed sleep).

Arterial Embolization of the Extremities

Look for a history of the following:

- Atrial fibrillation
- Recent MI with sudden-onset painful, pale, cold, pulseless, paresthetic, and paralytic lower extremity.

Get **Doppler studies** to locate the obstruction and consider **thrombolytics** (if early) or **embolectomy** (if later) with **fasciotomy.**

Patient Safety

Catheter-Associated Urinary Tract Infections (CAUTI)

CAUTI is the most common type of health care–associated infection and the leading cause of nosocomial bacteremia. The diagnosis of CAUTI is made when a patient has catheter-related bacteriuria combined with fever, suprapubic tenderness, costovertebral angle tenderness, and evidence of a systemic inflammatory response syndrome. The **most accurate test** is a urine culture. Treatment is prompt removal of the catheter and administration of antibiotics.

How is CAUTI prevented?

Answer: Early removal of the catheter has been shown to reduce the risk of CAUTI.

Prophylactic antibiotics have no role in the prevention of CAUTI and raise the risk of resistance and *C. diff.*

How should a patient with long-term indwelling bladder catheterization be managed?

Answer: Instruct the patient or caregiver on the use of intermittent catheterization.

Central Line-Associated Bloodstream Infection (CLABSI)

All catheters can introduce bacteria into the bloodstream and generate significant morbidity and mortality. If a patient with a central line develops signs of infection, blood cultures are taken from both the catheter and another peripheral vein. If the cultures yield similar results, the central line should be removed and antibiotics against *Staphylococcus aureus* should be started.

When should antibiotics be started in a patient with CLABSI?

Answer: Start antibiotics immediately after blood cultures are obtained. Base therapeutic choice upon sensitivities.

S. aureus, coagulase-negative staphylococci, and *Candida* species are the most commonly isolated organisms in CLABSI.

Should the catheter tip be cultured?

Answer: Yes. Central venous catheters should be cultured if the device has been in place for at least 7 to 10 days

Section 5
Pediatrics

contributing author Elizabeth August, MD

The Newborn

Management of the Newborn

At delivery, give the following:

- **0.5 percent erythromycin ophthalmic ointment**
- **1 mg of vitamin K IM** to prevent hemorrhagic disease

Basic Science Correlate

- Erythromycin is a bacteriostatic drug. Bacteriostatic drugs inhibit reproduction of the bacteria by blocking ribosomal formation of proteins.
- Penicillins are bactericidal. Bactericidal antibiotics kill bacteria by cell wall inhibition.

Basic Science Correlate

Factors II, VII, IX, and X are vitamin K–dependent clotting factors. Proteins C and S are vitamin K–dependent anticoagulants. Vitamin K adds a carboxyl group onto the glutamic acid on these factors. Protein C inhibits factor V.

Before discharge, do the following:

- Administer **hepatitis B vaccine** if mother is HBsAg **negative**
- If mother is HBsAg **positive**, administer **hepatitis IVIG** along with the hepatitis B vaccine
- **Perform hearing test** to rule out congenital sensorineural hearing loss (SNHL).
- Order neonatal screening tests. These are more reliable if done after 48 hours. Routine screening tests include the following:
  - **Phenylketonuria**
  - **Galactosemia**
  - **Hypothyroidism**

Apgar Score

The Apgar score is a measure of the need and effectiveness of resuscitation. The Apgar score does *not* predict outcome, but a persistently low Apgar (0–3) is associated with high mortality.

- The **1-minute** score gives an idea of what was going on **during labor and delivery.**
- The **5-minute** score gives an idea of **response to therapy** (resuscitation).

Abnormalities in the Newborn

The table below lists both benign findings in the newborn and disorders with their management.

Figure	Finding/ Description	Diagnosis	Association	Further Management
	Blue/gray macules on presacral back/ posterior thighs	Mongolian spots	Usually fade in first few years	Rule out child abuse
	Firm, yellow-white papules/ pustules with erythematous base, which peak on second day of life	Erythema toxicum		Self-limited
	Permanent, unilateral vascular malformation on head and neck	Port wine stain (nevus flammeus)	Sturge-Weber syndrome (AV malformation that results in **seizures, mental retardation, and glaucoma)**	Pulsed laser therapy For Sturge-Weber, evaluate for glaucoma and give anticonvulsives
	Red, sharply demarcated, raised lesions appearing in first 2 months, rapidly expanding, then involuting by age 5–9 years.	Hemangioma	Consider underlying organ involvement with deep hemangiomas. (If it involves the larynx, it can cause obstruction.) May cause high output cardiac failure when large.	Treat with steroids or pulsed laser if large or interferes with organ function.

(continued next page)

Figure	Finding/ Description	Diagnosis	Association	Further Management
	Preauricular tags/ pits	Preauricular tags/ pits	Hearing loss Genitourinary abnormalities	Hearing test Ultrasound of kidneys
	Defect in the iris	Coloboma of the iris	Other eye abnormalities CHARGE syndrome (**C**oloboma, **H**eart defects, **A**tresia of the nasal choanae, growth **R**etardation, **G**enitourinary abnormalities, and **E**ar abnormalities)	Screen for CHARGE syndrome
	Absence of the iris	Aniridia	Wilms tumor	Screen for Wilms tumor with **abdominal ultrasound** Q3 months until age 8
	Mass **lateral** to midline	Branchial cleft cyst	Remnant of embryonic development associated with infections	Infected cysts: Give antibiotics Surgical removal if large

(continued next page)

Basic Science Correlate

A thyroglossal duct cyst may be formed anywhere along the thyroglossal tract, which is formed from the descent of the primordial thyroid gland at the base of the tongue. The duct usually atrophies, but a cyst may form.

Basic Science Correlate

In embryology, the intestines are formed outside the abdomen and extend into the umbilical cord until 10 weeks. At that time, they migrate into the abdomen.

Figure	Finding/ Description	Diagnosis	Association	Further Management
	Mass in **midline** that moves with swallowing or tongue protrusion	Thyroglossal duct cyst (*see BSC above*)	Associated with infections May have thyroid ectopia	Surgical removal Thyroid scans and thyroid function test preoperatively
	GI tract protrusion through the umbilicus **with sac** (*see BSC above*)	Omphalocele (failure of GI sac to retract at 10–12 weeks gestation)	Malformations, **chromosomal disorders**	Screen for trisomy 13, trisomy 18, and trisomy 21
	Abdominal defect lateral to midline **without sac**	Gastroschisis	Intestinal atresia	Surgical correction (see Section 4 Surgery)
	Congenital weakness where vessels of the fetal and infant umbilical cord exited through the rectus abdominis muscle	Umbilical hernia	Congenital hypothyroidism	Screen with TSH May close spontaneously
	Scrotal swelling, transillumination	Hydrocele	Inguinal hernia	Differentiate from inguinal hernia
	Unilateral absence of testes in scrotal sac	Undescended testes	Associated with malignancy if > 1 year of age	No treatment **until 1 year of age** (1) Hormone injections (β-hCG or testosterone) (2) Surgery (orchiopexy)
	Urethral opening on ventral surface	Hypospadias	Other GU anomalies may be present (most common is undescended testes and inguinal hernias).	Do *not* circumcise
	Urethral opening on dorsal surface	Epispadias	Urinary incontinence (form of urinary exstrophy)	Surgical evaluation for bladder exstrophy
	Inguinal bulge or reducible scrotal swelling	Inguinal hernia (usually indirect)		Surgery

You are called to see a 9.5-pound newborn boy who is jittery 30 minutes after a bath. The pregnancy was complicated by prolonged delivery with shoulder dystocia. Physical exam reveals a large, plethoric infant who is tremulous. A pansystolic murmur is heard. Which of the following is the most appropriate diagnostic test?

a. Bilirubin level
b. Blood glucose
c. Galactose level
d. Serum calcium level
e. Serum TSH

Answer: **B.** Blood glucose is the best initial diagnostic exam to evaluate in infants that present large for gestation, plethora, and jitteriness. This child is most likely born an **infant of a diabetic mother (IODM).**

Look for **macrosomia** (all organs except the brain are enlarged), **history of birth trauma, and cardiac abnormalities** (cardiomegaly). The case may not give a history of diabetes in the mother. Treat with **glucose and small, frequent meals.**

Infant of a Diabetic Mother (IODM)

Lab abnormalities are the following:

- ***Hypo*glycemia (after birth)**
- ***Hypo*calcemia**
- ***Hypo*magnesemia**
- ***Hyper*bilirubinemia**
- ***Poly*cythemia**

IODM is associated with the following:

- **Cardiac abnormalities** (ASD, VSD, truncus arteriosus)
- **Small left colon syndrome** (abdominal distension)

IODM is associated with an **increased risk of developing diabetes and childhood obesity.**

Infants of diabetic mothers become hypoglycemic after delivery because of excess insulin. In utero, they acclimate to a high-glucose environment by producing more insulin, becoming hyperinsulinemic. At birth, upon leaving this high-glucose environment, IODMs' high insulin level makes them hypoglycemic.

Respiratory Distress in the Newborn

Keep the following in mind for ***all*** cases of respiratory distress in the newborn:

- Best initial diagnostic test: **Chest x-ray**
- Other diagnostic studies:
  - **ABG**
  - **Blood cultures** (sepsis)
  - **Blood glucose** (hypoglycemia)
  - CBC (anemia or polycythemia)
  - **Cranial ultrasound** (intracranial hemorrhage)
- Best initial treatment:
  - **Oxygen:** Keep $SaO_2 > 95$ percent.
  - Give **nasal CPAP** if high O_2 requirements to prevent barotrauma and bronchopulmonary dysplasia.
  - Consider **empiric antibiotics** for suspected sepsis.

CCS Tip: In cases of newborn respiratory distress, when hypoxia does not improve with oxygen therapy, evaluate the patient for cardiac causes of hypoxia (i.e., congenital heart defects).

Respiratory Distress Syndrome (RDS)

Clinical features are a **premature neonate** with the following:

- Tachypnea
- Nasal grunting
- Intercostals retractions within hours of birth

The hallmark finding is **hypoxemia.** Eventually **hypercarbia and respiratory acidosis develop.**

Diagnostic Testing

- Best initial tests: **Chest x-ray** (ground-glass appearance), **atelectasis, air bronchograms**
- Best predictive test: **Lecithin-sphingomyelin (L/S) ratio on amniotic fluid prior to birth**

Pneumonia and RDS look identical on chest x-ray. If in doubt, give antibiotics.

Treatment

- Best initial treatments: **Oxygen and nasal CPAP**
- Most effective treatment: **Exogenous surfactant administration** (proven to decrease mortality)

Lucinactant is the first synthetic peptide-containing surfactant approved for treatment of neonatal RDS.

Basic Science Correlate

Mechanism of Surfactant

- Surfactant prevents collapse of the aveoli by decreasing surface tension.
- Surfactant is produced by Type II pneumocytes, which start to develop around 24 weeks gestation. However, not enough surfactant is secreted until 35 weeks gestation.

Do the following for primary prevention:

- **Antenatal betamethasone:** This is *most* effective if > 24 hours before delivery and < 34 weeks gestation.
- **Avoid prematurity:** Give **tocolytics.**
- Give corticosteroids *immediately* to any **fetus** in danger of preterm delivery < 34 weeks.
- Postnatal corticosteroids do *not* help and are *not* indicated.

Possible complications:

- **Retinopathy of prematurity (ROP)** (hypoxemia)
- **Bronchopulmonary dysplasia** (prolonged high-concentration oxygen): Prevent with CPAP.
- **Intraventricular hemorrhage**

Transient Tachypnea of the Newborn (TTN)

This presents as tachypnea after a **term birth** of infant delivered by **cesarean section or rapid second stage of labor**, likely related to retained lung fluid. The condition usually resolves in 24–48 hours.

Basic Science Correlate

TTN is caused by retained lung fluid. That is, fluid present in the lungs in utero does not get squeezed out in passage through the birth canal. Increased fluid in the lungs causes *increased* airway resistance and *decreased* lung compliance.

Diagnostic Testing

Perform a **chest x-ray** to look for the following:

- **Air trapping**
- **Fluid in fissures**
- **Perihilar streaking**

Treatment

The best initial treatment is **oxygen** (minimal requirements needed), which results in rapid improvement within hours to days.

Meconium Aspiration

This presents as **severe respiratory distress and hypoxemia** in a **term neonate** with **hypoxia or fetal distress in utero.** (Meconium passed may be aspirated in utero or with the first postnatal breath.)

> **Basic Science Correlate**
>
> Meconium is the *first* stool a baby passes. It is sticky, like tar, and is composed of epithelial cells, lanugo, mucus, bile, and amniotic fluid. Fetuses in distress often pass meconium before birth. **Meconium aspiration** causes:
>
> - Blockage of aveoli
> - Decreased gas exchange
> - Irritation of airway, causing inflammation then pneumonia

Diagnostic Testing

Perform a **chest x-ray** to look for the following:

- **Patchy infiltrates**
- **Increased AP diameter** (barrel chest)
- **Flattening of diaphragm**

Treatment

- **Positive pressure ventilation**
- **High-frequency ventilation**
- **Nitric oxide therapy**
- **Extracorporeal membrane oxygenation**

Prevent by performing an **endotracheal intubation and airway suction** of depressed infants.

Possible complications:

- Pulmonary artery hypertension
- Air leak (pneumothorax, pneumomediastinum)
- Aspiration pneumonitis

Diaphragmatic Hernia

This presents as **respiratory distress and scaphoid abdomen** (distress related to pulmonary hypoplasia).

Diagnostic Testing

Perform a **chest x-ray** to **look for loops** of bowel visible in the chest.

Treatment

Perform **immediate intubation** (may require extracorporeal membrane oxygenation), followed by **surgical correction.**

Gastrointestinal and Hepatobiliary Disorders

Meconium Plugs (Lower Colon) and Meconium Ileus (Lower Ileum)

This presents initially with an intestinal obstruction. Associated conditions are the following:

- Plugs:
  - **Small left colon in IODM**
  - **Hirschsprung disease**
  - **Cystic fibrosis**
  - **Maternal drug abuse**
- Ileus: **Cystic fibrosis**

Diagnostic Testing

The best initial diagnostic test is an **abdominal x-ray.**

Treatment

Ileus with **Gastografin enema.**

Upper Gastrointestinal Malformation

A newborn is born by normal vaginal delivery without complication. There is no respiratory distress. Upon his first feed, he is noted to have prominent drooling; he gags and develops respiratory distress. Chest x-ray reveals an infiltrate in the lung. Which of the following will confirm the diagnosis?

a. Arterial blood gas
b. Blood cultures
c. CT scan of chest
d. Nasogastric tube placement
e. Gastrografin enema

Answer: **D.** This patient has a **tracheoesophageal fistula (TEF).** Classically, there is choking and gagging with the first feeding and then respiratory distress develops due to aspiration pneumonia. The feeding tube will be coiled in the chest. Don't forget to look for other abnormalities associated with VACTERL syndrome.

VACTERL abnormalities are the following:
- **V**ertebral defects
- **A**nal atresia
- **C**ardiac abnormalities
- **T**racheoesophageal fistula with **E**sophageal atresia
- **R**adial and **R**enal anomalies
- **L**imb syndrome

Basic Science Correlate

TEF is an embryological malformation: Division of the cranial part of the foregut into the respiratory and esophageal parts is incomplete. This occurs at week 4 of development.

A premature infant is born by normal vaginal delivery without complication. There is no respiratory distress. Upon her first feed, she begins vomiting gastric and bilious material. Chest x-ray is shown. What is the most likely diagnosis?

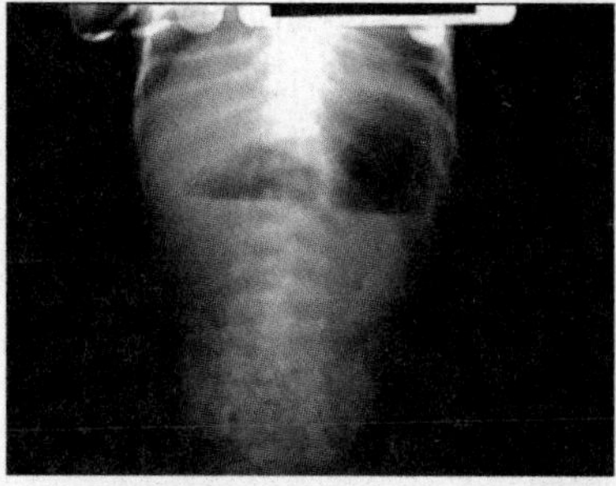

Answer: The most likely diagnosis is **duodenal atresia.** Half of infants with this condition are born prematurely, and the condition is associated with Down syndrome. Look for **polyhydramnios** in the prenatal exam. Treatment involves **nasogastric decompression and surgical correction.** You must search for other abnormalities (VACTERL association) with x-ray of the spine, abdominal ultrasound, and echocardiogram.

Differential diagnosis of double-bubble seen on x-ray includes duodenal atresia, annular pancreas, malrotation, and volvulus.

Basic Science Correlate

During duodenal development, the lumen is completely occluded by epithelium, then is re-formed. Failure to re-form a lumen = Duodenal atresia.

Necrotizing Enterocolitis (NEC)

NEC presents in a premature infant with **low Apgar scores** and **bloody stools, apnea, and lethargy** when feeding is started. **Abdominal wall erythema and distension are signs of ischemia.** NEC is a true medical/surgical emergency with 50 percent mortality related to ischemia, inflammation of the bowel, and ultimately perforation. The greatest risk factor for NEC is premature delivery.

Diagnostic Testing

Best initial diagnostic test: **Abdominal x-ray.** Ultrasound may also be useful in diagnosis.

There is an increased risk of NEC with formula feeding.

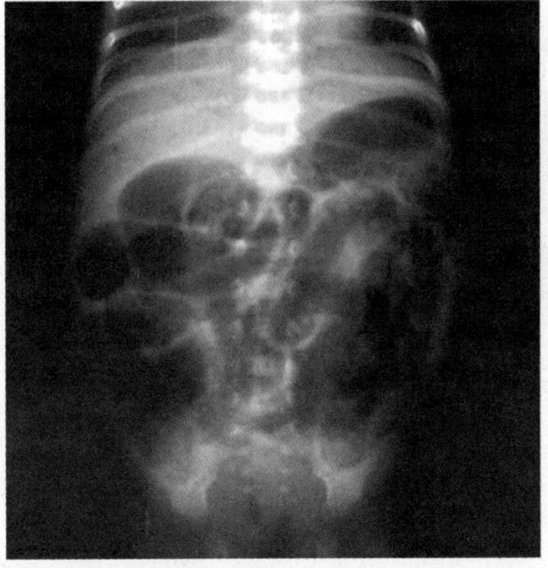

Pneumatosis intestinalis is associated with necrotizing enterocolitis.

Treatment

The best initial therapy is as follows:

- **Stop all feeds**
- **Decompress the gut**
- Begin **broad spectrum antibiotics**
- Evaluate for **surgical resection**

Pneumatosis intestinalis is the pathognomonic sign of NEC on radiograph, seen as gas cysts in the bowel wall instead of in the bowel lumen, which is normal.

Failure to Pass Meconium

- Best initial test: **Rectal examination.** A patent rectum with passage of a large voluminous stool after digital exam suggests **Hirschsprung disease.**
- Next step in the workup: **Barium enema** (megacolon proximal to obstruction)
- Best confirmatory test: **Rectal biopsy** (absent ganglionic cells). Treatment is **surgical resection.**

An absent anal opening on exam suggests **imperforate anus.** Treatment is **surgical reconstruction.**

Jaundice in the Newborn

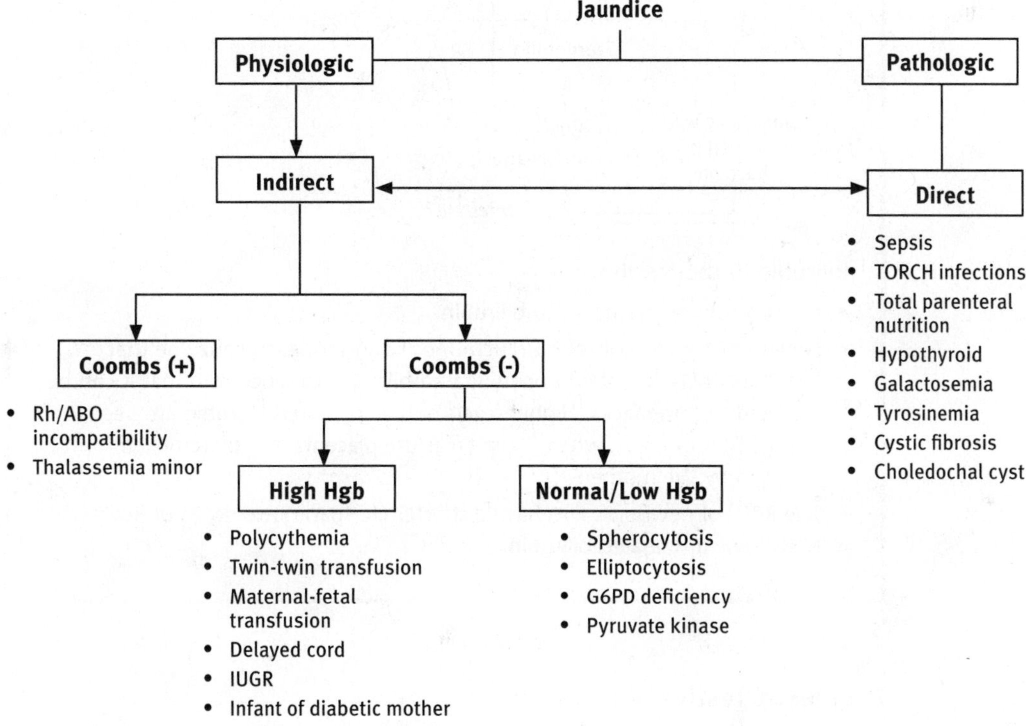

When is hyperbilirubinemia considered pathological?

- It appears on the first day of life.
- Bilirubin rises > 5 mg/dL/day.
- Bilirubin > 12 mg/dL in term infant.
- Direct bilirubin > 2 mg/dL at any time.
- It is present after the 2nd week of life.

Basic Science Correlate

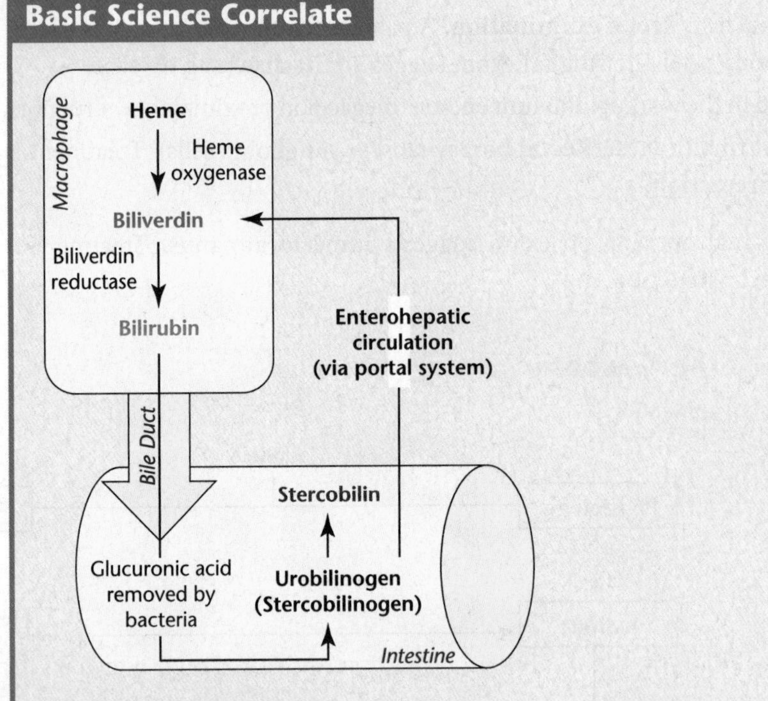

Bilirubin in the Newborn

- Hemoglobin breaks down to bilirubin.
- Newborns have low levels of glucuronosyltransferase, the enzyme that connects or "conjugates" unconjugated bilirubin to glucose so that it can be excreted through feces. Higher levels of unconjugated bilirubin are needed during development, when it can cross the placenta and be removed from the fetus by the mother.
- The RBCs of newborns also have a shorter life span. Breakdown of RBCs releases unconjugated bilirubin.

Diagnostic Testing

If jaundice presents in the first 24 hours, workup includes:

- Total and direct bilirubin
- Blood type of infant and mother: Look for ABO or Rh incompatibility.
- Direct Coombs test
- CBC, reticulocyte count, and blood smear: Assess for hemolysis.
- Urinalysis and urine culture if elevated direct bilirubin: Assess for sepsis.

If there is prolonged jaundice (> 2 weeks) and **NO elevation of conjugated bilirubin,** consider the following:

- **UTI or other infection**
- **Bilirubin conjugation abnormalities** (e.g., Gilbert's syndrome, Crigler-Najjar syndrome)
- **Hemolysis**
- **Intrinsic red cell membrane or enzyme defects** (spherocytosis, elliptocytosis, glucose-6-phosphate dehydrogenase deficiency, pyruvate kinase deficiency)

Where there is prolonged jaundice (> 2 weeks) **AND elevation of conjugated bilirubin,** consider **cholestasis:**

- Initial diagnostic tests: **liver function tests**
- Most specific tests: **ultrasound and liver biopsy**

Treatment

- **Phototherapy** when bilirubin > 10–12 mg/dL (normally decreases by 2 mg/dL every 4–6 hours)
- **Exchange transfusion** in any infant with suspected bilirubin encephalopathy or failure of phototherapy to reduce total bilirubin and risk of kernicterus

> The most feared complication of jaundice results from elevated indirect (*un*conjugated) bilirubin, which can cross the blood brain barrier, deposit in the basal ganglia and brainstem nuclei, and cause **kernicterus.**
> Watch out for hypotonia, seizures, opisthotonos, delayed motor skills, choreoathetosis, and sensorineural hearing loss. Management is **immediate exchange transfusion.**

Basic Science Correlate

Phototherapy isomerizes bilirubin, making it water-soluble.

Neonatal Sepsis

A 5-week-old infant is brought into the clinic with irritability, weight loss of 3 lbs over the past week, and "grunting." Physical examination reveals temperature of 102.5°F. There is a bulging anterior fontanel, delayed capillary refill. What is the next step in management?

Answer: Next step in management includes transferring the patient to the emergency room and initiating a ***full sepsis workup***. This includes: 1. CBC with differential, 2. blood culture, 3. urinalysis/urine culture, and 4. chest x-ray BEFORE antibiotics are given.

Basic Science Correlate

Gram-positive bacteria stain purple due to their *thick* peptidoglycan layer. Gram-negative bacteria stain red due to the *thin* peptidoglycan layer.

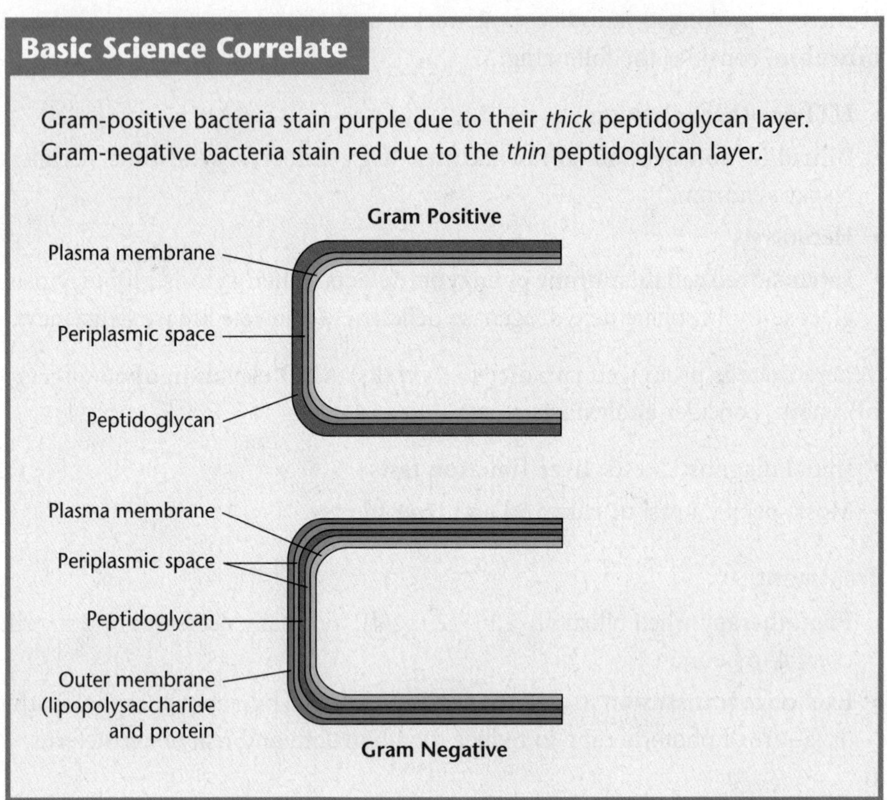

In cases of **early-onset sepsis** (within first 24 hours), **pneumonia** is the most common cause. The most common organisms involved are these:

- **Group B *Streptococcus*** (beta-hemolytic, gram-positive)
- ***E. coli*** (gram-negative, rod shaped)
- ***Haemophilus influenzae*** (gram-negative coccobacilli)
- ***Listeria monocytogenes*** (gram-positive, motile with flagella)

In cases of **late-onset sepsis** (after first 24 hours), meningitis and bacteremia are the most common causes. The most common organisms are these:

- ***Staphylococcus aureus*** (gram-positive cocci)
- ***E. coli***
- ***Klebsiella*** (gram-negative, oxidase-negative rod)
- ***Pseudomonas*** (gram-negative aerobic bacteria)

Treatment

- Empiric treatment of neonatal sepsis is to prescribe **ampicillin and gentamicin** until 48- to 72-hour cultures are negative.
- If meningitis is possible, **add cefotaxime**.

TORCH Infections Summary

Many of the TORCH infections have similar presentations. The following table highlights the distinguishing features to look for in the exam. (Refer to section 6 on obstetrics for more details.)

Infection	Classic Feature(s)	Diagnostic Workup
General features	Intrauterine growth retardation, hepatosplenomegaly, jaundice, mental retardation	Elevated total cord blood IgM
Toxoplasmosis	Hydrocephalus with generalized intracranial calcifications and chorioretinitis	IgM against toxoplasmosis
Rubella	Cataracts, deafness, and heart defects Blueberry muffin spots (extramedullary hematopoiesis)	Maternal rubella immune status negative or unknown—obtain IgM against rubella
CMV	Microcephaly with periventricular calcifications Petechiae with thrombocytopenia, sensorineural hearing loss	Urine or saliva CMV culture—if negative, excludes CMV Serum CMV IgM antibody in newborn suggests congenital CMV
Herpes	First week: Pneumonia/shock Second week: Skin vesicles, keratoconjunctivitis Third to fourth week: Acute meningoencephalitis	Best initial test: Tzanck smear/culture (does not exclude disease if negative) Most specific test: HSV PCR
Syphilis	Osteochondritis and periostitis; desquamating skin rash of palms and soles, snuffles (mucopurulent rhinitis)	Best initial test: VDRL screening Most specific test: IgM-FTA-ABS
Varicella	Neonatal: Pneumonia Congenital: Limb hypoplasia, cutaneous scars, seizures, mental retardation	Best initial test: IgM serology Most specific test: PCR of amniotic fluid

Seizures

In the newborn intensive care unit, an infant is noted to be "jittery" and has repetitive sucking movements, tongue thrusting, and brief apneic spells. Blood counts and chemistries are within normal limits. What is the initial workup of this patient?

Answer: Seizures classically present with **subtle repetitive movements,** such as chewing, tongue thrusting, apnea, staring, blinking, or desaturations. Classic tonic-clonic movements are uncommon. Look for **ocular deviation and failure of jitteriness to subside with stimulus** (e.g., passive movement of a limb). Complete diagnostic workup for seizures is listed below.

Diagnostic Testing

- **EEG:** May be normal
- **CBC, electrolytes, calcium, magnesium, glucose** (hypoglycemia is a common cause of seizures in infants of diabetic mothers)
- **Amino acid assay and urine organic acids** to detect inborn errors of metabolism and pyridoxine deficiency
- To look for infectious causes, perform the following:
  - TORCH infection studies: **Total cord blood IgM** for screening
  - **Blood and urine cultures**
  - **Lumbar puncture** if meningitis is suspected
- **Ultrasound of head in preterms** to look for intraventricular hemorrhage
  - Intracranial hemorrhage causes seizures typically 2–7 days after birth

Treatment

Correct the underlying cause, including electrolyte abnormalities. For acute seizure, use **lorazepam** *or* **diazepam** (rectally). Treatment for chronic seizures depends on type; with absence seizures, use **ethosuximide**.

Basic Science Correlate

Benzodiazepines bind the alpha-1 receptor site of the GABA receptor.

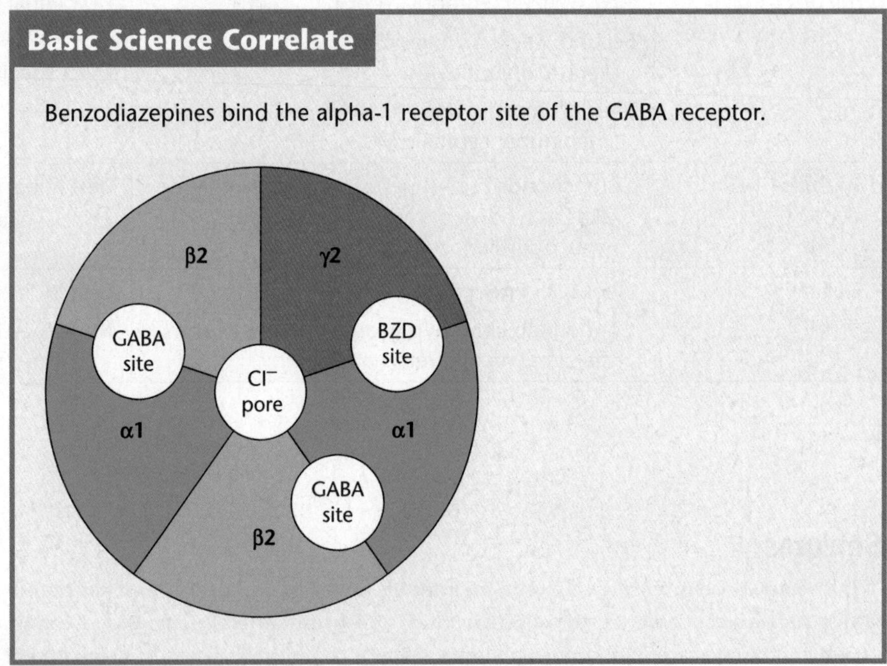

Substance Abuse and Neonatal Withdrawal

Neonatal withdrawal presents with the following:

- **Hyperactivity**
- **Irritability**
- **Fever**
- **Diarrhea**
- **Tremors/jitters**
- **High-pitched crying**
- **Sneezing**
- **Restlessness**
- **Vomiting**
- **Nasal stuffiness**
- **Poor feeding**
- **Seizures**
- **Tachypnea**

The timing of withdrawal:

- **Heroin, cocaine, amphetamine, and alcohol withdrawal:** Presents within the first 48 hours of life.
- **Methadone withdrawal:** Presents within the first 96 hours (up to 2 weeks). This drug is associated with a higher risk of seizures.

Complications

Infants of addicted mothers are at higher risk for the following complications:

- **Low birth weight**
- **Intrauterine growth restriction (IUGR)**
- **Congenital anomalies** (alcohol, cocaine)
- **Sudden infant death syndrome (SIDS)**

Also, watch out for complications of the mother's conditions, such as:

- **Sexually transmitted diseases**
- **Toxemia**
- **Breech**
- **Abruption**
- **Intraventricular hemorrhage** (cocaine use)

Treatment

The best initial treatment is to prescribe **opioids** (especially if specific prenatal opioid use was known) and **phenobarbital.**

> *Never* give naloxone to an infant born from mother with known narcotics use. It may precipitate sudden withdrawal, including seizures.

Teratogenesis and the Effect of Drugs on the Neonate

Drug	Effect	Drug	Effect
Anesthetics	Respiratory, CNS depression	**Isotretinoin**	Facial and ear anomalies, congenital heart disease
Barbiturates	Respiratory, CNS depression	**Phenytoin**	Hypoplastic nails, typical facies, IUGR
Magnesium sulfate	Respiratory depression	**Diethylstilbestrol (DES)**	Vaginal adenocarcinoma
Phenobarbital	Vitamin K deficiency	**Tetracycline**	Enamel hypoplasia, discolored teeth
Sulfonamides	Displaces bilirubin from albumin	**Lithium**	Ebstein's anomaly
NSAIDs	Premature closure of ductus arteriosus	**Warfarin**	Facial dysmorphism and chondrodysplasia
ACE inhibitors	Craniofacial abnormalities	**Valproate/ carbamazepine**	Mental retardation, neural tube defects

Genetics/Dysmorphology

Condition	Classic Feature(s)	Diagnostic Workup/Disease Associations
Trisomy 21: Down syndrome Risk associated with advanced maternal age (> 35 years)	Upward slanting palpebral fissures; speckling of iris (Brushfield spots); inner epicanthal folds; small stature; late fontanel closure; mental retardation	• Hearing exam • Echocardiogram: Endocardiac cushion defect > VSD > PDA, ASD; MVP (Cardiac abnormalities are a major cause of early mortality.) • Gastrointestinal: TEF, duodenal atresia • TSH: Hypothyroidism • With advancing age, have a low probability of developing acute lymphocytic leukemia and early-onset Alzheimer's disease
Trisomy 18: Edwards syndrome	Low-set, malformed ears; microcephaly; micrognathia; clenched hand—index over third, fifth over fourth; rocker-bottom feet and hammer toe; omphalocele	• Echocardiogram: VSD, ASD, PDA • Renal ultrasound: Polycystic kidneys, ectopic or double ureter • Most patients do not survive first year
Trisomy 13: Patau syndrome	Defect of midface, eye, and forebrain development: Holoprosencephaly, microcephaly, microphthalmia, cleft lip/palate	• Echocardiogram: VSD, PDA, ASD • Renal ultrasound: Polycystic kidneys • Single umbilical artery

(continued next page)

Basic Science Correlate

Trisomy is most commonly caused by nondisjunction during meiosis.

Condition	Classic Feature(s)	Diagnostic Workup/Disease Associations
Aniridia-Wilms tumor association (WAGR syndrome)	**W**ilms **A**niridia **G**U anomalies Mental **R**etardation	• When you see an infant with aniridia, do a complete workup for WAGR syndrome.
Klinefelter syndrome (XXY) 1:500 males	Low IQ, behavioral problems, slim with long limbs, gynecomastia	• Testosterone levels: Hypogonadism and hypogenitalism • Replace testosterone at 11–12 years of age.
Turner syndrome (XO) Sporadic; no association with maternal age	Small-stature female, gonadal dysgenesis, low IQ, congenital lymphedema, webbed posterior neck, broad chest, wide-spaced nipples	• Renal ultrasound: Horseshoe kidney, double renal pelvis • Cardiac: Bicuspid aortic valve, coarctation of the aorta • Thyroid function: Primary hypothyroidism • Can give estrogen, growth hormone, and anabolic steroid replacement
Fragile X syndrome Fragile site on long arm of X Molecular diagnosis—variable number of repeat CGG	Macrocephaly in early childhood, large ears, large testes Most common cause of mental retardation in boys	• Attention deficit hyperactivity syndrome
Beckwith-Wiedemann syndrome IGF-2 disrupted at 11p15.5	Multiorgan enlargement: Macrosomia, macroglossia, pancreatic beta cell hyperplasia (hypoglycemia), large kidneys, neonatal polycythemia	• Increased risk of abdominal tumors • Obtain ultrasounds and serum AFP every 6 months through 6 years of age to look for Wilms' tumor and hepatoblastoma
Prader-Willi syndrome Deletion of 15q11q13, which is paternally derived	Obesity, mental retardation, binge eating, small genitalia	• Decreased life expectancy related to morbid obesity
Angelman syndrome (happy puppet syndrome) Deletion of 15q11q13, which is maternally derived	Mental retardation, inappropriate laughter, absent speech or $<$ 6 words, ataxia and jerky arm movements resembling a puppet gait, recurrent seizures	• 80 percent develop epilepsy
Robin sequence (Pierre Robin) Associated with fetal alcohol syndrome, Edwards syndrome	Mandibular hypoplasia, cleft palate	• Monitor airway: Obstruction possible over first 4 weeks of life

Growth, Nutrition, and Development

Exam Tips on Pediatric Growth

Birth weight is normal in patients with *either* genetic short stature or constitutional delay of growth. Patients with either condition have normal growth velocity, which is below and parallel to the normal growth curve.

- Birth weight normally doubles by 6 months and triples by 1 year.
- Height percentile at 2 years of age normally correlates with final adult height percentile.
- Best indicator for acute malnutrition is weight/height < 5th percentile.
- Best indicator for under- and overweight is BMI.
- Skeletal maturity is related to sexual maturity (less related to chronologic age).
- The most common cause of failure to thrive in all age groups is psychosocial deprivation.
- All cases of underfeeding must be reported to child protective services (CPS).
- You must work up any child who has crossed 2 major growth percentiles.

Description of Growth Pattern	Differential Diagnosis	Workup
↓ weight gain more than ↓ length/height	• Undernutrition • Inadequate digestion • Malabsorption (infection, celiac disease, cystic fibrosis, disaccharide deficiency, protein-losing enteropathy)	Assess caloric intake Perform stool studies for fat Perform sweat chloride test
Normal weight gain ↓ length/height	• Growth hormone or thyroid hormone deficiency • Excessive cortisol secretion • Skeletal dysplasias	Growth hormone (GH) deficiency: • Insulin-like growth factor 1 (IGF-1) and IGF-binding protein 3 (IGF-BP3) Thyroid hormone: • TSH, free T4, free T3 Cushings: • 24-hour urinary cortisol or free cortisol Bone age (x-ray of hand and wrist): • Skeletal dysplasia: no delay in bone age and disproportionate bone length on exam
↓ weight gain equals ↓ length/height	Systemic illness: • Heart failure • Inflammation (e.g., inflammatory bowel disease or arthritis) • Renal insufficiency • Hepatic insufficiency Genetic short stature Constitutional delay in growth and development	Inflammatory markers: • CRP, ESR, CBC with diff Organ dysfunction: • LFT, creatinine, BUN • Electrolytes Bone age: • Genetic short stature: The bone age is close to the chronological age; puberty occurs at the normal time. • Constitutional delay of growth: The bone age is delayed, and puberty occurs later than in most children.

Breastfeeding

The advantages of breastfeeding:

- **Passive transfer of T-cell immunity:** Decreased risk of allergies and gastrointestinal and respiratory infections
- **Psychological/emotional:** Maternal-infant bonding

Basic Science Correlate

- IgM is secreted during early stages of humoral immunity. It is the first antibody secreted.
- IgG causes sustained immunity to pathogens. It is the only immunoglobulin that crosses the placenta.
- IgE binds to allergens and secretes histamine.
- IgA is found in mucosal areas (intestines, saliva, tears, breast milk). It is secreted during breastfeeding.

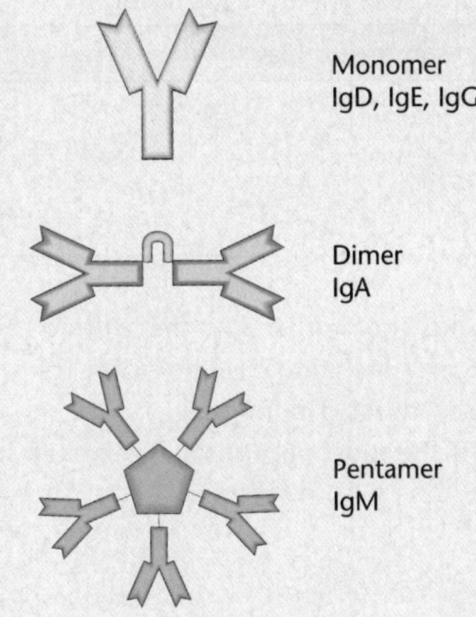

Following are the contraindications to breastfeeding:

- **Galactosemia in baby**
- **HIV**
- **HSV** *if* lesions on breast
- **Acute maternal disease if absent in infant** (e.g., tuberculosis, sepsis)
- **Maternal cancer receiving treatment**
- **Substance abuse**

Breastfeeding is *not* contraindicated in mastitis.

High-Yield Developmental Milestones

The absence of milestone behavior or persistence of it beyond a given time frame signifies **CNS dysfunction.** Exam questions typically describe an infant's/child's skills and ask for the corresponding age.

Age	Milestone
Newborn reflexes	Moro, grasp, rooting, tonic neck, and placing reflexes: Appear at birth and disappear at 4–6 months Parachute reflex (extension of arms when fall simulated): Present at 6–8 months and persists
9 months	Has pincer grasp, creeps and crawls, knows own name
12 months	Cruises, says 1 or more words, plays ball
15 months	Builds 3-cube tower, walks alone, makes lines and scribbles
18 months	Builds 4-cube tower, walks down stairs, says 10 words, feeds self
24 months	Builds 7-cube tower, runs well, goes up and down stairs, jumps with 2 feet, threads shoelaces, handles spoon, says 2–3 sentences
36 months	Walks downstairs alternating feet, rides tricycle, knows age and sex, understands taking turns
48 months	Hops on 1 foot, throws ball overhead, tells stories, participates in group play

Behavioral Disorders

A 4-year-old boy has problems with bedwetting. The mother says that during the day, he has no problems but is usually wet 6 of 7 mornings. He does not report dysuria or frequency and has not had increased thirst. The mother also says that he is a deep sleeper. Which of the following is the most appropriate next step in management?

a. Give anticholinergics.
b. Give desmopressin.
c. Give prophylactic antibiotics.
d. Perform renal ultrasound.
e. Reassure mother that bedwetting is normal.

Answer: **E.** Bedwetting before age 5 (before bladder control is anticipated) is normal.

Enuresis

Enuresis is the **involuntary voiding of urine, occurring at least twice a week for at least 3 months in children over 5 years** (when bladder control is anticipated). **Nocturnal enuresis** (nighttime wetting) is more common in boys who are usually continent, occurring within 2 years of daytime continence; address with behavior therapy. **Diurnal enuresis** (daytime wetting) is more common in girls and is associated with a higher rate of urinary tract infections (UTIs).

The most common causes of diurnal enuresis are diabetes insipidus, UTI, seizure, constipation, and abuse.

Diagnostic Testing

- Best initial test: **Urinalysis** in all patients
- If signs of infection are present: **Urine culture**
- If recurrent UTIs: **Bladder/renal ultrasound** (postvoid residual, anatomical abnormalities) or **voiding cystourethrogram**

Treatment

- Best initial treatment: Behavioral and motivational therapy (limit liquids, use a bed alarm, never punish the child) cures two thirds of patients.
- If behavioral therapy fails: **imipramine and desmopressin** (to decrease the volume of urine produced).

Encopresis

Encopresis is the **unintentional or involuntary passage of feces in inappropriate settings,** such as into clothing or onto the floor, **in children > 4 years** (the age by which most children control bowel movements).

Diagnostic Testing

- Best initial test: **Abdominal x-ray.** This distinguishes between retentive (most common; associated with constipation and overflow incontinence) and nonretentive (associated with abuse).
- Do *not* miss uncommon causes: Hirschsprung disease, anal fissure, ulcerative colitis, or spinal cord abnormalities.

Treatment

- Best initial therapies:
  - **Retentive** encopresis: **Disimpaction, stool softeners, and behavior intervention**
  - **Nonretentive** encopresis: **Behavior modification alone**

Immunizations

Exam Tips

- Premature infants or low-birth-weight babies:
  - Do *not* delay immunizations—immunize at chronological age.
  - Do *not* dose-adjust immunizations.
- Do *not* give live vaccines to immunocompromised patients.

- The following are *not* contraindications to immunization:
  - A reaction to a previous DPT of temperature < 105°F, redness, soreness, and swelling
  - A mild, acute illness in an otherwise well child
  - A family history of seizures or sudden infant death syndrome
- **MMR:** Documented egg allergy is *not* a contraindication.
- **Yellow fever vaccine:** Egg allergy *does* contraindicate.
- **Influenza vaccine:** Egg allergy *is no longer a contraindication.* Patients ≥ 6 months with a known egg allergy should receive **trivalent inactivated influenza vaccine (TIV)** followed by a 30-minute observation period in a facility prepared to recognize and treat anaphylaxis. Patients with a history of severe anaphylaxis to eggs should be referred to an allergy specialist to receive TIV.
- MMR does *not* cause autism or inflammatory bowel disease.
- Hepatitis B vaccine does *not* cause demyelinating neurologic disorders.
- Meningococcal vaccination is *not* related to development of Guillain-Barré.

Recommended immunization schedule for persons aged 0 through 18 years—**United States, 2014.**
(FOR THOSE WHO FALL BEHIND OR START LATE, SEE THE CATCH-UP SCHEDULE).

Vaccine	Birth	1 mo	2 mos	4 mos	6 mos	9 mos	12 mos	15 mos	18 mos	19–23 mos	2-3 yrs	4-6 yrs	7-10 yrs	11-12 yrs	13–15 yrs	16–18 yrs
Hepatitis B[1] (HepB)	1st dose	←2nd dose→			←3rd dose→											
Rotavirus[2] (RV) RV1 (2-dose series); RV5 (3-dose series)			1st dose	2nd dose	See footnote 2											
Diphtheria, tetanus, & acellular pertussis[3] (DTaP: <7 yrs)			1st dose	2nd dose	3rd dose			←4th dose→				5th dose				
Tetanus, diphtheria, & acellular pertussis[4] (Tdap: ≥7 yrs)														(Tdap)		
Haemophilus influenzae type b[5] (Hib)			1st dose	2nd dose	See footnote 5		←3rd or 4th dose, See footnote 5→									
Pneumococcal conjugate[6] (PCV13)			1st dose	2nd dose	3rd dose		←4th dose→									
Pneumococcal polysaccharide[6] (PPSV23)																
Inactivated poliovirus[7] (IPV) (<18 yrs)			1st dose	2nd dose	←3rd dose→							4th dose				
Influenza[8] (IIV; LAIV) 2 doses for some: See footnote 8					Annual vaccination (IIV only)						Annual vaccination (IIV or LAIV)					
Measles, mumps, rubella[9] (MMR)							←1st dose→					2nd dose				
Varicella[10] (VAR)							←1st dose→					2nd dose				
Hepatitis A[11] (HepA)							←2-dose series, See footnote 11→									
Human papillomavirus[12] (HPV2: females only; HPV4: males and females)														(3-dose series)		
Meningococcal[13] (Hib-MenCY ≥ 6 weeks; MenACWY-D ≥9 mos; MenACWY-CRM ≥ 2 mos)			See footnote 13											1st dose		Booster

- Range of recommended ages for all children
- Range of recommended ages for catch-up immunization
- Range of recommended ages for certain high-risk groups
- Range of recommended ages during which catch-up is encouraged and for certain high-risk groups
- Not routinely recommended

www.cdc.gov/vaccines/schedules/hcp/imz/child-adolescent.html

Active Immunizations after Exposure

Measles	0–6 months: Ig 6–12 months: Ig plus vaccine > 12 months: Vaccine only within 72 hours of exposure Pregnant or immunocompromised: Ig only
Varicella	Susceptible children and household contacts: VZIG and vaccine Susceptible pregnant women, newborns whose mothers had chickenpox within 5 days before delivery to 48 hours after delivery: VZIG
Hepatitis	Hepatitis B: Ig plus vaccine; given at birth, 1 month, and 6 months Hepatitis A: > 2 years only, Ig plus vaccine
Mumps and rubella	No postexposure protection available

Specific Routine Vaccinations

Hepatitis B	If mother is HBsAg negative: • First dose at birth. A total of 3 doses by **18 months.** If mother is HBsAg positive: • First dose of hepatitis B vaccine (HBV) plus hepatitis B Ig at 2 different sites within 12 hours of birth. A total of 3 doses by **6 months.**
DTaP	Total of 5 doses is recommended before school entry (last dose age 4–6 years). Pertussis booster vaccine *also* given during adolescence, regardless of immunization. Td is given at 11–12 years, then every 10 years.
HiB conjugated vaccine	Does not cover nontypeable *Haemophilus.* Not given after age of 5. Invasive disease does not confirm immunity; patients still require vaccines if < 5.
Varicella	Has been associated with the development of herpes zoster after immunization.
Meningococcal conjugate vaccine	Given at age 11–12 or at age 15. Indicated for all college freshmen living in dormitories. Menomune (MPSV4) indicated in children aged **2–10.**

Don't forget dilated eye exam by an ophthalmologist in cases of suspected infant abuse.

Child Abuse

Diagnostic Testing

- Laboratory studies: **PT, PTT, platelets, bleeding time, CBC**
- **Skeletal survey**
- If **severe injuries** (even with no neurological signs), perform the following:
  - **Head CT scan ± MRI**
  - **Ophthalmologic examination**
- If **abdominal trauma,** perform the following:
  - **Urine and stool for blood**
  - **Liver and pancreatic enzymes**
  - **Abdominal CT scan**
- Urine toxicology screen, especially if the case describes altered mental status

Treatment

1. The first step is *always* to **address medical and/or surgical issues.**
2. Then report any child suspected of being abused or neglected to **child protective services (CPS).** Initial action includes a phone report; in most states, a written report is then required within 48 hours.

The following are indications for hospitalization:

- **Medical condition requires it.**
- **Diagnosis is unclear.**
- **There is no alternative safe place.**

If parents refuse hospitalization or treatment, the physician must get an **emergency court order.**

You *must* explain to the parent why an inflicted injury is suspected abuse, that you are legally obligated to report it, that you have made a referral to protect the child, and that a CPS worker and law enforcement officer will be involved.

Respiratory Diseases

Condition	Classic Presentation	Diagnosis	Steps in Management	Complication(s)/ Prognosis
Croup *Parainfluenza 1 or 3, influenza A or B* **Notes:** *Parainfluenza* is an enveloped, single-stranded RNA virus. *Influenza* is an RNA virus of the family Orthomyxoviridae.	Child age 3 months to 5 years with URTI symptoms: rhinorrhea, sore throat, hoarseness and deep barking cough, inspiratory stridor, tachypnea Symptoms are worse at night.	Diagnosis is made clinically; however, neck x-ray positive for steeple sign can be diagnostic.	1. Humidified oxygen 2. Nebulized epinephrine and corticosteroids Antitussives, decongestants, sedatives, or antibiotics are *not* used in the management of croup.	Spontaneous resolution in 1 week Always suspect diagnosis of epiglottitis
Epiglottitis *H. influenzae type B* (now less common) *S. pyogenes, S. pneumoniae, S. aureus, Mycoplasma* **Notes:** *H. influenza* is a gram-negative coccobacillus. *S. pneumonia* is a gram-positive, alpha-hemolytic bacterium. *S. pyogenes* is a gram-positive coccus that causes group A streptococcal infection.	Sudden onset, muffled voice, drooling, dysphagia, high fever, and inspiratory stridor Patient prefers sitting in the tripod position. Patient has a toxic appearance.	This is a medical emergency. Go straight to management based on clinical diagnosis. Perform diagnostic workup *after* stabilization: • Neck x-ray (thumb-print sign) • Blood cultures • Nasopharyngoscopy in the OR • Epiglottic swab culture	1. Transfer to hospital/OR 2. Consult ENT and anesthesia 3. Intubate 4. Give antibiotics (ceftriaxone) and steroids 5. Give rifampin prophylaxis to household contacts if *H. influenzae* positive	Airway obstruction and death
Bacterial tracheitis *S. aureus* **Notes:** *S. aureus* is a gram-positive coccus that occurs in clusters.	Brassy cough, high fever, respiratory distress, but *no* drooling or dysphagia; child < 3 years; usually occurs after viral URTI	Clinical plus laryngoscopy: • Chest x-ray shows subglottic narrowing plus ragged tracheal air column • Blood cultures • Throat cultures	Antistaphylococcal antibiotics May require intubation if severe.	Airway obstruction

Differentiate epiglottitis from croup by the *absence* of a barking cough.

Clues to less common disorders:

- **Diphtheritic croup** (extremely rare in North America): Presents with a gray-white pharyngeal membrane; may cover soft palate; bleeds easily. Don't forget that diphtheria is a notifiable disease!
- **Foreign body aspiration:** Look for sudden choking/coughing without warning.
- **Retropharyngeal abscess:** Patient has drooling and difficulty swallowing.
- **Extrinsic compression** (vascular ring) or **intraluminal obstruction** (masses): Patient has continued symptoms and does not improve with treatment.
- **Angioedema:** This is due to a sudden allergic reaction. (Trigger is given in the case.) Manage with steroids and epinephrine. If severe, intubate for airway protection. Angioedema is mediated by bradykinin. This peptide increases the permeability of the vasculature, leading to the accumulation of fluid.
- **Pertussis:** Severe cough develops after 1–2 weeks with characteristic whoop and spells of cough (paroxysms). Look for child with incomplete immunization history.

The most common sites of foreign body aspiration are the following:

- In children > 1 year: Larynx
- In children < 1 year: Trachea or right mainstem bronchus

A toddler presents to the emergency center with sudden onset respiratory distress. The mother reports that the child was without symptoms, playing with LEGOS in the living room with her siblings. On physical examination, the patient is drooling and in moderate respiratory distress. There are decreased breath sounds on the right with intercostal retractions. Which of the following is the most appropriate next step in management?

a. Antibiotics
b. Bronchoscopy
c. Chest x-ray
d. Cricothyroidotomy
e. Throat cultures

Answer: **B.** Bronchoscopy is indicated both to visualize a suspected foreign body and for foreign body retrieval. If there is significant respiratory distress and hypoxemia, emergency cricothyroidotomy may be indicated. Foreign bodies are found most commonly in children < 4 years.

Recurrent infections in a young child should always raise the suspicion of **previously undiagnosed aspiration**. Get a chest x-ray to look for postobstruction atelectasis or visualization of the foreign body.

Best prevention against bronchiolitis is breastfeeding. Colostrum is particularly rich in IgA and protects against bronchiolitis.

Inflammation of the Small Airways

Bronchiolitis

The pathophysiology of bronchiolitis is as follows:

- Respiratory syncytial virus (RSV) (50 percent)
- Parainfluenza

- Adenovirus
- Other viruses

Bronchioles are the smallest parts of the airway (≤ 1 mm) and terminate at alveoli. They have ciliated cuboidal epithelium over a layer of smooth muscle. Bronchioles change in diameter and can reduce or increase airflow.

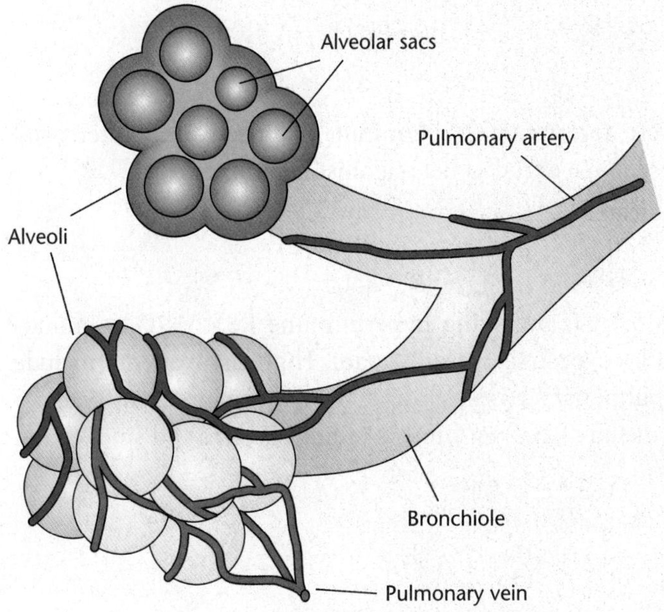

Anatomy of the Respiratory System

Bronchiolitis results in **inflammation,** which results in **ball-valve obstruction,** which results in **air trapping and overinflation.**

The classic presentation is in a **child < 2 years of age** (most severe in children 1–2 months old) with the following symptoms in fall and winter months:

- **Mild URI**
- **Fever**
- **Paroxysmal wheezy cough**
- **Dyspnea**
- **Tachypnea**
- **Apnea** (in young infants)
- On exam, there are **wheezing and prolonged expirations.**

Diagnostic Testing

Diagnosis is **clinical.** Following are diagnostic tests to perform:

- Best initial test: **Chest x-ray** shows hyperinflation with patchy atelectasis (may look like early pneumonia)
- Most specific test: **Viral antigen testing (IFA or ELISA)** of nasopharyngeal secretions

Treatment

Is **supportive only:**

> Ribavirin has not been shown to have clinical benefit and is generally not recommended.

- Hospitalize *if* severe tachypnea (> 60/minute), pyrexia, and intercostal retractions are present. Give trial of beta-agonist nebulizers.
- Steroids are *not* indicated.

Prevention

In high-risk patients *only,* is by giving hyperimmune RSV IVIG or monoclonal antibody to RSV F protein (palivizumab). High-risk patients include those with bronchopulmonary dysplasia and those born preterm. General prevention methods include hand-washing, avoiding secondhand smoke, and avoiding sick contacts.

Pneumonia

Classic presentations:

- **Viral:** Most common cause in children < 5 years. Most commonly RSV.
  - **URI symptoms**
  - **Low-grade fever**
  - **Tachypnea** (most consistent finding)
- **Bacterial:** Most common cause in children > 5 years. Most commonly *S. pneumoniae, M. pneumoniae,* or *C. pneumoniae* (*not* trachomatis).
  - **Acute-onset, sudden, shaking chills**
  - **High fever**
  - **Prominent cough**
  - **Pleuritic chest pain**
  - **Markedly diminished breath sounds**
  - **Dullness to percussion**
- **Chlamydia trachomatis:** Infants 1–3 months of age with insidious onset (usually > 3 weeks).
  - *No* fever or wheezing (distinguishes from RSV) ± conjunctivitis at birth
  - Classic findings are **staccato cough** and **peripheral eosinophilia.**

Diagnostic Testing

- **Chest x-ray:**
  - **Viral:** Hyperinflation with bilateral interstitial infiltrates and peribronchial cuffing
  - **Pneumococcal:** Confluent lobar consolidation
  - **Mycoplasma/Chlamydia:** Unilateral lower-lobe interstitial pneumonia; looks worse than presentation
- **CBC with differential:**
  - Viral usually < 20,000
  - Bacterial 15,000–40,000
- **Viral antigens:** IgM titers for mycoplasma
- **Blood cultures**

CCS Tip: In cases of pneumonia, do *not* order sputum cultures. They are of no help in the management of pneumonia in children.

Treatment

- **Outpatient (mild cases): Amoxicillin** is the best choice. (Alternatives are cefuroxime and amoxicillin/clavulanic acid.)
- **Hospitalized: IV cefuroxime.** (If *S. aureus,* add **vancomycin.**)
- If viral origin suspected, may withhold antibiotics. However, give antibiotics if the child deteriorates. (Up to 30 percent may have coexisting bacterial pathogens.)
- ***Chlamydia* or *Mycoplasma*: Erythromycin** or other macrolide

Cystic Fibrosis (CF)

A 3-year-old white female presents with rectal prolapse. She is noted to be in the less-than-5th percentile for weight and height. The parents also note that she has a foul-smelling bulky stool each day that "floats." They also state that the child has developed a repetitive cough over the last few months. What is the first step in workup in this patient?

a. Genetic testing
b. Pulmonary function tests
c. Rectal biopsy
d. Sweat chloride
e. Stool studies

Answer: **D.** Sweat chloride is the best initial test to diagnose cystic fibrosis.

CF is an **autosomal, recessively inherited disease** caused by a mutation in the **CFTR gene**. The body regulates sweat and mucus by channeling water and chloride through a specific protein. The CFTR gene controls expression of this protein. In CF, the malfunctioning protein does not allow the chloride to flow through, and the blocked channel causes a buildup of **thick mucus**.

Meconium ileus occurs in 10 percent of patients. Look for abdominal distention at birth, failure to pass meconium, and bilious vomiting.

The most common initial presentation of cystic fibrosis is **meconium ileus.** Other signs and symptoms that warrant workup for CF are the following:

- **Failure to thrive** from malabsorption (steatorrhea due to pancreatic exocrine insufficiency, vitamin A, D, E, and K deficiency)
- **Rectal prolapse:** Most often in infants with steatorrhea, malnutrition, and cough
- **Persistent cough** in first year of life with copious purulent mucus production

Other associated conditions are undescended testes, **infertility (absent vas deferens), and allergic bronchopulmonary aspergillosis.**

Diagnostic Testing

- Best initial and most specific test: **2 elevated sweat chloride concentrations (> 60 mEq/L) obtained on separate days.**
- **Genetic testing** is highly accurate but does not detect all chromosome-7 mutations. It is done to detect carrier status and for prenatal diagnosis.
- **Newborn screening:** Determine immunoreactive trypsinogen in **blood spots** and then confirm with **sweat** or **DNA testing.**
- **Chest x-ray** is useful in monitoring course of disease and acute exacerbations.
- **Pulmonary function testing** is not done until age 5 or 6 to evaluate disease progression (obstructive → restrictive).

Treatment

Supportive care consists of aerosol treatment, albuterol/saline, chest physical therapy with postural drainage, and pancrelipase (aids digestion in patients with pancreatic dysfunction).

G551D mutation is present in 5% of CF patients and interferes with activation of CFTR chloride channel.

All CF patients should undergo genotyping to determine whether they carry the G551D mutation.

Ivacaftor (VX-770) is the first approved cystic fibrosis (CF) therapy that restores the function of a mutant CF protein. It is recommended for all patients age 6 and older who carry at least one copy of the **G551D mutation**. It has been shown to decrease sweat chloride levels, improve FEV_1, decrease pulmonary symptoms and exacerbations, and improve weight gain.

The most common organisms that cause infection in cystic fibrosis are *Staphylococcus aureus*, *Haemophilus influenzae*, and *Pseudomonas aeruginosa*.

The following treatment has been shown to improve survival:

- **Ibuprofen** reduces inflammatory lung response, slows patient's decline
- **Azithromycin** slows rate of decline in FEV_1 in patients < 13 years
- **Antibiotics** during exacerbations delay progression of lung disease

Antibiotics to treat CF:

- **Mild disease:** Give macrolide, trimethoprim-sulfamethoxazole (TMP-SMX), or ciprofloxacin.
- **Documented infection with *Pseudomonas* or *S. aureus*:** Treat aggressively with piperacillin plus tobramycin or ceftazidime.
- **Resistant pathogens:** Use inhaled tobramycin.

Other important management considerations:

- Give all routine vaccinations *plus* pneumococcal and yearly flu vaccines.
- *Never* delay antibiotic therapy (even if fever and tachypnea are absent).
- Steroids improve PFTs in the short term, but there's no persistent benefit when steroids are stopped.
- Expectorants (guaifenesin or iodides) are *not* effective in the removal of respiratory secretions.

Cardiology

Congenital Heart Disease (CHD)

The most common symptom of **acyanotic defects** is **congestive heart failure.** The most common acyanotic lesions are these:

- **Ventricular septal defect**
- **Atrial septal defect**
- **Atrioventricular canal**
- **Pulmonary stenosis**
- **Patent ductus arteriosus**
- **Aortic stenosis**
- **Coarctation of the aorta**

In infants with **cyanotic defects,** the primary concern is **hypoxia.** The most common defects associated with cyanosis are these:

- **Tetralogy of Fallot**
- **Transposition of the great arteries (TGA)**

Because functional closure of the ductus arteriosis may be delayed in CHD:

- CHDs that rely on the ductus will present within 1 month
- Infants with left-to-right shunting lesions will present at 2–6 months of age

Do *not* be reassured by normal antenatal ultrasounds; the majority of CHD cases are diagnosed after delivery.

Consider CHD in any child presenting with the following:

- **Shock, tachypnea, cyanosis** (especially if fever is absent): Note that cyanosis and hypoxemia classically do *not* respond to oxygen as is seen in pulmonary conditions.
- Infants: **Feeding difficulty, sweating while feeding, rapid respirations, easy fatigue**
- Older children: **Dyspnea on exertion, shortness of breath, failure to thrive**
- Abnormalities on exam:
  - **Upper extremity hypertension** or **decreased lower extremity blood pressures**
  - **Decreased femoral pulses** (obstructive lesions of the left side of the heart)
  - **Facial edema, hepatomegaly**
  - **Heart sounds:** Pansystolic murmur, grade 3/6 murmurs, PMI at upper left sternal border, harsh murmur, early midsystolic click, abnormal S2

When is a murmur on the exam innocent?

- When the question includes fever, infection, or anxiety
- When it is *only* systolic (never diastolic)
- When it is < grade 2/6

The presence or absence of a heart murmur is *not* used to suggest CHD.

CCS Tip: Because sepsis and CHD present very similarly, begin antibiotic therapy at the same time as workup for CHD.

Diagnostic Testing

- Best initial tests: **Chest x-ray and EKG.** Increased pulmonary vascular markings are the following:
  - Transposition of the great arteries (TGA)
  - Hypoplastic left heart syndrome
  - Truncus arteriosus
- Most specific test: **Echocardiography**

High-Yield Congenital Heart Defects	
Acyanotic lesions	
Heart Defect	**Comments**
Ventricular septal defect	Harsh holosystolic murmur over lower left sternal border ± thrill; loud pulmonic S2 Almost half of cases have spontaneous closure within the first 6 months. Surgical repair if failure to thrive, pulmonary hypertension, or right-to-left shunt > 2:1
Atrial septal defect	Loud S1, wide fixed splitting of S2, systolic ejection murmur along left upper sternal border. Majority are asymptomatic, are of secundum types, and close by age 4. Primary and sinus types require surgery. Most common type: patent foramen ovale A patent foramen ovale needs to be closed if a paradoxical embolus has gone through it. Late complications: Mitral valve prolapse, dysrhythmias, and pulmonary hypertension
Atrioventricular canal	Combination of the primum type of atrial septal defect, ventricular septal defect, and common atrioventricular valve Presentation similar to ventricular septal defect Perform surgery in infancy *before* pulmonary hypertension develops.
Pulmonary stenosis	May be asymptomatic or may result in severe congestive heart failure. Give prostaglandin E1 infusion at birth. Attempt balloon valvuloplasty.
Patent ductus arteriosus	More common in girls (2:1), babies where maternal rubella infection was present, and premature infants Wide pulse pressure, bounding arterial pulses, and characteristic sound of "machinery" (to-and-fro murmur) Indomethacin-induced closure helpful in premature infants. Term infants often require surgical closure.
Aortic stenosis	Early systolic ejection click at apex of left sternal border Valve replacement and anticoagulation may be required.
Coarctation of the aorta	Of all cases, 98 percent occur at origin of left subclavian artery. Blood pressure higher in arms than legs, bounding pulses in arms and decreased pulses in legs Ductus dependant: Give PGE1 infusion to maintain ductus patent (ensures lower extremity blood flow) Surgery repair after stabilization

(continued next page)

Basic Science Correlate

Ventricular septal defect results from incomplete formation of the interventricular septum, leaving an incomplete closure of the interventricular foramen.

The **ductus arteriosus** connects the pulmonary artery and descending aorta during development. It allows the blood to bypass the lungs, since the fetus is not receiving any oxygen from them in utero.

Aortic stenosis occurs when the leaflets of the valves fuse together. It can be congenital or acquired over time.

Cyanotic lesions	
Heart Defect	**Comments**
Tetralogy of Fallot	Most common CHD beyond infancy Defects include ventricular septal defect, right ventricular hypertrophy, right outflow obstruction, and overriding aorta Substernal right ventricular impulse, systolic thrill along the left sternal border Intermittent hyperpnea, irritability, cyanosis with decreased intensity of murmur Treatment: Give oxygen, beta blocker, PGE1 infusion for cyanosis present at birth Surgical repair at 4–12 months
Transposition of the great arteries	Most common cyanotic lesion presenting in the immediate newborn period. More common in infant of diabetic mother. S2 usually single and loud, murmurs usually absent Ductus-dependent: Give PGE1 to keep ductus open. Definitive surgical switch of aorta and pulmonary artery needed as soon as possible.

Antibiotic Prophylaxis and Prevention of Endocarditis

Antibiotics prior to genitourinary or gastrointestinal procedures are no longer recommended, *even* in high-risk patients. Giving antibiotics prior to dental procedures is no longer recommended *except* with the following:

- Prosthetic valves
- Previous endocarditis
- Congenital heart disease (unrepaired or repaired with persistent defect)
- Cardiac transplantation patients with cardiac valve abnormalities

Hypertension

Hypertension in pediatrics is based on the nomogram and falls into 4 categories:

- Normal: ≤ 90 percent
- Pre-hypertension: > 90 to ≤ 95 percent
- Stage I: > 95 to ≤ 99 percent
- Stage II: ≥ 99 percent + BP 5 mm Hg

Routine blood pressure checks are recommended beginning at age 3. On exam, be sure to check all 4 extremities (to look for coarctation).

Always work up for secondary hypertension under the following circumstances:

- **Newborns:** Umbilical artery catheters → renal artery/vein thrombosis.
- **Early childhood:** Renal parenchymal disease, coarctation, endocrine, medications
- **Adolescents:** Essential hypertension is associated with obesity.
  - Evaluate for renal and renovascular hypertension.
  - Majority of causes of renovascular hypertension may be due to urinary tract infection (secondary to an obstructive lesion), acute glomerulonephritis, Henoch-Schönlein purpura with nephritis, hemolytic uremic syndrome, acute tubular necrosis, renal trauma, leukemic infiltrates, mass lesions, and renal artery stenosis.

Consider renal causes of hypertension in **every** pediatric patient presenting with hypertension.

Diagnostic Testing

- Screening tests:
  - **CBC**
  - **Urinalysis**
  - **Urine culture**
  - **Electrolytes**
  - **Glucose**
  - **BUN**
  - **Creatinine**
  - **Calcium**
  - **Uric acid**
  - **Lipid panel** with essential hypertension and positive family history
- **Echocardiogram** for chronicity (left ventricular hypertrophy)
- Kidney evaluation:
  - **Renal ultrasound**
  - **Voiding cystourethrogram,** if there is a history of repeated UTIs (especially < 5 years)

- **24-hour urine collection** for protein excretion and creatinine clearance
- **Plasma renin activity (PRA):** Best screen for renovascular and renal disorders

- Endocrine causes:
  - **Urine and serum catecholamines,** if pheochromocytoma is suspected
  - **Thyroid and adrenal hormone levels**
- **Drug screening** (in adolescents), if drug abuse is suspected

Treatment

If the patient is obese, order **lifestyle changes:**

- **Weight control**
- **Aerobic exercise**
- **No-added-salt diet**
- **Monitoring of blood pressure**

If there is no response to lifestyle changes, give **antihypertensives:**

- The best initial antihypertensive is a **diuretic** or **beta blocker.**
- Then add **calcium channel blocker and ACE inhibitor** (good in high-renin hypertension secondary to renovascular or renal disease or high-renin essential hypertension)

Gastrointestinal Disease

Diarrhea

Acute Diarrhea

The most common cause of acute diarrhea in infancy is a **rotavirus.** The most common causes of bloody diarrhea are ***Campylobacter*, amoeba (*E. histolytica*), *Shigella*, *E. coli*,** and ***Salmonella*.**

Following are characteristics of selected microbes causing acute diarrhea:

- **Rotavirus:** double-stranded DNA virus
- **Shigella:** gram-negative, non-spore-forming rod
- **Campylobacter:** gram-negative spiral that is motile with flagella
- **Salmonella:** gram-negative rod that is motile
- ***Clostridium difficile*:** gram-positive, spore-forming bacteria
- **Giardia:** anaerobic protozoan with flagella
- **Cryptosporidium:** protozoan that mostly affects immunocompromised patients

The best initial test is a stool examination for the following:

- **Stool cultures** with blood, leukocytes, suspected hemolytic uremic syndrome
- ***Clostridium difficile* toxin** if a recent history of antibiotics
- **Ovum and parasites**

The best initial therapy is **hydration and fluid and electrolyte replacement.** Do *not* use antidiarrheals in children. Antibiotics are rarely used (even in bacterial diarrhea), except for the following cases:

- ***Shigella*:** Trimethoprim/sulfamethoxazole
- ***Campylobacter*:** Self-limiting. Erythromycin speeds recovery and reduces carrier state and is recommended for patients with severe disease or dysentery.
- ***Salmonella*:** Treatment indicated only for patients < 3 months old, who are toxic, who have disseminated disease, or who have *S. typhi.*
- ***C. difficile*:** Metronidazole or PO vancomycin and discontinuation of other antibiotics
- ***E. histolytica* or *Giardia*:** Metronidazole
- ***Cryptosporidium*:** Antiparasitics. Watch for malnutrition in pediatric patients.

Hemolytic Uremic Syndrome (HUS)

- HUS is a complication of acute invasive (bloody) diarrhea, most commonly caused by *E. coli* O157:H7 (also *Shigella, Salmonella, Campylobacter*).
- *Never* give antibiotics in suspected cases of *E. coli* O157:H7—there is an increased risk of developing HUS.
- Young children present 5–10 days after infection with pallor (microangiopathic hemolytic anemia), weakness, oliguria, and acute renal insufficiency or acute renal failure (ARF). HUS is the most common cause of ARF in young children.
- Look for anemia, helmet cells, burr cells, fragmented cells, elevated WBCs, negative Coombs, low platelets (< $100{,}000/mm^3$), low-grade microscopic hematuria, and proteinuria.
- Treatment: Supportive care, treatment of hypertension, aggressive nutrition, early dialysis
- Prognosis: More than 90 percent of patients survive the acute stage; a small number develop end-stage renal disease (ESRD).
- Monitor blood pressure for 5 years.
- Monitor renal function with BUN/creatinine for 2–3 years after HUS.

Chronic Diarrhea

Chronic, nonspecific diarrhea presents with **normal weight, height, and nutritional status with no fat in stool.** History usually includes **excessive intake of fruit juice or carbonated fluids** or **low fat intake.** If there is weight loss and stool with high fat, screen for malabsorption syndromes (see below).

- Pancreatic insufficiency presents with prominent steatorrhea. Get a sweat chloride test to rule in/out cystic fibrosis.
- Giardiasis is the only infection that causes chronic malabsorption. If giardiasis is suspected, order a duodenal aspirate/biopsy or immunoassay.
- Malrotation can present with malabsorption and incomplete bowel obstruction.

Malabsorption

Malabsorption may appear from birth or after introduction of new foods.

Diagnostic Testing

- **Fat malabsorption:**
  - Best initial screening test: **Sudan black stain**
  - Best confirmatory test: **72-hour stool for fecal fat** (gold standard for steatorrhea)
  - **Serum trypsinogen screens** for pancreatic function
- **Protein malabsorption:** *Cannot* be evaluated directly.
  - Best initial test: **Spot stool alpha-1 antitrypsin level**
- **Vitamins/minerals:** Measure serum Fe, folate, Ca, Zn, and Mg and vitamins B12, D, and A.

Celiac Disease

Celiac disease presents with the following within the first 2 years:

- Chronic diarrhea
- Failure to thrive
- Growth retardation
- Anorexia

Symptoms occur with exposure to **gluten, rye, wheat, and barley.** Intolerance is lifelong.

Celiac patients have an increased lifetime risk of osteoporosis and GI malignancies (most commonly enteropathy-associated T-cell lymphoma).

Diagnostic Testing

- Best initial diagnostic test: **Antitransglutaminase antibodies**
- Most specific test: **Histology on biopsy**

Treatment

Celiac disease is managed with a **lifelong strictly gluten-free diet.**

Gastroesophageal Reflux Disease (GERD)

A 4-month-old girl presents with several weeks of chronic wheeze and apneic episodes 20–30 minutes after feeds. She has been spitting up after feeds since birth. The infant has presented to the office on several occasions with the same complaint despite adjustments in feed technique and formula consistency. She is at the 5th percentile for weight. Which of the following is the most appropriate intervention?

a. Erythromycin
b. Fundoplication
c. Metoclopramide
d. Omeprazole
e. Ranitidine

Answer: **E.** GERD results from incompetent esophageal sphincter tone early in life. Symptoms typically resolve by 12–24 months. Diagnosis is **clinical.** However, the best initial test is **esophageal pH monitoring. Endoscopy** is used to evaluate for erosive gastritis or other complications. The best initial management is a **change in feeding technique and thickened feeds. H2-receptors** are considered first line in children because of the safety profile. However, **proton pump inhibitors** tend to be more effective in suppressing gastric acid production.

Pyloric Stenosis

A 4-week-old boy presents with recurrent vomiting after feeds. Vomitus is nonbilious in nature. Laboratory findings include chloride 88 mEq, potassium 3.1 mEq, sodium 146 mEq, and pH 7.48. What is the best initial test in the workup of this infant?

a. Abdominal x-ray
b. Barium enema
c. CT scan of the abdomen
d. Esophageal pH monitoring
e. Ultrasound

Answer: **E.** The case will describe a first-born European-Caucasian male with nonbilious projectile vomiting typically in first 6 weeks of life. There is hypochloremic and metabolic alkalosis, and a firm, mobile, 1-inch mass is often palpated in the epigastrium. The best initial test is **ultrasound of the abdomen.** Treatment is **pyloromyotomy.** Abdominal x-ray is less useful in identifying pyloric stenosis and is not the test of choice in cases where clinical suspicion is high. CT scan is not indicated to prevent exposure to radiation when a more appropriate test is available.

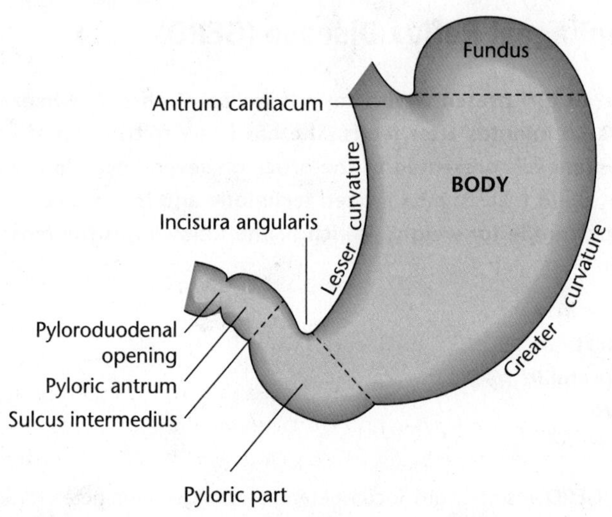

Anatomy of the Stomach

Hypertrophy: enlarged cells, but the same number of cells

Hyperplasia: normal cell size, but more cells

Pyloric stenosis is caused by a hypertrophied pylorus. The hypertrophied pylorus obstructs the outlet, so nothing passes to the duodenum and projectile vomiting ensues. The vomitus *does not* contain bile. (Food must be able to get to the duodenum in order to come in contact with bile.)

The absence or presence of bile in vomitus is the key difference between duodenal atresia (no bile) and pyloric stenosis (bile). Hypochloremic metabolic alkalosis is pathognomonic of pyloric stenosis. Vomiting causes loss of the gastric acid (i.e., hydrochloric acid). The low chloride level prevents the kidneys from excreting bicarbonate, leading to alkalosis.

Malrotation and Volvulus

Look for an infant with **bilious emesis** and **recurrent abdominal pain** with **vomiting.** Always suspect volvulus when the patient has an acute small-bowel obstruction without a history of bowel surgery.

Diagnostic Testing

- Best initial test: **Ultrasound** (inversion of superior mesenteric artery and vein and duodenal obstruction) or **barium enema** (cecum is not in the right lower quadrant)
- Abdominal x-ray is *not* helpful (only helpful in duodenal destruction; shows "double-bubble" sign).

Treatment

Treatment is with **surgery.**

Hematochezia

A 2-year-old boy is brought to the office because his mother has noticed bleeding in his diaper for 1 week. The child has had no complaints. Physical examination is unremarkable. Which of the following is the best initial test?

a. Guaiac exam
b. Push enteroscopy
c. Red blood cell tagged scan
d. Tc-99m pertechnetate scan
e. Upper endoscopy

Answer: **D.** The Tc-99m pertechnetate scan is also known as the Meckel radionuclide scan, the diagnostic exam for **Meckel diverticulum.** Intermittent, painless rectal bleeding is the classic presentation due to acid-related bleeding of aberrant mucosa (remnant of embryonic yolk sac). May present with intussusception (remnant may become a lead point) or diverticulitis or look like acute appendicitis.

Meckel diverticulum is a remnant of the omphalomesenteric duct. It follows the rule of 2's:

- 2 percent of the population have it
- 2 feet from the ileocecal valve
- 2 inches in length
- 2:1 male to female
- 2 types of tissue (gastric and pancreatic)

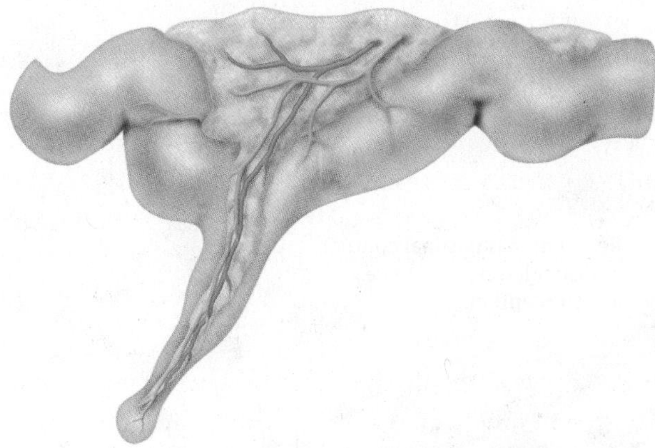

Meckel Diverticulum

Intussusception

A 16-month-old child is seen for cramping and colicky abdominal pain for the past 12 hours. He has a 1-week history of diarrhea but developed episodes of vomiting and passed black-bloody stool today. Physical examination is remarkable for a lethargic child; abdomen is tender to palpation. Temperature is 101.3°F. White blood count is 18,000. Which of the following is the most important next step in management?

a. Antibiotic prophylaxis
b. Bowel resection
c. Electrolyte replacement
d. Embolectomy
e. Reduction of bowel

Answer: **E.** Reduction of telescoped bowel is the priority of management in patients presenting **intussusception.**

Intussusception is the **telescoping of bowel that classically occurs in children < 2 years,** often following gastrointestinal or upper respiratory infection, or it may occur spontaneously in patients with a "lead point" (Meckel diverticulum, polyp, neurofibroma, hemangioma) or with a history of Henoch-Schönlein purpura.

The case will describe **sudden paroxysms of colicky abdominal pain in a lethargic child along with shock and fever.** The classic **"black currant jelly"** stool results from mucosal necrosis due to venous obstruction.

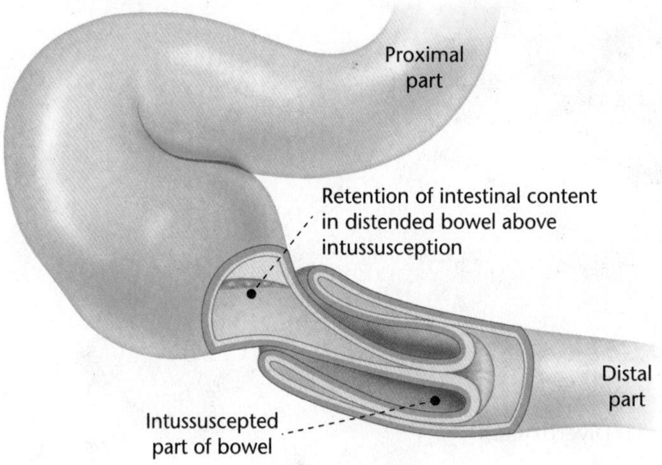

Intussusception

Diagnostic Testing and Treatment

- Best initial test: **Plain film of the abdomen** to rule out obstruction
- Next steps: **Air enema,** which is both diagnostic and curative. **Manual reduction** may be needed if radiographic reduction is not successful.

Renal and Urologic Disorders

Urinary Tract Infections (UTIs) in Pediatrics

UTIs are more common in **boys ≤ 1 year** and **girls > 2.** Most girls develop their first UTI by age 5 (peaks are during infancy and toilet training). The most common agent is **Gram-negative rods.** Diagnosis is as with adults.

Diagnostic Testing

- Best initial test: Urinalysis
- Most accurate test: Urine culture

Treatment

- **Cystitis** (dysuria): Amoxicillin, trimethoprim-sulfamethoxazole
- **Pyelonephritis** (fever, flank pain): IV ceftriaxone or ampicillin plus gentamicin

Do *not* give the following:

- Sulfonamides or nitrofurantoin in infants < 1 month old (give ceftriaxone)
- Tetracyclines in children < 7 years
- Quinolones in children < 16 years

Note that children are at greatest risk of **kidney damage,** including kidney scars, poor kidney growth, poor kidney function, and high blood pressure, especially if an underlying urinary tract abnormality exists.

Further Management

- Do **urine culture** 1 week after stopping antibiotics to confirm sterile urine; reassess periodically for next 1–2 years.
- Obtain **voiding cystourethrogram** (VCUG) and **renal ultrasound** in:
  - Children of any age with ≥ 2 febrile UTI **or**
  - First febrile UTI with any of the following:
    - Family history of renal or urological disease
    - Poor growth
    - Hypertension
    - Organism other than *E. coli*

Vesicoureteral Reflux (VUR)

A 2-year-old girl presents with a urinary tract infection. She has had multiple urinary tract infections since birth but has never had any follow-up studies to evaluate these infections. Physical examination is remarkable for an ill-appearing child who has a temperature of 40°C (104°F) and is vomiting. Voiding cystourethrogram reveals abnormal urinary backflow from the bladder. Which of the following is the most important step to prevent permanent damage?

a. ACE inhibitors
b. Trimethoprim-sulfamethoxazole
c. NSAIDs
d. Regular creatinine measurement
e. Surgical reconstruction

Answer: **B.** Antibiotic prophylaxis (trimethoprim-sulfamethoxazole or nitrofurantoin) is used for the 1st year following diagnosis for any grade of VUR, particularly in younger infants, to prevent kidney scarring from recurrent infections.

VUR is abnormal movement of urine from the bladder into the ureters/kidneys. Urine usually travels from the kidneys through the ureters, then into the bladder. In VUR, urine flow is reversed.

VUR predisposes the child to **pyelonephritis,** which leads to **scarring,** which leads to **reflux nephropathy** (hypertension, proteinuria, renal insufficiency to end-stage renal disease [ESRD], impaired kidney growth).

Diagnostic Testing

Perform a **voiding cystourethrogram (VCUG) and renal scan.** If scarring is present, follow creatinine periodically.

Treatment

- **Antibiotic prophylaxis**
- **Surgery** under the following conditions:
  - Any breakthrough UTI
  - New scars
  - Failure to resolve

Obstructive Uropathy

The first presentation of obstructive uropathy is often infection or sepsis. The most common causes of obstructive uropathy are the following:

- **Boys: Posterior urethral valves** are the most common cause of bladder obstruction. Look for walnut-shaped mass (bladder) above pubic symphysis and weak urinary stream.
- **Newborns: Hydronephrosis and polycystic kidney disease** are the most common causes of a palpable abdominal mass.

The best initial diagnostic tests are **VCUG and renal ultrasound.**

Hematuria

Acute Poststreptococcal Glomerulonephritis (APGN)

A 10-year-old boy presents with lower extremity swelling. He has had a sore throat for 2 weeks and fever. His mother has noticed very dark, brownish-red urine over the past couple of days. He has no known allergies. On physical examination, his blood pressure is 185/100 mm Hg. Which of the following is indicated for management?

a. ACE inhibitors
b. Diuretics
c. Erythromycin
d. Oral prednisone
e. Penicillin

Answer: **E.** The most appropriate therapy for **APGN** is antibiotics to eradicate the underlying infection. Penicillin is the drug of choice. Erythromycin is used on patients who are penicillin-allergic.

APGN presents in **children 5–12 years old, 1–2 weeks after strep pharyngitis or 3–6 weeks after skin infection (impetigo).** The classic triad of symptoms is **edema, hypertension, and hematuria.**

Diagnostic Testing

- **Urinalysis:** RBCs, RBC casts, protein, polymorphonuclear cells
- **Low C3** (Returns to normal in 6–8 weeks.)
- Need **positive throat culture** or **increasing antibody titer to streptococcal antigens**
- Most specific test: **Anti-DNase antigen**

Treatment

- **Penicillin** (erythromycin if penicillin-allergic)
- **Supportive care:** Sodium restriction, diuresis, fluid and electrolyte management
- Antihypertensives are *not* indicated in acute management.
- Steroids do *not* have a role in management.

There is complete recovery in > 95 percent of patients.

Other Conditions Presenting with Hematuria

- **IgA nephropathy (Berger's disease):** This is the most common chronic glomerular disease worldwide. It can present in adolescents but most commonly presents in a patient in her **20s or 30s** with **gross hematuria after upper respiratory infection or gastrointestinal infection.** There will be **mild proteinuria and hypertension** and a *normal* C3 on lab workup. The most important step in management is **blood pressure control.**

- **Alport syndrome:** This will present in a **young boy** with **hearing difficulties** and **asymptomatic microscopic hematuria and intermittent gross hematuria after upper respiratory infections.** Family history is significant for males with renal problems and sensorineural hearing loss. Look for **ocular abnormalities** in workup.

Polycystic Kidney Disease: Autosomal-Recessive Type (Infantile)

Polycystic kidney disease is suggested when an infant presents with **bilateral flank masses and hypoplasia.** Look for the following in the case:

- **Hypertension**
- **Oliguria**
- **Acute renal failure**

Diagnostic Testing

Perform an **ultrasound of the kidneys** (cysts through cortex and medulla) and **the liver** (bile duct proliferation and hepatic fibrosis).

Treatment

Treatment is with **dialysis and transplantation.** Of all patients, 80 percent have 10-year survival.

Proteinuria

- **Transient:** From **fever, exercise, dehydration, or cold exposure**
- **Orthostatic:** This is the most common form of persistent proteinuria in school-aged children and adolescents. Look for history of **normal proteinuria in supine position but greatly increased proteinuria in upright position.** Rule this out *before* any other evaluation is done.
- **Glomerular or tubular disorders:** Suspect a glomerular disorder with **proteinuria > 1 g/24 hours** or if the case describes **hypertension, hematuria, or renal dysfunction.**

Nephrotic Syndrome: Minimal Change Disease

A 3-year-old child presents to the physician with puffy eyes. The mother reports diarrhea 2 weeks ago. On physical examination, there is no erythema or evidence of trauma, insect bite, cellulitis conjunctival injection, or discharge. Urinalysis reveals 3+ proteinuria. Laboratory profile is significant for albumin 2.1 mg/dL creatinine is 0.9; and C3 and C4 are normal. Which of the following is the next step in management?

a. Outpatient prednisone
b. Hospitalize and observe
c. Heparin
d. High-dose methylprednisone
e. Intravenous antibiotics

Answer: **A.** Outpatient prednisone is the first step in management of patients presenting with **mild cases of minimal change disease.** Prednisone is continued daily for 4–6 weeks, then tapered to alternate days for 2–3 months without initial biopsy.

Nephrotic syndrome is most common at 2–6 years of age, often arising after minor infections. It presents with the following:

- **Proteinuria** (> 40 mg/m^2/hour) (Creatinine is usually normal.)
- **Hypoalbuminemia** (< 2.5 g/dL)
- **Edema** (initially around eyes and lower extremities)
- **Hyperlipidemia**
- C3 and C4 are normal.

Treat this condition as follows:

- **Supportive care:** Sodium restriction, fluid restriction
- **Oral prednisone**
- Relapses on steroids may indicate that patient is steroid dependent or resistant. The patient should receive **cyclophosphamide, cyclosporine, high-dose pulsed methylprednisolone.**

Following are possible complications of nephrotic syndrome:

- **Infection:** Most frequent is spontaneous bacterial peritonitis. You *must* immunize against *Pneumococcus* and *Varicella.*
- Increased risk of **thromboembolism** due to increased prothrombotic factors and decreased fibrinolytic factors

Endocrine Disorders

Congenital Adrenal Hyperplasia (CAH)

CAH refers to a group of autosomal recessive disorders that result in inadequate cortisol and/or aldosterone synthesis. The most common is **21-hydroxylase deficiency**, in which

- decreased production of cortisol →
- increased ACTH →
- adrenal hyperplasia →
- shunting to androgen synthesis →
- masculinization of external genitalia in females.

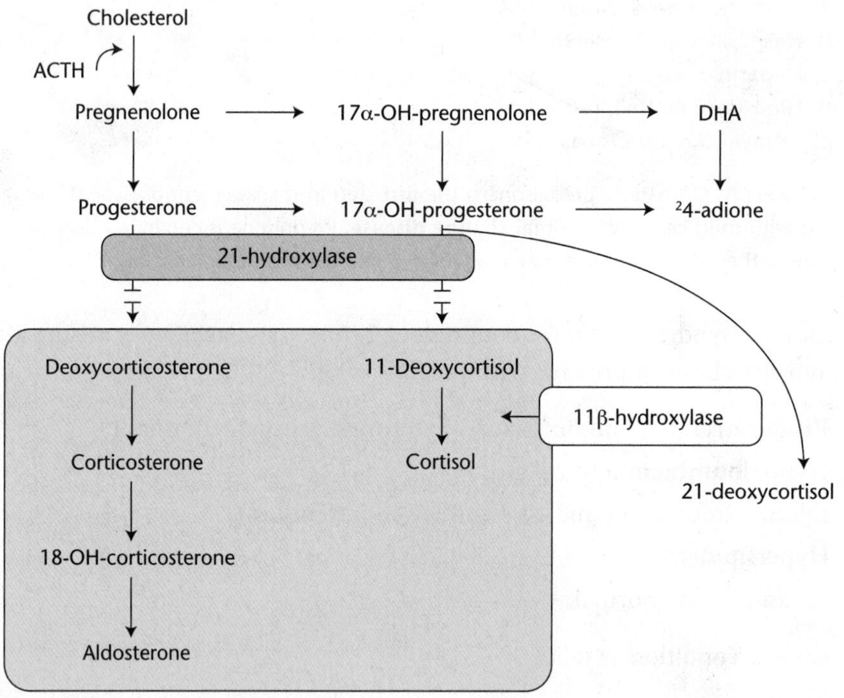

Steroidogenesis in 21-Hydroxylase Deficiency

In 21-hydroxylase deficiency, the patient cannot convert progesterone to deoxycorticosterone, leading to a deficiency in corticosterone. The patient also cannot convert 17 alpha-hydroxyprogesterone into 11-deoxycortisol, leading to a low cortisol level that stimulates the ACTH to produce more. The result is a buildup of progesterone and androgens, causing masculinization of the genitalia.

CAH presents in an infant with the following signs:

- **Vomiting**
- **Dehydration**
- **Hyponatremia** (salt losing)
- **Hypoglycemia**
- **Hyperkalemia**
- Females have **ambiguous genitalia** at birth.

Diagnostic Testing

- Best initial test: **Increased 17-OH progesterone** (Also find low cortisol levels, increased renin, and decreased aldosterone.)
- Definitive diagnostic test: **17-OH progesterone before and after an intravenous bolus of ACTH.**

Treatment

- **Hydrocortisone**
- **Fludrocortisone** if salt losing
- Increased doses of **both** hydrocortisone **and** fludrocortisone in times of stress
- **Corrective surgery for females**

Rheumatic and Vasculitic Disorders

Kawasaki Disease

An 18-month-old presents with a fever for 1 week and a rash on his hands with desquamation that developed today. On examination, he is noted to have conjunctival injection, erythematous tongue, cracked lips, and edema of the hands. He has palpable and painful lymph nodes in the neck. What is the next step in management?

a. Anticoagulation
b. Echocardiogram
c. IVIG
d. Methylprednisolone
e. Prednisone

Answer: **C. Kawasaki disease** is an acute vasculitis of medium-sized arteries and the leading cause of acquired heart disease in the United States and Japan. IVIG and high-dose aspirin should be started immediately to prevent coronary artery involvement (reduces risk from 25 percent to < 5 percent). Echocardiogram should be performed at diagnosis for baseline measurement; however, coronary artery abnormalities occur in the 2nd to 3rd week.

Of patients with Kawasaki disease, 80 percent are < 5 years. The condition presents with **fever for ≥ 5 days, plus 4 of the following 5 criteria:**

- **Bilateral bulbar conjunctivitis without exudate**
- **Intraoral erythema, strawberry tongue, dry and cracked lips**
- **Erythema and swelling of hands and feet; desquamation of fingertips 1–3 weeks after onset**
- **Nonvesicular rash**
- **Nonsuppurative cervical lymphadenitis**

Diagnostic Testing

- Increased ESR, C-reactive protein (CRP) at 4–8 weeks
- Platelets increase in weeks 2–3 (often > 1 million)
- Cardiac findings:
  - Early myocarditis, pericarditis
  - Coronary artery aneurysms in the 2nd to 3rd week

Treatment

- **Best initial step:** Intravenous immunoglobulin (IVIG) and high-dose aspirin as soon as possible, based on clinical diagnosis
- **2D echocardiogram and EKG:** Get baseline at diagnosis; repeat at 2–3 weeks and at 6–8 weeks
- Add **anticoagulant (warfarin)** for high-risk thrombosis (e.g., when platelet count is very high)
- Steroids have *not* shown benefit

The prognosis is as follows:

- Only IVIG has been shown to reduce incidence of cardiovascular complications.
- There is a 1–2 percent mortality due to coronary artery thrombosis secondary to coronary artery aneurysms.

Henoch-Schönlein Purpura (HSP)

HSP is the diagnosis when the case describes a young child (2–8 years) with the following:

- **Maculopapular lesions** (palpable purpura) on the legs and buttocks (more common in adults)
- **Fever**
- **Abdominal pain** (more common in pediatric patients)
- A recent history of **upper respiratory viral illness**

HSP is small vessel vasculitis caused by IgA and C3 deposits in arterioles, capillaries, and venules. IgA levels are high in HSP. Renal biopsy has identical findings as IgA nephropathy. The key difference is that HSP occurs in children and is a systemic disease affecting the skin, connective tissues, GI, kidneys, and joints.

HSP is associated with the following conditions:

- **Intussusception**
- **Arthritis**
- **Glomerulonephritis/nephrosis** (develops in 25 percent of patients)

Diagnostic Testing

HSP is diagnosed from the clinical presentation. Tests show the following:

- **Increased platelets, WBCs, ESR, anemia**
- **Increased IgA, IgM**
- **Anticardiolipin** or **antiphospholipid antibodies**
- Urine: **RBCs, WBCs, casts, albumin**
- Definitive diagnosis: **Skin biopsy** (rarely done)

Treatment

Treatment is **supportive:**

- Intestinal or renal complications are treated with **corticosteroids,** which help prevent renal insufficiency and bowel perforation.
- Give **aspirin** (acetylsalicylic acid, ASA) if anticardiolipin or antiphospholipid antibodies are positive and/or thrombotic events occur.

Hematology

Anemia

When is anemia considered physiological?

Answer: In **term infants,** normal hemoglobin nadir occurs at **12 weeks at 9–11 mg/dL.** The anemia results from a progressive drop in RBC production (due to erythropoietin suppression at birth) until tissue oxygen needs are greater than at delivery. *No* treatment is needed.

Response is exaggerated and earlier in **preterm infants.** In preterms, hemoglobin nadir occurs at **3–6 weeks** at **7–9 mg/dL.** Some patients may require transfusions.

Iron-Deficiency Anemia

A normal newborn has sufficient stores of iron to meet requirements for 4–6 months, but iron stores and absorption are variable.

Breast milk has less iron than most formulas but has higher bioavailability. Iron in breast milk is more readily absorbed in the proximal intestine.

Decreased dietary iron results in anemia at **9–24 months.**

Treatment

- **Give oral ferrous salts.**
- **Limit cow's milk.**
- **Continue iron replacement for 8 weeks after blood value normalizes** to replete bone marrow iron stores.

Lead Poisoning

Consider lead poisoning when the case describes **hyperactivity, aggression, and learning disability** (may be mistaken for ADHD). Other clues include **impaired growth, constipation, and mental lethargy.**

Diagnostic Testing

- Best initial screening: **Blood lead testing at 12 and 24 months** in high-risk children. Blood lead level (BLL) ≤ **5 mcg/dL** is acceptable.
- Labs: **Microcytic, hypochromic anemia, increased free erythrocyte porphyrins (FEP), and basophilic stippling**
- **X-rays of long bones** (dense lead lines)

Treatment

- **Refer to department of health** when blood lead level > 15 mcg/dL.
- Begin **chelation** when blood lead level > 45 mcg/dL.

Hemoglobin (Hb) Disorders

A 6-month-old, previously well African-American infant presents to the pediatrician with painful swollen hands and swollen feet. What are the most common causes of mortality in pediatric cases with sickle cell disease?

Answer:

- **Infection** (autosplenectomy by age 5) leads to increased susceptibility to infection, particularly with encapsulated bacteria (*S. pneumococcus, H. influenzae, N. meningitidis*).
- **Acute chest syndrome** (this and sepsis are most common causes of mortality).
- **Acute splenic sequestration** (peak incidence from 6 months to 3 years of age).

Diagnostic Testing

- Best diagnostic test: **Hb electrophoresis** (also used in newborn screening)
- **Prenatal diagnosis** for parents with trait:
  - **Chorionic villus sampling at 10–12 weeks gestation;** or
  - **Amniocentesis at 14–18 weeks**

Treatment

- **Transfuse** in the following situations:
  - Symptomatic anemia (shortness of breath or chest pain)
- **Exchange transfusion** in the following situations:
  - Life-threatening complications (stroke, acute chest syndrome, splenic crisis)
  - Before high-risk surgery

Recurrent painful crises are *not* an indication for transfusion.

- Give **aggressive antibiotic therapy for infections.**
- **Hydroxyurea:** Increases HbF levels. Reduces recurrent painful crises and number of transfusions. Does *not* reduce risk of stroke. Indicated in the following situations:
  - ≥ 3 crises per year
  - Symptomatic anemia
  - Life-threatening complications

- Routine care consists of the following measures:
  - **Penicillin prophylaxis** beginning at 3 months until 5 years of age
  - **Immunizations:** Regular *plus* pneumococcal at age 2 months, influenza at 6 months then yearly, and meningococcal at 2 years
  - **Daily folate supplementation**
- **Bone marrow transplant** is the only definitive treatment. It has a mortality rate of 10 percent.

Beta Thalassemia Major (Cooley Anemia)

Beta thalassemia results from absent or reduced synthesis of beta chains of hemoglobin. Two alleles are responsible for production of the beta globulin protein. Beta thalassemia minor is caused by a mutation in one allele; beta thalassemia major is caused by mutations in both. Beta thalassemia major presents in second month of life with the following:

- Progressive **anemia, hypersplenism, and cardiac decompensation** (Hb < 4 mg/dL)
- **Expanded medullary space** with increased expansion of face and skull
- **Extramedullary hematopoiesis**
- **Hepatosplenomegaly**

Diagnostic Testing

- Best initial and most specific test: **Hemoglobin electrophoresis—HbF** increased, variable increased HbA_2, absent or reduced HbA. (Excess alpha globin chains → alpha tetramers form → increase in HbF.)
- **Severe anemia, low reticulocytes, increased nucleated RBCs, microcytosis (MCV 55–80 FL), markers of hemolysis** (increased indirect bilirubin, LDH, decreased haptoglobin)
- **Increased serum ferritin and transferrin saturation**

Treatment

- **Transfusion therapy** to maintain Hb > 9 g/dL
- **Iron chelation: Deferoxamine** (usually started before 8 years) plus **vitamin C**
- **Splenectomy:** Hypersplenism is common. Splenectomy is usually deferred until age 5.
- Routine care consists of the following measures:
  - **Folate supplementation**
  - **Vaccinations:** Pneumococcal vaccine, hepatitis B vaccine, daily penicillin prophylaxis
  - **Growth hormone:** Excess iron is related to deficiency in growth hormone.
- **Bone marrow transplantation** is curative.

Hemorrhagic Disorders

The type of bleeding is a clue to the underlying condition:

- **Von Willebrand's disease (VWD)** or **platelet dysfunction** leads to the following:
  - **Mucous membrane bleeding**
  - **Petechiae**
  - **Small ecchymoses**
  - **Menorrhagia**
  - **Postoperative bleeding** (autosomal-dominant but more common in females)

Basic Science Correlate

Von Willebrand's factor (VWF) is important in platelet adhesion. When endothelial damage occurs, VWF binds to collagen, causing platelet activation: Once the glycoprotein IIb/IIIa binds with VWF, it stimulates platelet aggregation forming the beginning of a platelet plug.

VWF also acts as a carrier protein for factor VIII.

- **Clotting factor deficiencies** (e.g., hemophilia A or B) lead to **deep bleeding (hemarthrosis)** with more extensive ecchymoses and hematoma.

Diagnostic Testing

- Best initial tests:
  - **Platelets:** Thrombocytopenia is the most common cause of bleeding in children.
  - **Bleeding time:** Evaluates qualitative platelet defects or vWD
  - **PT (extrinsic pathway) and PTT (intrinsic pathway):** PTT is 2–3 times elevated in hemophilia A and B; von Willebrand's disease has increased bleeding time and PTT.
- Confirmatory tests:
  - **Mixing studies:** Add normal plasma to the patient's plasma and repeat PT/PTT/1NR.
  - **Specific clotting factor assay:** Look for decreased levels of Factor VIII (hemophilia A), Factor IX (hemophilia B)
  - **Quantitative assay for vWF Ag, vWF activity** (ristocetin cofactor activity [decreased in vWF])
- If platelet dysfunction is suspected, perform **platelet aggregation studies.**

Evaluate mixing studies as follows:

- If lab prolongation is corrected, there is a deficiency of clotting factor.
- If lab prolongation is not corrected or is only partially corrected, an inhibitor is present (most common inhibitor with in-hospital patients is heparin).
- If it is more prolonged with clinical bleeding, an antibody against a clotting factor is present (mostly factors VIII, IX, or XI).
- If there is no clinical bleeding but both the PTT and mixing study are prolonged, lupus anticoagulant (predisposition to excessive clotting).

If the case describes a hemophilia patient, previously well controlled, who presents with sudden bleeding diathesis, order mixing studies (coagulation factor inhibitor—usually factor VIII inhibitor).

Treatment

- **Hemophilia A**
  - **Minor bleeding** is treated with **desmopressin** (releases endogenous factor) **plus aminocaproic acid** or **tranexamic acid** (minimize fibrinolysis). For maximal effectiveness, antifibrinolytic medications should be given *before* oral surgical procedures. Cryoprecipitate is *not* used.
  - **Major bleeding** (bleeding into joint, iliopsoas muscle, other large bleed) is *always* treated by giving **factor VIII.**
- **Hemophilia B**
  - Treatment of **major or minor bleeding** is with **factor IX concentrates** because of the thrombotic potential of prothrombin complex concentrates.
- **von Willebrand's Disease (vWD)**
  - *Avoid* cryoprecipitate.
  - **Minor bleeding and subtype 1** are treated with **desmopressin** (promotes release of preformed vWF from endothelial cells).
  - **Major bleeding and subtypes 2 and 3** are treated with **plasma-derived vWF-containing concentrates with factor VIII.**

A 4-year-old child is brought in by her mother because of red "spots and rashes" on her lower extremities. Today she fell from her bicycle and was bleeding for 30 minutes. She has no known medical problems, and the only significant history is a recent upper respiratory viral illness. Examination reveals petechiae in lower extremities and purpura on her buttocks. There are no signs of active bleeding. PT, PTT, and bleeding time are within normal limits. Platelet count is 32,000. Hemoglobin is 12 mg/dL. What is the next step in the workup?

a. Bone marrow biopsy
b. Factor levels
c. Mixing study
d. Peripheral smear
e. Ristocetin assay

Answer: **D.** This case is a classic presentation of **immune thrombocytopenic purpura (ITP)** in childhood. The most common age of onset is 1–4 years, usually after a nonspecific viral infection. The defect is autoantibodies against the platelet surfaces. Diagnosis is by exclusion. Always get a peripheral smear to rule out TTP and HUS.

- **Immune thrombocytopenic purpura (ITP):** Most patients recover platelet counts within 6 months. Transfusion is contraindicated, *unless* there is life-threatening bleeding. Do *not* treat platelet count; treatment is based on clinical bleeding.
  - 1st choice: **Prednisone**
  - 2nd choice: **IVIG**
  - 10–20 percent of patients develop **chronic ITP,** and **immune therapy with rituximab** or **splenectomy** can be considered

Except for petechiae and ecchymosis, the physical exam should be normal in ITP. If there is hepatosplenomegaly or lymphadenopathy, consider doing a workup for other disorders (e.g., acute leukemia).

Neurology

Seizures

You are asked to see a previously well 13-month-old boy who is brought in after a generalized tonic-clonic seizure 1 hour ago. The seizure lasted several minutes. The mother remembers that a similar episode occurred when she was a child. On examination vitals are BP 100/52, HR 110, Temp 101.4°F, RR 32. She wishes to know if her child has epilepsy. What is the most appropriate response to the parents?

a. Reassure mother that there is no risk of epilepsy.
b. There is a slightly increased risk of epilepsy.
c. There is a high risk of epilepsy developing in the next year.
d. The patient has epilepsy but medications will be withheld until second episode of seizure.
e. The patient has epilepsy and will require anti-seizure medications

Answer: **A.** This patient presents with ***simple febrile seizure***—generalized tonic-clonic seizure < 10 min duration occurring with rapid onset high fever (when > 39°C [102°F]) in child 9 months to 5 years of age. There is usually positive family history. There is no risk of epilepsy. Management includes evaluation for meningitis and controlling fever. DO NOT order EEG or neuroimaging.

The risk of epilepsy is increased in a case presenting as febrile seizure under any of the following conditions:

- **Atypical seizure:** > 15 minutes, more than 1 in a day, and focal findings
- **Family history of epilepsy and initial seizure before 9 months of age**
- **Abnormal development**
- **Preexisting neurologic disorder**

Seizure Disorder

Epilepsy is present when **at least 2 unprovoked seizures occur more than 24 hours apart.**

Early treatment with antiseizure medication reduces the risk of subsequent seizures and improves time to remission. Antiseizure medications may be stopped after the patient has been seizure-free for 2 years.

Seizure Disorder	Classic Features	EEG Findings	Treatment
Absence seizures	Frequent seizures with cessation of motor activity or speech, blank facial expression, and flickering of eyelids More common in girls, rare in children < 5 years, rarely lasts longer than 30 seconds No aura or postictal state	3-second spike and generalized wave discharge	First line: Ethosuximide Alternative: Valproic acid
Juvenile myoclonic epilepsy (JME)	Jerky movement occurring in the morning Onset around adolescence	Irregular spike-and-wave pattern	First line: Valproic acid
West syndrome (infantile spasms)	Infantile spasms during the first year of life Clusters of mixed flexor and extensor spasms of trunk and extremities, persisting for minutes with brief intervals between each spasm Of children with West syndrome, 75 percent have an underlying central nervous system disorder (Down syndrome is most common).	Hypsarrhythmia (very high-voltage slow waves, irregularly interspersed with spikes and sharp waves)	First line: ACTH, prednisone, vigabatrin, pyridoxine (vitamin B6)
Partial seizure	Simple: Tonic or clonic movements involving most of the face, neck, and extremities and lasting 10–20 seconds. There is no postictal period. Generalized: Includes impaired consciousness	Spike and sharp waves or multifocal spikes	First line: Carbamazepine and valproic acid
Generalized seizure	Aura, loss of consciousness, eyes roll back, tonic contraction, apnea then clonic rhythmic contractions alternating with relaxation of all muscle groups Tongue biting, loss of bladder control Prominent postictal state	Anterior temporal lobe shows sharp waves or focal spikes	First line: Valproic acid

Infectious Disease

Fever without a Focus in the Young Child

Fever (temperature of > 38°C/100.4°F rectally) without focus **lasts < 1 week** and occurs in **children < 36 months old.** It is *not* the same as "fever of unknown origin," which has been present for > 3 weeks.

Treatment

Give **empiric antibiotics** under the following conditions:

- Documented **rectal temperature > 38°C/100.4°F**
- **WBC > 15,000, neutrophils > 1,500 with band forms**
- **Neonate:** Hospitalize, pan-culture (blood, urine), and give **prophylactic antibiotics** to cover for group B *Streptococcus, E. coli,* and *Listeria*
- **Infant:** Most common organism is *Streptococcus pneumoniae*
    - **Well appearing:** Give **single-dose IM ceftriaxone** and follow up in 24 hours
    - **Toxic appearing:** Start **empiric IV antibiotics**

Meningitis

A 5-month-old child presents with lethargy, poor feeding, and irritability. He has been vomiting for 2 days and has had a temperature of 101.3°F. On exam, the fontanelles are noted to be bulging, and there is paralysis of the lateral gaze on the left side. The mother reports that he is up-to-date on all vaccinations. Which of the following is the next step in management?

a. CT scan of the head
b. Empiric antibiotics
c. Lumbar puncture
d. Steroids
e. Urine culture

Answer: **B.** This history is **highly suggestive of meningitis.** However, the patient is also exhibiting signs of increased intracranial pressure, a contraindication to lumbar puncture (workup of meningitis includes blood culture and lumbar puncture, unless there are signs of ICP). CT scan is not sensitive in diagnosing increased ICP or meningitis. It is not required for the initiation of antibiotics when clinical suspicion is high. The most important next step in management is to begin empiric antibiotics based on clinical suspicion. Intravenous dexamethasone has been shown to be of value in management of meningitis due to HiB. However, HiB is uncommon in the United States with the advent of vaccines, which protect infants against HiB infections.

Treatment

- Initial empiric treatment: **Vancomycin** plus either **cefotaxime** or **ceftriaxone**
- Specific treatment:
  - *S. pneumoniae:* **Penicillin or 3rd-generation cephalosporin** for 10–14 days
  - *N. meningitidis:* **Penicillin** for 5–7 days
  - HiB: **Ampicillin** for 7–10 days plus **IV dexamethasone**
  - Pretreated and no organism identified: **3rd-generation cephalosporin** for 7–10 days
  - Gram-negative (*E. coli*): **Third-generation cephalosporin** for 3 weeks

The following are possible complications of meningitis:

- **Neurologic dysfunction, thrombosis, and mental retardation** may occur, especially if therapy is delayed
- The most common complication is **hearing loss** (especially with pneumococcus)
- Subdural effusion, common with HiB → **seizures and persistent fever**
- Meningococcus: **Septic shock, disseminated intravascular coagulation, acidosis, adrenal hemorrhage, renal and heart failure**

Meningitis can be prevented with chemoprophylaxis with **rifampin** for *N. meningitidis* and HiB but not for *S. pneumoniae.* Prophylaxis should be given to *all* close contacts regardless.

Section 6
Obstetrics

contributing author Elizabeth August, MD

The Uncomplicated Pregnancy

Diagnosing Pregnancy

Pregnancy is suggested in a patient with amenorrhea, enlargement of the uterus, and a (+) urinary β-hCG. Pregnancy is confirmed with the following:

- **Presence of a gestational sac:** This is seen by transvaginal ultrasound at 4 to 5 weeks. This corresponds to a serum β-hCG level of about 1,500 mIU/mL.
- **Fetal heart motion:** Seen by ultrasound at 5 to 6 weeks.
- **Fetal heart sounds:** Heard with Doppler ultrasonography at 8 to 10 weeks.
- **Fetal movements:** Felt by the examining physician after 20 weeks.

CCS Tip: Order pregnancy counseling (e.g., "Avoid alcohol and tobacco.") in newly diagnosed pregnant patients via the ORDER icon. Type in, "Counsel patient, pregnancy."

Gravidity: number of pregnancies
Parity: number of births with a gestational age > 24 weeks

Routine Prenatal Screening Tests

First Trimester

A 21-year-old primigravida, para 0 (G1 P0) presents for her first prenatal visit at 11 weeks' gestation, which is confirmed by obstetric sonogram. She has no risk factors. What screening tests will you perform?

Answer: See the following chart.

Screening	Test	Diagnostic Significance	Next Step in Management
FIRST TRIMESTER ROUTINE TESTS			
Anemia, blood disorders	CBC	• Anemia = Hb < 10 g/dL (normal: 10–12 g/dL). The most reliable indicator of true anemia is MCV. • Most common cause of anemia is iron deficiency. (See BSC below) • WBC > 16,000/mm³ is abnormal.	• ↓ hemoglobin ↓ MCV: Give iron. Test for thalassemia if anemia does not improve. • ↓ hemoglobin ↑ MCV ↑RDW: Give folate. • Thrombocytopenia (< 150,000/ mm³): Correlate clinically for ITP or HELLP syndrome.
Blood type, Rh, and antibody	Type and screen Direct and indirect Coombs	• Rh negative mothers may become sensitized (anti-D Ab) → risk of erythroblastosis fetalis in the next pregnancy. • Indirect Coombs test (or atypical antibody test [AAT]) detects atypical RBC Ab's.	• Give RhoGAM to Rh negative mothers at 28 weeks *after* first rescreening for absence of anti-D antibodies. • Give RhoGAM in Rh negative mothers after any procedure (CVS, amniocentesis) and after delivery.
Genitourinary screening	Cervical PAP smear	• Detects cervical dysplasia or malignancy.	• See Gynecology section for management.
	Urinalysis/ Urine culture	• UA: Screen for underlying renal disease and infection. • UCx: Screen for asymptomatic bacteriuria (ASB).	• Always treat ASB in pregnancy to prevent pyelonephritis (30% risk when untreated). • Rx: Nitrofurantoin (before 30 weeks), cephalosporins, amoxicillin
Immunization status	Rubella antibody	• (–) Rubella IgG Ab's means ↑ risk of primary rubella infection.	• Do *not* give *Rubella* immunization in pregnancy. • Immunize seronegative patients *after* delivery.
	Hepatitis B surface antigen	• (+) HBsAg: Indicates risk for vertical transmission of HBV	• (+) HBsAg: Order HBVe antigen. • (+) HBeAg signifies a highly infectious state.
Infection: Syphilis	VDRL or RPR	Confirm (+) VDRL/RPR with treponema-specific tests (MHATP or FTA).	• (+) confirmatory test: Treat with intramuscular penicillin. • Penicillin allergic: Desensitize and then treat with penicillin.

Ab's = antibodies; FTA: fluorescent treponema antibody absorption; Hb = hemoglobin; IM = intramuscular; MHATP: microhemagglutination assay for antibodies to *T. pallidum*; PO = oral

(continued next page)

Basic Science Correlate

Anemia in pregnancy is caused by increased levels of hepcidin, which inhibits iron transport. Pregnancy increases iron demand, but hepcidin prevents absorption.

Screening	Test	Diagnostic Significance	Next Step in Management
Infection: HIV	ELISA	• Confirm (+) ELISA screen with Western blot test (presence of HIV core and envelope antigens).	• Always get consent for HIV testing. • All babies born to HIV (+) women will be HIV antibody (+) (passive transport of maternal Ab's). (+) Ab's do not indicate infection in infant. • Antiretrovirals are not contraindicated in pregnancy. • See Perinatal Infections for further treatment.
Infection: Chlamydia/ Gonorrhea	Cervical culture	• Gram stain • Chlamydia and gonorrhea culture (see BSC below) • Also treat *Trichomonas vaginalis* (can cause premature labor).	(+) Chlamydia/gonorrhea • PO azithromycin + IM ceftriaxone (treatment of choice) • Alternative: PO amoxicillin (+) Bacterial vaginitis • PO metronidazole or clindamycin (+) *Trichomonas vaginalis* • PO metronidazole
FIRST TRIMESTER OPTIONAL TESTS			
Tuberculosis	PPD	• Test for exposure to TB in high risk mothers. • (+) test is induration, not erythema.	• (–) PPD: No further follow-up is needed. • (+) PPD: Order chest x-ray to rule out active disease. Treatment for positive screen: • (+) PPD/ (–) CXR: INH and B6 for 9 months. • (+) PPD/ (+) CXR (+) sputum: Begin triple therapy antituberculosis Rx if sputum stain positive. Obtain sputum for culture. • Avoid streptomycin in pregnancy because of the risk of ototoxicity in the fetus.
Trisomy 21: Early testing	β-hCG Pregnancy-associated plasma protein A (PAPP-A) Fetal nuchal translucency	• Offered to high-risk pregnancies (females above the age of 35 at delivery, women with a history of prior trisomy 21).	• (+) screening test is confirmed with chorionic villus sampling in the first trimester.

Basic Science Correlate

Chlamydia trachomatis is an obligate intracellular parasite: It needs a host cell to survive.

Neisseria gonorrhea is a gram-negative diplococcus that grows on chocolate agar. Nuclear acid amplification (NAAT) is the test of choice.

Maternal serum alpha fetoprotein **(MS-AFP)** increases with gestational age, and is expressed in **multiples of the median (MoM).**

- > 2.2 MoM is considered *elevated.*
- < 2.5 MoM is considered *normal.*

Inhibin A is made by the placenta during pregnancy and normally remains constant during 15th–18th week of pregnancy. The level of **inhibin A** is increased in the blood of mothers of fetuses with Down syndrome.

Second Trimester

A 23-year-old woman (G3 P1 Abortion 1) is seen at 17 weeks gestation. She recently underwent a triple marker screen with the maternal serum alpha fetoprotein (normal < 2.2 MoM). Her test showed an elevation in maternal serum alpha fetoprotein. On examination, her uterus is at the umbilicus. What is the next step in management?

a. Amniocentesis
b. Chorionic villus sampling
c. Inhibin A
d. Recommendation of termination of pregnancy
e. Ultrasound

Answer: **E.** The most common cause of an abnormal maternal serum alpha fetoprotein (MS-AFP) is gestational dating error. The first step in evaluating any pregnancy with an abnormal MS-AFP is to get ***an obstetric ultrasound*** to confirm the gestational date.

Screening	Test	Diagnostic Significance	Next Step in Management
SECOND TRIMESTER OPTIONAL TESTS			
Triple Marker Screen *Testing window is 15–20 weeks gestation.*	1. MS-AFP 2. β-hCG 3. Estriol 4. Add Inhibin A in high-risk women (↑ sens to 80%).	• Never test MS-AFP alone: Only 20% sensitivity → ↑ to 70% sensitivity with triple screen. • **↑ MS-AFP:** Neural tube defect (NTD), ventral wall defect, twin pregnancy, placental bleeding, renal disease, sacrococcygeal teratoma • **↓ MS-AFP:** – **Trisomy 21 (Down syndrome)** ∘ **↓ MS-AFP** ∘ **↓ Estriol** ∘ **↑ β-hCG** – **Trisomy 18** ∘ **↓ MS-AFP** ∘ **↓ Estriol** ∘ **↓ β-hCG**	**1) Abnormal MS-AFP:** First step in management: • Perform ultrasound to confirm dating. • If dating error, repeat MS-AFP. • A normal repeat MS-AFP is reassuring. Note: Accurate gestational dating is needed for interpretation of results. **2) Dates confirmed by ultrasound:** Next step in management: For ↑ MS-AFP: a) Amniocentesis for amniotic fluid alpha fetoprotein (AF-AFP) level and acetylcholinesterase activity For ↓ MS-AFP: b) Amniocentesis for karyotyping Note: Elevated levels of amniotic fluid-acetylcholinesterase activity are specific to open NTD.

AF-AFP = amniotic fluid alpha fetoprotein; MS-AFP = maternal serum alpha fetoprotein

Third Trimester

A 38-year-old woman (G2 P1) is at 27 weeks' gestation. She weighs 227 pounds. She has gained 30 pounds during her pregnancy but reports that most of this is "fluid retention." She was diagnosed with gestational diabetes during her last pregnancy. Which of the following is the next step in management?

a. Begin insulin therapy
b. Begin glipizide therapy
c. Obtain 1-hr 50 g OGTT
d. Obtain 3-hr 75 g OGTT
e. Obtain 3-hr 100 g OGTT

Answer: **C.** The first step in evaluating for gestational diabetes is with the 1 hr ***50 g OGTT in weeks 24–28***. When this is positive, the patient must then undergo the confirmatory ***3 h 100 g OGTT.***

Screening	Test	Diagnostic Significance	Next Step in Management
THIRD TRIMESTER ROUTINE TESTS			
Diabetes	1 hr 50 g OGTT given between weeks 24–28.	• Abnormal result: 1hr blood glucose > 140 mg/dL	• (+) screening: perform 3-hr 100 g OGTT (the definitive test for glucose intolerance in pregnancy). Requires overnight fast.
Anemia	CBC Measured at weeks 24–28.	• Hemoglobin < 10 g/dL = anemia. • The most common cause is iron deficiency (even if not present in 1st trimester).	• Give iron supplementation for iron deficiency.
Atypical antibodies	Indirect Coombs test	• Performed in Rh-negative women to look for atypical antibodies (anti-D Ab) before giving RhoGAM.	• RhoGAM is not indicated in Rh negative women who have developed anti-D antibodies.
GBS screening	Vaginal and rectal culture for group B streptococci at 35–37 weeks	• (+) GBS is a high risk for sepsis in newborn. • Treat with intrapartum IV antibiotics.	• Intrapartum antibiotic – IV penicillin G – IV clindamycin or erythromycin in penicillin-allergic patient

GBS = Group B Streptococcus; IV = intravenous; OGTT = oral glucose tolerance test

Gestational diabetes does not present with typical symptoms of diabetes. The vast majority of patients are diagnosed on OGTT screening.

The confirmatory test for diabetes in pregnancy is the **3 hr 100 g OGTT.**

- If the plasma glucose is > 125 mg/dL at the beginning of the test (i.e., fasting blood glucose), **diabetes mellitus** is the diagnosis.
- *Abnormal* plasma glucose measurements are: > 140 mg/dL at 3 hr, > 155 mg/dL at 2 hr, and > 180 mg/dL at 1 hr.
- If only 1 postglucose load measurement is abnormal, the diagnosis is **impaired glucose tolerance.**
- If 2 or more of the postglucose load measurements are abnormal, the diagnosis is **gestational diabetes.**
- The 1 hr 50 g OGTT is a sensitive test; it must catch *all* patients that *may* have the disease.
- The 3 hr 100 g OGTT is a specific test; it must catch *all* the people that *actually* have the disease.

Basic Science Correlate

Sensitivity = true positives/true positives + false negatives.

Specificity = true negatives/true negatives + false positives.

Give Rh(D) immunoglobulin in Rh negative mothers:
- at 28 weeks.
- within 72 hours of delivery.
- after miscarriage or abortion.
- during amniocentesis or CVS.
- with heavy vaginal bleeding.

Nausea and Vomiting During Pregnancy

The following antiemetics can be used safely to relieve nausea and vomiting during the first trimester:

- Doxylamine
- Metoclopramide
- Ondansetron
- Promethazine
- Pyridoxine (vitamin B6)

Third Trimester Bleeding

CCS Tip: Initial steps in management of late pregnancy bleeding:

- Perform **initial management**:
  - Get the patient's vitals
  - Place external fetal monitor
  - Start IV fluids with normal saline

- Order **lab tests**:
  - CBC
  - DIC workup (platelets, PT, PTT, fibrinogen, and D-dimer)
  - Type and cross-match
  - Obstetric ultrasound to rule out placenta previa

- Perform **further steps in management**:
  - Give blood transfusion for large volume loss.
  - Place Foley catheter and measure urine output.
  - Perform vaginal exam to rule out lacerations.
  - Schedule delivery if fetus is in jeopardy or gestational age is ≥ 36 weeks.

Never perform a digital or speculum examination in a patient with late vaginal bleeding until a vaginal ultrasound *first* rules out placenta previa.

Abruptio Placenta

When there is **sudden onset vaginal bleeding** and **severe, constant pelvic pain** in a patient with a history of **hypertension** or **trauma (e.g., motor vehicle accident),** bleeding results from avulsion of anchoring placental villi from the lower uterine segment.

Less commonly, the hematoma does not dissect through the margin of the placenta, and bleeding remains concealed (concealed hemorrhage). The clue to the diagnosis is **severe, constant pain** with only a **scant amount of bleeding.**

Disseminated intravascular coagulation (**DIC**) is a feared complication following the release of tissue thromboplastin into the circulation.

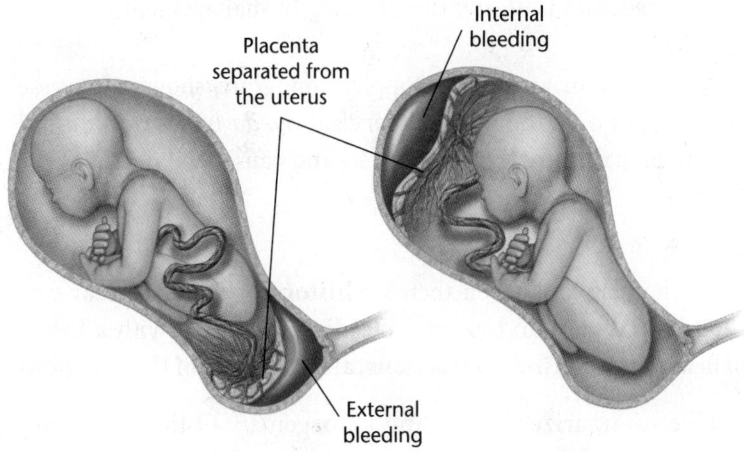

Abruptio Placenta (Placental Abruption)

Placenta Previa

Classically, **sudden-onset painless bleeding occurs** at rest or during activity without warning. The case may include a **history of trauma, coitus,** or **pelvic examination** before bleeding starts.

Placenta previa occurs when the placenta is implanted in the **lower uterine segment.** Types of placenta previa are complete previa (the placenta covers the entire os), incomplete previa (the cervical os is only partially covered), and marginal (the placenta is near but does not cover the os).

Placenta Accreta

The 3 forms of placenta accreta are distinguished by the depth of penetration:

- **Placenta accreta:** does not penetrate the entire thickness of the endometrium
- **Placenta increta:** extends further into the myometrium
- **Placenta percreta:** when the placenta penetrates the entire myometrium to the uterine serosa

If placental implantation occurs over a previous uterine scar, the **villi may invade** into the deeper layers of the decidua basalis and myometrium (called placenta accreta, increta, or percreta). In this scenario, intractable bleeding may require a **cesarean hysterectomy.**

Vasa Previa

Vasa previa is **life-threatening for the fetus.** It occurs when velamentous cord insertion results in umbilical vessels crossing the placental membranes over the cervix. When membranes rupture, the fetal vessels are torn, and blood loss is from the fetal circulation. **Fetal exsanguination** and **death** occur rapidly.

The classic triad is as follows:

1. **Rupture of membranes**
2. **Painless vaginal bleeding**
3. **Fetal bradycardia**

Emergency cesarean section is *always* the first step in management.

If the question describes an antenatal Doppler sonogram showing a vessel crossing the membranes over the internal cervical os, *do not perform amniotomy.* Amniotomy may rupture the fetal vessels and cause fetal death.

Uterine Rupture

Uterine rupture is the diagnosis when there's a **history of a uterine scar** with sudden-onset **abdominal pain** and **vaginal bleeding** associated with a **loss of electronic fetal heart rate, uterine contractions,** and **recession of the fetal head.**

The following table summarizes causes and management of third-trimester bleeding.

	Abruptio Placenta	Placenta Previa	Vasa Previa	Uterine Rupture
Pain	Yes	No	No	Yes
Risk factors	Previous abruption Hypertension Trauma Cocaine abuse	Previous previa Multiparity Structural abnormalities (e.g., fibroids) Advanced maternal age	Velamentous insertion of the umbilical cord Accessory lobes Multiple gestation	Previous classic uterine incision Myomectomy (fibroids) Excessive oxytocin Grand multiparity
Diagnosis: Sonogram	Placenta in normal position ± retroplacental hematoma	Placenta implanted over the lower uterine segment	Vessel crossing the membranes over the internal cervical os	N/A
Management	1. Emergent c-section: Best choice for placenta previa or if patient/fetus is deteriorating. 2. Vaginal delivery if ≥ 36 weeks or continued bleeding. May be attempted in placenta previa if placenta is > 2 cm from internal os. 3. Admit and observe if bleeding has stopped, vitals and fetal heart rate (FHR) stable, or < 34 weeks.		Immediate c-section	Immediate surgery and delivery
Complication	Disseminated intravascular coagulation	Placenta accreta/increta/percreta → hysterectomy	Fetal exsanguination	Hysterectomy for uncontrolled bleeding

Perinatal Infections

Group B β-Hemolytic Streptococci (GBS)

A 28-year-old woman presents at 36 weeks' gestation with rupture of membranes. On examination she is found to have 7 cm cervical dilatation. She received all of her prenatal care, and her only complication was a course of antibiotics for asymptomatic bacteriuria. GBS screening was negative. Her first baby was hospitalized for 10 days after delivery for GBS pneumonia and sepsis. What is the most appropriate management?

a. Administer intrapartum IV penicillin.
b. Administer intramuscular azithromycin.
c. Rescreen for group B streptococci.
d. Schedule cesarean section.
e. No intervention is needed.

Answer: **A.** Intrapartum IV penicillin is indicated because the patient's previous birth was complicated with neonatal GBS sepsis.

- Thirty percent of women have **asymptomatic vaginal colonization** with GBS.
- Vertical transmission results in **pneumonia** and **sepsis in the neonate** within hours to days of birth.
- There is a **50 percent mortality rate** with neonatal infection.

GBS-related meningitis occurs after the first week and is a hospital-acquired infection that is unrelated to vertical transmission.

Treatment

- Intrapartum IV ampicillin
- Penicillin allergy: IV cefazolin, clindamycin, or erythromycin

When are antibiotics the answer?

- GBS (+) urine, cervical, or vaginal culture at any time during pregnancy
- Presence of high-risk factors:
  - Preterm delivery
  - Membrane rupture > 18 hours
  - Maternal fever
  - Previous baby with GBS sepsis

When are antibiotics NOT the answer?

- **Planned c-section without rupture** of membranes (even if culture is [+])
- Culture (+) on a previous pregnancy, but **culture (–) in the current pregnancy**

IgG antibodies in the mother indicate past exposure and are protective. IgM antibodies suggest recent exposure and risk of exposure to the fetus.

Toxoplasmosis

Infection with *Toxoplasma gondii* parasite is the most common diagnosis when the case describes a patient handling **cat feces or litter boxes,** drinking **raw goat milk,** eating **raw meat**, or possibly gardening.

Basic Science Correlate

Toxoplasmosis is present in **undercooked meat and cat feces** (after the cat eats an affected rodent). Toxoplasmosis can live in the environment > 1 year.

Classic triad of congenital toxoplasmosis:
1. Chorioretinitis
2. Intracranial calcifications
3. Hydrocephalus

Vertical transmission only occurs with **primary infection of the mother.** Most serious infections occur during the first trimester.

Suspect primary infection of toxoplasmosis when the question gives a history of a **mild mononucleosis-like syndrome** and **presence of a cat** in the household. Intrauterine growth retardation may be seen on ultrasound.

Prevention

- The most important preventive measure against toxoplasmosis infection is to advise pregnant women to avoid handling cat feces, raw goat milk, and undercooked meat.

Management

- Test for toxoplasma IgG and IgM levels.
- Give **pyrimethamine** and **sulfadiazine** for the treatment of serologically confirmed fetal/neonatal infection via amniocentesis.

Varicella

Transplacental infection results from **primary varicella infection** in the mother (25–40 percent infection rate).

The greatest risk to the fetus is if a **rash** appears in the mother **between 5 days antepartum and 2 days postpartum.**

Neonatal infection presents with "zigzag" skin lesions, limb hypoplasia, microcephaly, microphthalmia, chorioretinitis, and cataracts.

> **Basic Science**
>
> Varicella is in the family Herpesviridae, **human herpesvirus type 3.**
>
> Primary infection causes varicella. After clinical symptoms disappear, the virus lies dormant in the dorsal root ganglia. It may reactivate late in life, causing shingles. Herpesvirus commonly reactivates in immunocompromised patients.

Prevention

- **Vaccination:** Live-attenuated varicella virus to **nonpregnant** women.
- **Postexposure prophylaxis: VariZIG** (purified human immunoglobulin with high levels of antivaricella antibodies) within 10 days of exposure. VariZIG does not prevent infection but only attenuates the clinical effects of the virus. (Note: VZIG is no longer available.)

Treatment

- **Maternal** varicella (uncomplicated): Oral **acyclovir** to mother *plus* **VariZIG** to mother *and* neonate
- **Congenital varicella: VariZIG** *and* **IV acyclovir** to the neonate

Rubella

Vertical transmission of rubella virus (causative virus of German measles) occurs with primary infection during pregnancy (70–90 percent).

Neonates with congenital rubella present with **congenital deafness** (most common sequelae), congenital heart disease (e.g., patent ductus arteriosus, or PDA), **cataracts, mental retardation, hepatosplenomegaly, thrombocytopenia,** and **"blueberry muffin" rash.** Adverse effects occur with primary infection in the first 10 weeks of gestation.

> **Basic Science**
>
> Rubella is a single-stranded RNA virus of the family Togaviridae.

Prevention

- Perform **first-trimester screening** and have mother **avoid infected individuals.**
- Immunize seronegative women *after* delivery.
- No postexposure prophylaxis is available.

A 24-year-old child-care worker is 29 weeks pregnant and is currently working. One of the children was diagnosed with rubella last week. Rubella antigen testing is performed and her IgG titer is negative. What is the risk of neonatal transmission in this patient? What is the next step in management?

a. Give anti-rubella antibodies
b. Give betamethasone
c. Give rubella vaccine now
d. Give rubella vaccine after delivery
e. Ultrasound of the fetus

Answer: **D.** There is no postexposure prophylaxis available, and immunization during pregnancy is contraindicated (live vaccine). The only correct management is to await normal delivery and give vaccination to the mother after delivery.

Basic Science

CMV is another member of the family Herpesviridae, **HHV-5.**

Cytomegalovirus (CMV)

Congenital CMV syndrome is the *most* common congenital viral syndrome in the United States. CMV is the *most* common cause of sensorineural deafness in children. CMV is spread by **infected body fluid secretions.**

The greatest risk for vertical transmission occurs with **primary infection** (infection rate is 50 percent).

Most mothers develop **asymptomatic infections** or describe **mild, mononucleosis-like symptoms.** About 10 percent of infants with congenital CMV infection are symptomatic at birth.

Manifestations include **intrauterine growth restriction, prematurity, microcephaly, jaundice, petechiae, hepatosplenomegaly, periventricular calcifications, chorioretinitis,** and **pneumonitis.**

Diagnostic Testing

- Send CMV IgM and IgG levels from the mother:
  - IgG (+) / IgM (–) indicates past exposure and no risk for primary infection.
  - IgG (+) / IgM (+) or IgG (–) / IgM (+) indicates recent infection.

Prevention

- Follow universal precautions with all body fluids. Avoid transfusion with CMV-positive blood.

Treatment

- Antiviral therapy with **ganciclovir** or foscarnet prevents viral shedding and prevents hearing loss but does not cure the infection.
- CMV hyperimmune globulin may reduce the risk of congenital infection in pregnant women with primary CMV infection.

Herpes Simplex Virus (HSV)

A 21-year-old multipara is admitted to the birthing unit at 39 weeks gestation in active labor at 6 cm dilation. Membranes are intact. She has a history of genital herpes preceding the pregnancy. Her last outbreak was 8 weeks ago. She now complains of pain and pruritus. On examination, she had localized, painful, ulcerative lesions on her right vaginal wall. Which of the following is the next step in management?

a. Administer IV acyclovir
b. Administer terbutaline
c. Obtain culture of ulcer
d. Proceed with vaginal delivery
e. Schedule cesarean section

Answer: **E.** Active genital herpes is an indication for cesarean section.

The *most* common cause of transmission is **contact with maternal genital lesions** during an active HSV episode. Transplacental infection can also occur with **primary infections** during pregnancy (50 percent risk). *Greatest risk* is primary infection in the third trimester. Suspect primary HSV infection if the case describes **fever, malaise,** and **diffuse genital lesions** during pregnancy.

Neonatal infection acquired during delivery has **50 percent mortality rate.** Surviving infants develop meningoencephalitis, mental retardation, pneumonia, hepatosplenomegaly, jaundice, and petechiae.

Diagnostic Testing

- (+) HSV culture from vesicle fluid or ulcer or HSV PCR

Prevention

- Perform c-section in women with lesions suspicious for **active genital HSV** at the time of labor.
- Do *not* use fetal scalp electrodes for monitoring (increased risk of HSV transmission if mother has active HSV lesion).
- Advise standard precautions (avoid intercourse if partner has active lesions, avoid oral sex in presence of oral lesions, avoid kissing neonate in presence of oral lesions).

Treatment

- **Acyclovir** to patient for primary infection during pregnancy

Human Immunodeficiency Virus (HIV)

Basic Science Correlate

HIV is a single-stranded, positive, enveloped RNA virus, a member of the family Retroviridae, genus Lentivirus. Once the virus enters a host cell, *viral* reverse transcriptase converts the viral RNA genome into double-stranded DNA. This allows integration of the *viral DNA* into the host *cellular DNA*.

A 24-year-old HIV positive female (G2 P1) presents in her 16th week of pregnancy. Her previous child was diagnosed HIV positive after vaginal delivery. What is the most effective method of decreasing the risk of vertical transmission?

a. Avoidance of artificial rupture of membranes
b. Avoidance of breastfeeding
c. Antiretroviral triple therapy
d. Cesarean section
e. Zidovudine monotherapy

Answer: **C.** All of the strategies are recommended, however. Zidovudine (ZDV) monotherapy is not as effective as triple therapy in decreasing the risk of HIV transmission to the fetus (25 percent to 8 percent). Triple antiretroviral therapy is indicated for more effective management of HIV in the mother to drive the viral load to < 1,000. ZDV monotherapy alone is never indicated. Cesarean section (***before rupture of membranes***), avoidance of breastfeeding or intrapartum invasive procedures (artificial ROM, fetal scalp electrodes) also decreases transmission rate. Combination of all of the above strategies listed above reduces the transmission rate to 1 percent.

Zidovudine monotherapy is no longer indicated for anyone.

Major route of vertical transmission is contact with infected genital secretions at the time of vaginal delivery. Without treatment, the vertical transmission rate is 25–30 percent.

Continue antiretrovirals in all pregnant patients.

Elective cesarean is of most benefit in women with low CD4 counts and high RNA viral loads (> 1,000). All neonates of HIV-positive women will have positive HIV tests from transplacental passive IgG passage.

Prevention and Treatment

HIV-infected pregnant women should receive ART therapy regardless of HIV RNA level.

- **Triple-drug therapy** (which *must* include ZDV):
  - Start triple therapy immediately, regardless of CD4 and viral load, to decrease risk of transmission.
  - Intravenous intrapartum ZDV if viral load is high at time of delivery
  - Combination ZDV-based ART for 6 weeks after delivery

- Give the infant prophylaxis against HIV, with 6 weeks of **zidovudine**
- Schedule c-section at 38 weeks *unless* < 1,000 viral copies/mL.
- Advise the mother **not to breastfeed** (breast milk transmits the virus).
- **Avoid invasive procedures** (e.g., artificial rupture of membranes, fetal scalp electrodes).

Do a c-section of the mother's viral load is > 1,000 at the time of delivery.

Syphilis

If the case describes a previously treated syphilis infection, *never* assume immunity. There is **no immunity** from prior infection with syphilis, and reinfection can occur over and over again.

Transplacental infection results from primary and secondary infection (60 percent risk of transmission). The lowest risk of transmission is with latent or tertiary infection.

Early acquired (first trimester) congenital syphilis includes the following symptoms/outcomes:

- Nonimmune hydrops fetalis
- Maculopapular or vesicular peripheral rash
- Anemia, thrombocytopenia, and hepatosplenomegaly
- Large and edematous placenta
- Perinatal mortality rates ~ 50 percent

Late-acquired congenital syphilis is diagnosed after 2 years of age and includes the following symptoms:

- Hutchinson teeth
- "Mulberry" molars
- "Saddle" nose
- "Saber" shins
- Deafness (cranial nerve 8 palsy)

Always order an HIV test in any pregnant patient who has tested positive for an STD.

C-section will not prevent vertical transmission of syphilis, because it happens through the placenta before birth.

Diagnostic Testing

- VDRL or RPR screening in first trimester. Confirm (+) screen with FTA-ABS.
- Screening test will be falsely negative in primary syphilis.
  - When the case describes a woman with a painless genital ulcer, order **darkfield microscopy** for diagnosis of primary syphilis.

Treatment

- Benzathine penicillin IM × 1 for (+) mothers
- Penicillin allergy: Oral desensitization followed by full dose benzathine penicillin

A 34-year-old multigravida presents for prenatal care in the second trimester. She admits to a past history of substance abuse but states she has been clean for 6 months. With her second pregnancy, she experienced a preterm delivery at 34 weeks' gestation of a male neonate who died within the first day of life. She states that at delivery, the baby was swollen with skin lesions and that the placenta was very large. She was treated with antibiotics, but she does not remember their name or other details. On a routine prenatal panel with this current pregnancy, she is found to have a positive VDRL test. What is the next step in management?

a. FTA-ABS
b. Intramuscular penicillin
c. Lupus anticoagulant
d. Oral penicillin
e. RPR
f. Ultrasound

Answer: **A.** The next step after any positive screening test is the confirmatory test before starting therapy. **FTA-ABS** or **MHA-TP** are the confirmatory tests for syphilis. Once syphilis is confirmed, the most appropriate management is intramuscular penicillin.

Hepatitis B Virus (HBV)

Neonatal infection results from **primary infection in third trimester** or **ingestion of infected genital secretions** during vaginal delivery.

Of those neonates who get infected, **80 percent will develop chronic hepatitis,** compared with only 10 percent of infected adults.

HBeAg (+) prenatal transmission = 80–90%

A 29-year-old multigravida was found on routine prenatal laboratory testing to be positive for hepatitis B surface antigen. She is an intensive care unit nurse. She received 2 units of packed red blood cells 2 years ago after experiencing postpartum hemorrhage with her last pregnancy. Which of the following indicates the greatest risk of transmission?

a. Anti-HBc
b. Anti-HBs
c. HBe Ag
d. HBs Ag
e. IgM anti-HBc

Answer: **C.** Mothers who are (+) for HBsAg, anti-HBe antibody, and IgM anti-HBc are acutely infected. There is only a 10 percent vertical transmission risk. Mothers who are also (+) for **HBeAg** have an **80 percent risk** of transmission to fetus. Anti-HBs (antibody to surface antigen) indicates immunity to infection from previous immunization. Hepatitis B surface antibody is an IgG antibody that can cross the placenta.

Prevention

- Hepatitis B infection is *not* an indication for cesarean delivery.
- Avoid invasive procedures during pregnancy (e.g., amniocentesis).
- Breastfeeding is *not* contraindicated *after* the neonate has received active immunization and HBIG.
- Immunization:
  - **HBsAg-negative:** Give active immunization during pregnancy
  - **Postexposure prophylaxis for the mother:** HBIG (antibodies to hepatitis B) passive immunization and vaccine

Treatment

- Hepatitis immunization and HBIG in neonate
- Chronic HBV can be treated with either interferon or lamivudine

Hypertension in Pregnancy

Hypertension (BP ≥ 140/90 mm Hg) during pregnancy can be classified as **chronic hypertension** or **gestational hypertension.** Both types of hypertension predispose the mother and the fetus to more serious conditions.

When hypertension is accompanied by signs and symptoms of end-organ damage or neurological sequelae, the diagnosis is **preeclampsia, eclampsia,** or the **HELLP syndrome.**

With sustained hypertension, the fetus may be **growth restricted** and **hypoxic** and is at risk for **abruptio placenta.**

Diagnosis is as follows:

- **Chronic hypertension** is the diagnosis when there is a **history of elevated blood pressure before pregnancy** or **before 20 weeks' gestation.**
- **Gestational hypertension** is the diagnosis when blood pressure develops after **20 weeks' gestation** and **returns to normal baseline by 6 weeks** postpartum. It occurs more commonly in multifetal pregnancy.
- **Preeclampsia** is the diagnosis when there is **proteinuria** and/or **presence of "warning signs."**

Warning signs of maternal jeopardy:
- Hallmark symptoms:
  - **Headache**
  - **Epigastric pain**
  - **Changes in vision**
- Signs: **Pulmonary edema, oliguria** (Peripheral edema is *not* a warning sign.)
- Labs: **Thrombocytopenia, elevated liver enzymes**

Preeclampsia and Eclampsia

Mild preeclampsia is indicated with:

- Sustained BP elevation > **140/90 mm Hg**
- Proteinuria of **1–2+** (on dipstick) or > **300 mg** (on a 24-hour urine)

Severe preeclampsia is indicated by mild preeclampsia plus one of the following:

- Sustained BP elevation **>160/110 mm Hg**
- Proteinuria of **3–4+** (on dipstick) or **> 5 g** (on 24-hour urine)
- Presence of **"warning signs"**

Primiparas are *most* at risk. Other risk factors are multiple gestation, hydatidiform mole, diabetes mellitus, age extremes, chronic hypertension, and chronic renal disease.

A 19-year-old primigravida presents at 32 weeks' gestation for routine follow-up. She denies headache, epigastric pain, or visual disturbances. She has gained 2 pounds since her last visit 2 weeks ago. On examination, her blood pressure is 155/95, which is persistent on repeat BP check 10 minutes later. She has only trace pedal edema. Which of the following is the next step in management?

a. **Begin methyldopa.**
b. **Begin labetalol.**
c. **Perform an electrocardiogram.**
d. **Perform a fetal ultrasound.**
e. **Perform urinalysis.**

Answer: **E.** Always rule out preeclampsia in a hypertensive pregnant patient. Even if she is asymptomatic, proteinuria indicates preeclampsia and a worse prognosis.

Further diagnosis:

- **Chronic hypertension with superimposed preeclampsia** is the diagnosis when there is chronic hypertension with **increasingly severe hypertension, proteinuria,** and/or **"warning signs."**
- **Eclampsia** is the diagnosis when the case describes **unexplained grand mal seizures** in a **hypertensive** and/or **proteinuric** pregnant woman in the last half of pregnancy. Patients present with same signs and symptoms as in preeclampsia with the addition of unexplained tonic-clonic seizures. Seizures from **severe diffuse cerebral vasospasm** cause cerebral perfusion deficits and edema.
- **HELLP syndrome** is the diagnosis when there is hemolysis (H), elevated liver (EL) enzymes, and low platelets (LP).

Seizure disorder is *not* a risk factor for eclampsia.

Diagnostic Testing

- Order **CBC, chem-12 panel, coagulation panel,** and **urinalysis with urinary protein.**
- Labs will show the following:
  - **Hemoconcentration:** ↑hemoglobin, ↑hematocrit, ↑blood urea nitrogen (BUN), ↑serum creatinine, and ↑serum uric acid
  - **Proteinuria**
  - In severe preeclampsia, **disseminated intravascular coagulation** and **liver enzyme elevation**

The *only* definitive cure is delivery and removal of all fetal-placental tissue.

Treatment

- **Blood pressure control:**
  - Don't treat *unless* BP > 160/100 mm Hg (antihypertensives decrease utero-placental blood flow)
  - Goal SBP is 140–150 mm Hg and DBP is 90–100 mm Hg
  - **Maintenance therapy:**
    - First line therapy is methyldopa or labetalol (alpha and beta blocker that preserves blood flow to uterus and placenta).
    - Second line therapy is nifedipine (calcium channel blocker).
  - **Acutely elevated BP**/treatment of severe preeclampsia or eclampsia:
    - Intravenous hydralazine or labetalol
  - **Never give ACE inhibitors, ARBs, or renin inhibitors, or start thiazide diuretics during pregnancy.**
- **Seizure management and prophylaxis**:
  - Protect the patient's airway and tongue
  - **Give IV $MgSO_4$ (magnesium sulfate)** bolus for seizure and infusion for continued prophylaxis
- **Monitoring**:
  - Serial sonograms (evaluate for intrauterine growth restriction [IUGR])
  - Serial BP monitoring and urine protein
- **Labor:**
  - Induce labor if ≥ 36 weeks with mild preeclampsia: attempt vaginal delivery with IV oxytocin if mother and fetus are stable.
  - Aggressive, prompt delivery is the best step for severe/superimposed preeclampsia or eclampsia at *any* gestational age.
  - Give intrapartum IV $MgSO_4$ and hydralazine and/or labetalol to manage BP.

A 32-year-old multigravida at 36 weeks' gestation was found to have BP 160/105 on routine prenatal visit. Previous BP readings were normal. She complained of some right-upper-quadrant abdominal pain. Urinalysis showed 3+ proteinuria. She is emergently induced for labor and delivers an 8 lb. 3 oz. boy. Two days after delivery, routine labs reveal elevated total bilirubin, lactate dehydrogenase, alanine aminotransferase (ALT), and aspartate aminotransferase (AST). Platelet count is 85,000. Postpartum evaluation reveals that she has no complaints of headache or visual changes. Which of the following is the most likely diagnosis?

a. Cholecystitis
b. HELLP syndrome
c. Hepatitis
d. Gestational thrombocytopenia
e. Preeclampsia

Answer: **B**. Patient has evidence of hemolysis (elevated LDH), elevated liver enzymes, and thrombocytopenia.

Gestational thrombocytopenia:
- Most common cause of thrombocytopenia in pregnancy
- Mild: Counts > 70,000
- Not associated with other abnormalities, and no symptoms
- Usually develops in third trimester

HELLP Syndrome

HELLP syndrome occurs in 5–10 percent of preeclamptic patients. It typically presents in the **third trimester** but may occur in the postpartum period, commonly presenting **2 days after delivery.** Risk factors differ from preeclampsia, since HELLP syndrome is more common in whites, multigravids, and women of older maternal age.

Treatment

- Schedule **immediate delivery** at any gestational age.
- Give **IV corticosteroids** (dexamethasone) when platelets < 100,000/mm^3 *both* antepartum and postpartum; continue until platelet count is > 100,000/mm^3 and liver function normalizes.
- Give **platelet transfusion** if platelet count < 20,000/mm^3 *or* platelet count < 50,000/mm^3 if cesarean section will be performed.
- **IV $MgSO_4$** for seizure prophylaxis, even if BP is normal.
- Steroids may also need to be considered for assistance with fetal lung maturation if prior to 36 weeks.

Complications of HELLP syndrome are as follows:

- DIC
- Abruptio placenta
- Fetal demise
- Ascites
- Hepatic rupture

Medical Complications in Pregnancy

Cardiac Abnormalities

- Heart disorders account for about **10 percent of maternal obstetric deaths.**
- Women with high-risk disorders (e.g., pulmonary hypertension, Eisenmenger syndrome, severe valvular disorders, prior postpartum cardiomyopathy) should be advised *not* to become pregnant due to risk of sudden death.
- Cardiovascular changes in pregnancy (30–50 percent ↑ cardiac output [CO]) may unmask or worsen underlying cardiac conditions. These changes are maximal at **28 and 34 weeks' gestation.**

Peripartum Cardiomyopathy

- Heart failure with no identifiable cause can develop between the last month of pregnancy to 5 months postpartum.
- Risk factors include multiparity, age ≥ 30, multiple gestations (i.e., twins or triplets, etc.), and preeclampsia.
- The 5-year mortality rate is 50 percent.

No seizure medication is proven safe in pregnancy. Valproate is the most dangerous.

Management of Specific Cardiac Conditions

Heart Failure

- Risk of maternal or fetal death is associated with class III or IV heart failure.
- *Never* use an ACE inhibitor or aldosterone antagonist in pregnancy.
- Loop diuretics, nitrates, and β-blockers may be continued.
- Digoxin may be used in pregnancy to improve symptoms, but it does not improve outcome.

Arrhythmias

- Continue rate control as with nonpregnant patients.
- Do *not* give amiodarone or warfarin.

Endocarditis Prophylaxis

- Indications are the same as for nonpregnant patients (see "Endocarditis" in Infectious Diseases).
- Give daily prophylaxis in patients with rheumatic heart disease.
- Do *not* give prophylactic antibiotics during uncomplicated vaginal/cesarean delivery in patients with valvular disease or prosthetic valves.

Valvular Disease

- Regurgitant lesions are well tolerated and do *not* require therapy.
- Stenotic lesions have an increased risk of maternal/fetal morbidity and mortality.
- Mitral stenosis has an increased risk of pulmonary edema and atrial fibrillation.

Hypercoagulable States

- **Pulmonary embolus** is the leading cause of maternal death in the United States. Fifty percent of pregnant women who develop thromboemboli have an underlying thrombophilic disorder. Virchow's triad consists of endothelial injury, vascular stasis, and hypercoagulability.
- When is anticoagulation the answer on the test?
  - **DVT** or **PE** in pregnancy
  - Atrial fibrillation (AF) **with underlying heart disease,** but not atrial fibrillation alone
  - **Antiphospholipid syndrome**
  - **Severe heart failure** (ejection fraction [EF]) < 30 percent)
  - **Eisenmenger syndrome**
- The anticoagulant of choice is low molecular weight heparin **(LMWH),** which does not cross the placenta (warfarin does cross the placenta and is contraindicated in pregnancy) and isn't associated with osteopenia (unfractionated heparin causes osteopenia).
  - Warfarin is contraindicated, as it causes fetal abnormalities and even death.

> Most common underlying thrombophilias:
> - Factor V Leiden mutation
> - Prothrombin gene mutation
> - Antiphospholipid syndrome
> - Hyperhomocysteinemia (MTHFR)
> - Antithrombin III deficiency

- Patients with a history of **DVT** or **PE** in a previous pregnancy or a history of **underlying thrombophilic condition** should receive **prophylactic LMWH** throughout pregnancy, **unfractionated heparin** during labor and delivery, and warfarin for 6 weeks postpartum.

Thyroid Disorders

- Hyperthyroidism in pregnancy causes **fetal growth restriction** and **stillbirth.**
- Hypothyroidism in pregnancy causes **intellectual deficits** in offspring and **miscarriage.**
- Pregnancy does *not* change the symptoms of hypothyroidism or hyperthyroidism or the normal values and ranges of free serum thyroxine (T4) and thyroid-stimulating hormone (TSH).
- Continue hormone replacement in patients with hypothyroidism during pregnancy. Increase the dose by 25–30 percent when hypothyroid patients become pregnant.
- Do not give thyroid replacement with triiodothyronine or desiccated thyroid. The drug of choice is **levothyroxine.**
- **Beta blockers** are the drug of choice for symptomatic hyperthyroidism. Radioactive iodine is never given in pregnancy.

Graves' Disease

- **Propylthiouracil (PTU)** is the drug of choice during the first trimester (methimazole is the second-line therapy). PTU crosses the placenta and may cause goiter and hypothyroidism in the fetus, so methimazole is used in the second and third trimesters. Congenital Graves' disease in the fetus may be **masked until 7 to 10 days after birth,** when the drug's effect subsides.
- Maternal thyroid-stimulating immunoglobulins (Igs) and thyroid-blocking Igs can cross the placenta and cause **fetal tachycardia, growth restriction,** and **goiter.**

Basic Science Correlate

PTU and methimazole are Class D drugs that harm the fetus by **inhibiting thyroperoxidase**, an enzyme needed to produce T3 and T4.

Diabetes in Pregnancy

- Target values of **FBS < 90 mg/dL** and **< 120 mg/dL** 1 hour after a meal.
- **Gestational diabetes (GDM)** is managed initially with diet and light exercise.
- If target glucose measurements are not met, the drug of choice is insulin. Insulin requirements increase throughout the course of the pregnancy but decrease as soon as the placenta is delivered.

- Glyburide and metformin have been used by some in pregnancy.
- Avoid oral hypoglycemics while breastfeeding, as they can cause hypoglycemia in neonates.

Routine Monitoring in Diabetic Patients

- **HbA1c in each trimester.** If HbA1c elevated in first trimester,
  - obtain targeted ultrasound at 18–20 weeks to look for structural anomalies; and
  - obtain fetal echocardiogram at 22–24 weeks to assess for congenital heart disease.
- **Triple-marker screen at 16–18 weeks** to assess for neural tube defects (NTD)
- **Monthly sonograms** to assess fetal macrosomia or IUGR
- **Monthly biophysical profiles**
- **Start weekly nonstress test (NST) and amniotic fluid index (AFI) at 32 weeks** if taking insulin, macrosomia, previous stillbirth, or hypertension.
- **Start NSTs and AFIs at 26 weeks** if small vessel disease is present or there is poor glycemic control.
- For gestational diabetes mellitus (GDM) patients, order a **2-hour 75 g OGTT** 6–12 weeks postpartum to determine if diabetes has resolved.
  - Thirty-five percent of women with GDM will develop overt diabetes within 5 to 10 years after delivery.
- **Caudal regression syndrome** is an uncommon congenital abnormality associated with overt DM.

Congenital malformations (especially NTDs) are strongly associated with HbA1c > 8.5 in the first trimester.

GDM is *not* associated with congenital anomalies, since hyperglycemia is not present in the first half of pregnancy.

Labor in Diabetic Patients

- Target delivery gestational age is **40 weeks** because of delayed fetal maturity.
- Induce labor at **39–40 weeks if < 4,500 g** or earlier if there is poor glycemic control. A lecithin/sphingomyelin (L/S) ratio of 2.5 and presence of phosphatidyl glycerol ensures fetal lung maturity.
- Schedule cesarean section if > **4,500 g** because of the risk of **shoulder dystocia.**
- Maintain maternal blood glucose levels between **80 and 100 mg/dL** using 5 percent dextrose in water **and** an insulin drip.
- Turn off any insulin infusion after delivery, because insulin resistance decreases with rapidly falling levels of hPL after delivery of the placenta. Maintain blood glucose levels with a sliding scale.

Liver Diseases

A 31-year-old primigravida woman presents at 20 weeks' gestation with dizygotic twins of different genders. She is of Swedish descent and complains of intense skin itching. Her sister experienced similar complaints when she was pregnant and delivered her baby prematurely. No identifiable rash is noted on physical examination. She states that her urine appears dark colored. What is the diagnosis?

Answer: The diagnosis is **intrahepatic cholestasis of pregnancy.** It occurs in genetically susceptible women (of European heritage) and is associated with multiple pregnancies.

- **Symptoms:** Classic symptoms include **intractable nocturnal pruritus** on the palms and soles of the feet without skin findings.
- **Diagnosis:** 10- to 100-fold increase in serum **bile acids**
- **Treatment: Ursodeoxycholic acid** is the treatment of choice. Symptoms may be relieved by antihistamines and cholestyramine. Ursodeoxycholic acid reduces cholesterol absorption and dissolves gallstones; however, gallstones re-form when the patient stops taking the medication.

Urinary Tract Infections, Pyelonephritis, and Bacteriuria

Asymptomatic Bacteriuria	Acute Cystitis	Pyelonephritis
1. Urine culture (+) 2. No urgency, frequency, or burning 3. No fever	1. Urine culture (+) 2. Urgency, frequency, or burning 3. No fever	1. Urine culture (+) 2. Urgency, frequency, or burning 3. Fever and CVA tenderness
Tx: *Outpatient* PO antibiotics (Nitrofurantoin is drug of choice; alt: Cephalexin or amoxicillin)		**Tx:** Admit to hospital; IV hydration, IV cephalosporins or gentamicin, and tocolysis
Cx: 30% of cases develop acute pyelonephritis when untreated		**Cx:** Preterm labor and delivery; Severe cases → sepsis, anemia, and pulmonary dysfunction

Termination of Pregnancy

Induced Abortion

The more advanced the gestation, the higher the rate of complications.

First-Trimester Methods

- **Dilation and curettage (D&C)** is the *most* common first trimester abortion procedure and is performed **before 13 weeks' gestation.** Give prophylactic antibiotics, conscious sedation, and paravertebral block local anesthetic. Rarely complicated by endometritis (outpatient antibiotic) and/or retained products of conception (repeat curettage).

- **Medical abortion** through the use of **oral mifepristone** (Mifeprex, a progesterone antagonist) and **oral misoprostol** (Cytotec, prostaglandin E1) is an alternative to surgical abortion. It may only be used in the **first 63 days of amenorrhea.** Approximately 2 percent abort incompletely and require D&C. *Clostridium sordellii* sepsis can occur in rare cases.

Spontaneous Abortion/Fetal Demise

Death of an embryo or fetus has various different terms based on the gestational age or weight at the time of in utero death.

- **Spontaneous abortion** is the expulsion of an embryo/fetus < **500 g** or < **20 weeks'** gestation. It most commonly initially presents with uterine pain and vaginal bleeding.
- **Fetal demise** is the in utero death of a fetus **after 20 weeks'** gestation. The most common symptom is a **loss of fetal movements.**

Spontaneous Abortion

Type	Ultrasound Finding	Treatment
Complete	No products of conception; cervix closed	Follow up with β-hCG
Incomplete	Some products of conception present; cervix closed	Dilation and curettage (D&C)
Inevitable	Products of conception present; intrauterine bleeding; dilation of cervix	Medical induction or D&C
Threatened	Products of conception present; intrauterine bleeding; no dilation of cervix	Bed rest
Missed	Fetus is dead but remains in uterus	Medical induction or D&C
Septic	Infection of the uterus	D&C *and* IV levofloxacin *and* metronidazole

Etiology

- **Chromosomal abnormalities of the embryo or fetus** are the most common cause of spontaneous abortion. Risk factors are strongly related to advanced maternal age, previous spontaneous abortion, and maternal smoking.
- **Fetal demise is most commonly idiopathic.** Risk factors include antiphospholipid syndrome, overt maternal diabetes, maternal trauma, severe maternal isoimmunization, and fetal infection.

Diagnostic Testing

1. **Speculum exam** to evaluate for cervical/vaginal sources of bleeding and presence of vaginal dilation. Speculum exam is never the first step in management of late trimester bleeding because of the risk of bleeding in a low implanted placenta.
2. **Ultrasound** to evaluate fetal cardiac activity and ± of products of conception.

Complications

- When the case describes prolonged fetal demise (> 2 weeks), the most serious complication to look out for is **disseminated intravascular coagulation (DIC)**, resulting from release of **tissue thromboplastin** from deteriorating fetal organs.

CCS Tip: *Always* rule out coagulopathy by ordering platelet count, D-dimer, fibrinogen, PT, and PTT in patients presenting with fetal demise. If DIC is identified, immediate delivery is needed.

A 24-year-old woman visits the clinic with left-sided abdominal and flank pain and vaginal spotting. Her last menstrual period was 7 weeks ago. She denies fevers, nausea, or vomiting. She has one prior pregnancy with spontaneous vaginal delivery. She has used OCPs in the past but currently uses an intrauterine device for contraception. Pelvic examination, reveals a slightly enlarged uterus, closed cervix. No palpable adnexal mass is identified however there is tenderness on bimanual exam. A quantitative serum ß-hCG value is 2,650 mIU. What is the diagnosis?

a. Ectopic pregnancy
b. Hydatidiform mole
c. Incomplete abortion
d. Missed abortion
e. Threatened abortion

Answer: A. The classic presentation of ectopic pregnancy is 1) amenorrhea, 2) vaginal bleeding, and 3) unilateral pelvic-abdominal pain. When the case also describes abdominal guarding or rigidity, hypotension and tachycardia, ***ruptured ectopic pregnancy*** is the diagnosis.

Ectopic Pregnancy

The *most* common risk factor is **pelvic inflammatory disease** (PID). However, any cause of tubal scarring or adhesions increases risk: infections (PID, IUD), history of surgery (tubal ligation, tubal surgery), or congenital risks (diethylstilbestrol [DES] exposure).

One percent of pregnancies are ectopic pregnancies. Incidence increases to 15 percent if the patient has had a previous ectopic pregnancy.

Diagnosis

- Diagnosis is presumed when
  - β-hCG > 1,500 mIU; and
  - no intrauterine pregnancy is seen on vaginal sonogram.
- Note: The absence of an adnexal mass does *not* rule out ectopic pregnancy.
- Presume ectopic pregnancy has **ruptured** when the patient is unstable (hypotension, tachycardia) and there are symptoms of peritoneal irritation (abdominal guarding or rigidity).

You cannot rule out a normal intrauterine pregnancy when ß-hCG is < 1,500 mIU. The next step is to repeat ß-hCG and repeat the sonogram when ß-hCG is > 1,500 mIU.

Treatment

- Ruptured ectopic pregnancy (look for an unstable patient): Immediate **laparotomy/salpingectomy**
- Unruptured ectopic pregnancy: **Methotrexate** or **laparoscopy** (salpingostomy)
- Give **RhoGAM** to Rh negative women
- Follow up with β-hCG to ensure there has been complete destruction of the ectopic trophoblastic villi.

Intrauterine pregnancy is normally seen on the following:

- **Vaginal sonogram** at 5 weeks gestation when serum ß-hCG > 1,500 mIU
- **Abdominal sonogram** at 6 weeks gestation when ß-hCG > 6,500 mIU

Salping**ostomy** = Open the fallopian tube
Salping**ectomy** = Remove the fallopian tube

Indications for methotrexate are as follows:

- Pregnancy mass < 3.5 cm diameter
- Absence of fetal heart motion
- ß-hCG level < 6,000 mIU
- No history of folic supplementation

Basic Science

Methotrexate is a folate antagonist. Folate is needed for the synthesis of thymidine (remember that nucleoside?), which is essential for the formation of DNA.

Cervical Insufficiency

A 29-year-old primigravida presents to the emergency department at 19 weeks' gestation with lower pelvic pressure without contractions. She reports increased clear vaginal mucus discharge. Fetal membranes are found to be bulging into the vagina, and the cervix cannot be palpated. Fetal feet can be felt through the membranes. What is the next step in management?

a. Abdominal cerclage
b. Prophylactic antibiotics
c. Tocolysis
d. Vaginal cerclage
e. Rule out chorioamnionitis

Answer: **E.** Although emergency cerclage (vaginal or abdominal) is indicated in women who present with cervical dilation in the absence of labor or abruption, ***it can only be performed when chorioamnionitis is first ruled out***. Tocolysis is not appropriate in management of cervical insufficiency. Prophylactic antibiotics and tocolytics are not recommended.

Risk factors for cervical insufficiency are a history of any of the following:

- Second-trimester abortion
- Cervical laceration during delivery
- Deep cervical conization
- Diethylstilbestrol (DES) exposure

Cervical Cerclage:
- Performed at 14–16 weeks
- Suture encircles cervix to prevent cervical canal from dilation
- Indicated electively or emergently in cervical insufficiency

Treatment

- Perform **elective cerclage placement** at 13–16 weeks' gestation for patients with ≥ 3 unexplained midtrimester pregnancy losses.
- Only perform **urgent cerclage** after first ruling out labor and chorioamnionitis.
- Perform **cerclage removal** at 36–37 weeks, after fetal lung maturity.

What is the next step in management of an asymptomatic woman with no prior history of preterm labor, found to have short cervix on routine transvaginal ultrasound before 16–20 weeks?

Answer: Transvaginal ultrasound surveillance to evaluate for persistent cervical shortening, and to evaluate for changes in cervical dilation; however, cerclage is not indicated unless dilation is present and chorioamnionitis or signs of labor are not present. Repeat the exam after 20 weeks if short cervix is still present.

Disproportionate Fetal Growth

Intrauterine Growth Restriction (IUGR)

- **IUGR** is the diagnosis when the estimated fetal weight (EFW) is < **5–10 percentile** for gestational age or < **2,500 g** (5 lb, 8 oz). Accurate, early pregnancy dating is essential for making the diagnosis.
- An **early sonogram** (< 20 weeks) is the next step in management if accurate dates are not known.
- *Never* change the gestational age based on a late sonogram.

	Symmetric IUGR	Asymmetric IUGR	
	Fetal Causes	Maternal Causes	Placental Causes
	↓ *growth potential*	↓ *placental perfusion*	
Etiology	– Aneuploidy – Infection (e.g., TORCH) – Structural anomalies (e.g., congenital heart disease, NTD, ventral wall defects)	– Hypertension – Small vessel disease (e.g., SLE) – Malnutrition – Tobacco, alcohol, street drugs	– Infarction – Abruption – Twin-twin transfusion – Velamentous cord insertion
Ultrasound	↓ *in all measurements*	↓ *abdomen measurements; normal head measurements*	
Workup	– Detailed sonogram – Karyotype – Screen for fetal infections	– Monitor with serial sonograms, nonstress test, amniotic fluid index (AFI), biophysical profile, and umbilical artery Doppler – AFI is often decreased, especially with severe uteroplacental insufficiency	

Basic Science Correlate

Symmetric IUGR is caused by *intrinsic* factors (e.g., genetic issue, fetal infection).

Asymmetric IUGR is caused by *extrinsic* factors, such as **low oxygen** and **nutrient transfer from the placenta** leading to hypoxia in the fetus. These conditions can lead to hypoglycemia (from ↓ glycogen and fat stores) and polycythemia (from ↑ erythropoietin).

Macrosomia

Macrosomia is indicated by a fetus with estimated fetal weight (EFW) > 90–95 percentile for gestational age or birth weight of 4,000–4,500 g.

Risk factors include the GDM, overt diabetes, prolonged gestation, obesity, ↑↑ in pregnancy weight gain, multiparity, and male fetus.

Complications include:

- **Maternal:** Injury during birth, postpartum hemorrhage, and emergency cesarean section
- **Fetus:** Shoulder dystocia, birth injury, asphyxia
- **Neonate:** Hypoglycemia, Erb palsy

Management: Elective cesarean (if EFW > 4,500 g in diabetic mother or > 5,000 g in nondiabetic mother)

Labor, Delivery, and the Postpartum Period

Fetal Testing

- **Obstetric ultrasound**
  - Crown-rump length determines gestational age at 10–13 weeks.
  - High-resolution ultrasonography is indicated when maternal serum markers are abnormal or there is a family history of congenital malformations.
- **Chorionic villous sampling (CVS)**
  - Performed at 12–14 weeks.
  - Chorionic villi is sampled for karyotyping.
  - Pregnancy loss rate is 0.7 percent.
- **Amniocentesis**
  - Performed after 15 weeks with ultrasound guidance.
  - Amniocytes are used for karyotyping.
  - AF-AFP and acetylcholinesterase from amniotic fluid screens for neural tube defects.
  - Pregnancy loss rate is 0.5 percent.
- **Percutaneous umbilical blood sample**
  - Involves ultrasound guided aspiration of fetal blood from the umbilical vein after 20 weeks' gestation.
  - Is both diagnostic (e.g., blood gases, karyotype, IgG and IgM antibodies) and therapeutic (e.g., intrauterine transfusion with fetal anemia).
  - Pregnancy loss rate is 1–2 percent.
- **Fetoscopy**
  - Transabdominal fiberoptic scope performed after 20 weeks under regional or general anesthesia.
  - Indications include intrauterine surgery or fetal skin biopsy (ichthyosis).
  - Pregnancy loss rate is 2–5 percent.

Premature Rupture of Membranes (PROM)

This is rupture of the fetal membranes before the onset of labor. *Ascending infection* from the lower genital tract is the *most common* risk factor for PROM.

Diagnosis

- Sterile speculum examination reveals the following:
  - There is posterior fornix pooling of **clear amniotic fluid** (AF).
  - Fluid is **nitrazine positive.**
  - Fluid is **ferning positive.**
- Ultrasound: **Oligohydramnios**

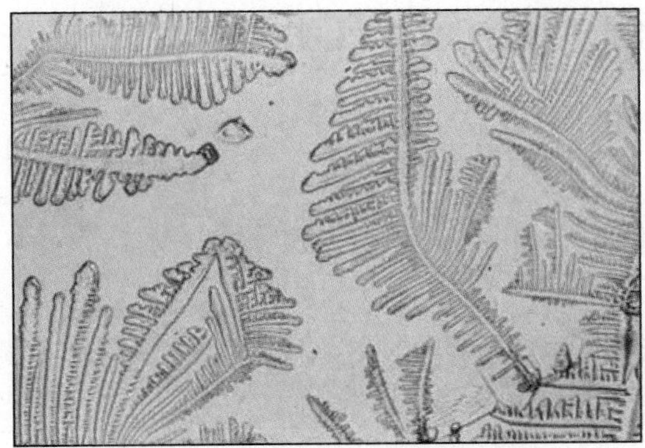

Ferning pattern of amniotic fluid

Chorioamnionitis is the feared complication. It is diagnosed clinically as:

- Maternal fever and uterine tenderness
- Confirmed PROM
- Absence of a URI or UTI

Management

- If uterine contractions are present, do *not* give tocolysis.
- If **chorioamnionitis** is present,
  - get cervical cultures;
  - start IV antibiotics; and
  - schedule delivery.
- If **infection is absent,** manage as follows:
  - **Before viability (< 24 weeks):** Manage patient with bed rest at home.
  - **Preterm viability (24–33 weeks):** Hospitalize. Give IM betamethasone if < 32 weeks. Obtain cervical cultures. Begin prophylactic ampicillin and erythromycin for 7 days.
  - **At term (> 34 weeks):** Initiate delivery.

An adequate uterine contraction
- occurs every 2–3 minutes;
- lasts 45–60 seconds; and
- has 50 mm Hg intensity.

Normal and Abnormal Labor

Stages of Labor

Labor Stage	Definition	Duration	Abnormalities
Stage 1—Latent phase effacement	Begins: Onset of regular UC Ends: Acceleration of cervical dilation	< 20 hours (primipara) < 14 hours (multipara)	**Prolonged latent phase:** 1) Cervix dilated < 3 cm 2) No cervical change in 20 h (primipara)/14 h (multipara) **Cause:** Most common cause is analgesia. **Management:** Rest and sedation
Stage 1—Active phase dilation	Prepares cervix for dilation Begins: Acceleration of cervical dilation Ends: 10 cm (complete) Rapid cervical dilation	> 1.2 cm/hour (primipara) > 1.5 cm/hour (multipara)	**Active phase prolongation or arrest:** 1) Cervix dilated ≥ 3cm 2) *Prolongation:* Cervical dilation of < 1.2 cm/h (primipara) / < 1.5 cm/h (multipara) 3) *Arrest:* No cervical change in ≥ 2h **Cause:** Abnormalities with passenger (fetal size or abnormal presentation), pelvis, or power (dysfunctional contractions) **Management:** • Hypotonic contractions → IV oxytocin • Hypertonic contractions → morphine sedation • Adequate contractions → emergency cesarean section
Stage 2—Descent	Begins: 10 cm (complete) Ends: delivery of baby Descent of the fetus	< 2 hours (primipara) < 1 hour (multipara) + 1 hour if epidural	**Second-stage arrest** • Failure to deliver within 2 hours (primipara) or 1 hour (multipara) • Add additional 1 hour if epidural **Cause:** Abnormalities with passenger, pelvis, or power **Management:** • Fetal head is not engaged → emergency cesarean • Fetal head is engaged → trial of obstetric forceps or vacuum extraction
Stage 3—Expulsion	Begins: delivery of baby Ends: delivery of placenta Delivery of placenta	< 30 minutes	**Prolonged third stage** • Failure to deliver placenta within 30 minutes **Cause:** Consider placenta accreta/increta/percreta **Management:** • IV oxytocin • If oxytocin fails, attempt manual removal • Hysterectomy may be needed

Umbilical Cord Prolapse

An obstetric emergency because a compressed cord has **jeopardized fetal oxygenation,** cord prolapse most often occurs with rupture of membranes before the head is engaged in breech of transverse lie. A **fetal heart rate (FHR) rate that suggests hypoxemia** (e.g., severe bradycardia, severe variable accelerations) may be the only clue.

Management

- *Never* attempt to replace the cord.
- Place the patient in knee-chest position, elevate the presenting part, and give **terbutaline** to decrease force of contractions.

> **Basic Science Correlate**
>
> Terbutaline is a beta-adrenergic agonist that causes myometrial relaxation. It binds to the beta-2 receptors, increasing intracellular adenylyl cyclase.

- Perform **immediate cesarean delivery.**

> Reassuring FHR tracing:
> - Baseline FHR 110–160 beats/minute
> - (+) Accelerations
> - (–) Decelerations
> - (+) Beat-to-beat variability
>
> Nonreassuring FHR tracing:
> - Baseline FHR shows tachycardia or bradycardia
> - (–) Accelerations
> - (+) Variable or late decelerations
> - (–) Beat-to-beat variability

Evaluating Fetal Heart Rate (FHR) Tracings

Baseline heart rate is the mean FHR during a 10-minute segment of time, excluding periodic changes. Changes in fetal heart rate and normal periodic changes of FHR are related to the following:

- Uterine hyperstimulation (commonly caused by medications)
- Fetal head compression
- Umbilical cord compression
- Placental insufficiency

Normal baseline FHR = 110–160 beats/minute.

- **Tachycardia** (> 160 beats/minute) is most commonly related to medications (β-agonist: terbutaline, ritodrine).
- **Bradycardia** (< 110 beats/minute) is most commonly related to medications (β-blockers or local anesthetics).

Periodic changes in heart rate include the following:

- **Accelerations:** *Abrupt* increases in FHR lasting < 2 minutes that are *unrelated* to contractions. They always occur in response to fetal movements and are **always reassuring.**
- **Early decelerations:** *Gradual* decreases in FHR beginning and ending *simultaneously* with contractions. They occur in response to **fetal head compression.**

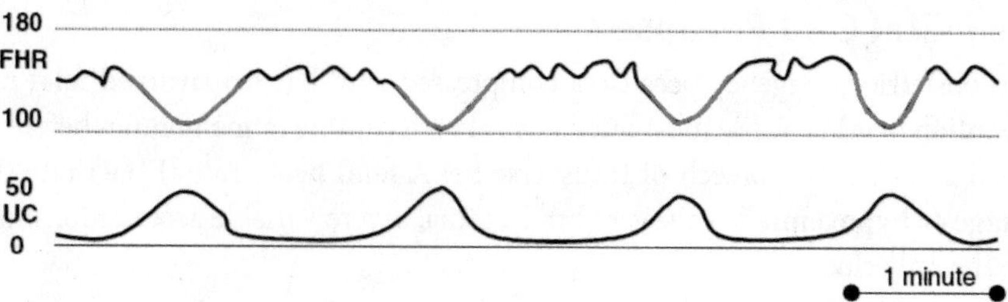

Early Decelerations — head compression

- **Variable decelerations:** *Abrupt* decreases in FHR that are *unrelated* to contractions. These are related to umbilical cord compression. Severe variables are nonreassuring and indicate **fetal acidosis.**

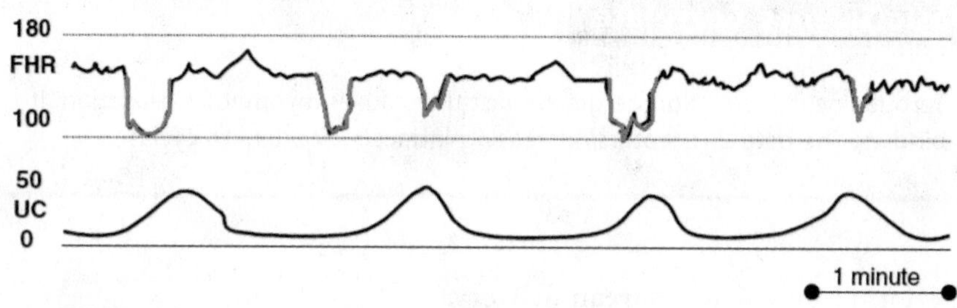

Variable Decelerations — umbilical cord compression

- **Late decelerations** are *gradual* decreases in FHR and *delayed* in relation to contractions. These are related to **uteroplacental insufficiency.** All late decelerations are nonreassuring and indicate **fetal acidosis.**

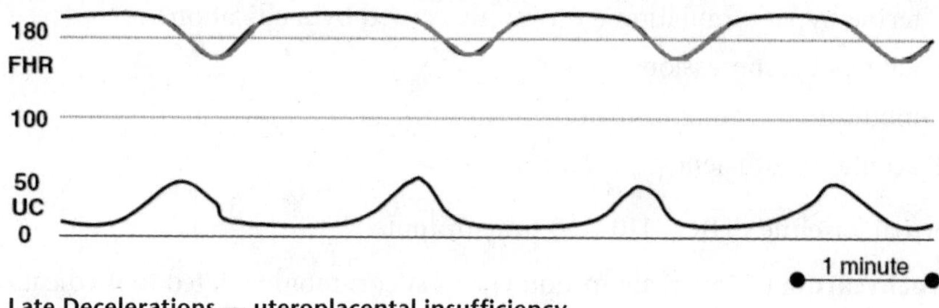

Late Decelerations — uteroplacental insufficiency

- **Variability:** Beat-to-beat fetal heart rate normally has variability. Normal variability is 6–25 beats/minute. **Absence of variability** is a nonreassuring pattern.

A 31-year-old primigravida at term is in the maternity unit in active labor. She is 6 cm dilated, 100 percent effaced 0 station, with the fetus in cephalad position. IV oxytocin is being administered because of arrest of cervical dilation at 6 cm. Fetal membranes are intact. The nurse informs you that the external fetal monitor tracing now shows the fetal heart rate baseline at 175/minute with minimal variability and repetitive late decelerations. There is no vaginal bleeding. What is the most appropriate next step in management?

a. Change maternal position
b. Discontinue oxytocin
c. Immediate cesarean section
d. Perform obstetric ultrasound
e. Obtain fetal scalp pH

Answer: **B.** Medications are a common cause of baseline fetal tachycardia or bradycardia. For management of nonreassuring fetal tracing, follow the following stepwise approach.

Stepwise Approach to Nonreassuring Fetal Tracings

1. Examine the electronic fetal monitoring (EFM) strip: Look for nonreassuring patterns.
2. Identify nonhypoxic causes that can explain the abnormal findings. (Most common are medications, particularly β-agonists or β-blockers.)
3. Begin intrauterine resuscitation as follows:
   a. Discontinue medications (e.g., oxytocin)
   b. Give IV normal saline bolus
   c. Provide high-flow oxygen
   d. Change patient's position (left lateral)
   e. Vaginal exam to rule out prolapsed cord
   f. Perform scalp stimulation to observe for accelerations (reassuring)
4. Prepare for delivery if the EFM tracing does not normalize.
5. If the EFM is unequivocal, obtain fetal scalp pH (requires dilated cervix and ruptured membranes). Normal fetal pH > 7.20.

Operative Obstetrics

Forceps- or Vacuum-Assisted Delivery

When is it the answer?

- Prolonged second stage (most common indication)
- Nonreassuring EFM strip in absence of contraindications
- To avoid maternal pushing when mother has cardiac and/or pulmonary conditions that would increase her risk.

When is it *not* the answer?

- Mother has small pelvis
- Cervix is not fully dilated

- Membranes have not ruptured
- Fetal head is not engaged
- Orientation of the head is not certain

Cesarean Delivery

- The cesarean section rate is approximately **33 percent** in the United States (including both primary and repeat procedures).
- **Risks** include the following: Increased risk of hemorrhage, infection, visceral injury (bladder, bowel, ureters), and DVTs.
- **Low segment transverse incision:** This is the most common procedure. It can only be performed with longitudinal lie of the fetus.
- **Classic vertical incision:** Can be performed with any fetal lie. Because of the increased risk of uterine rupture in subsequent pregnancies, cesarean must be initiated before labor begins.

When is it the answer?

- **Cephalopelvic disproportion (CPD):** With failure of progression or arrest in labor
- **Fetal malpresentation:** Most commonly preterm breech and nonfrank breech
- **Nonreassuring EFM strip**
- **Placenta previa** (unless placental edge > 2 cm from internal os)
- **Infection:** Mother who is HIV-positive or has active vaginal herpes
- **Uterine scar:** Prior myomectomy (fibroid) or prior classic incision c-section

External cephalic version (ECV) is done to change a baby from breech or other non-cephalic presentation to the cephalic position. The physician pushes on the baby through the mother's abdomen to attempt to roll the baby into position.

Trial of vaginal birth after cesarean (VBAC) should be attempted in patients in the absence of c-section indications when the previous cesarean was a low segment uterine incision. The success rate is 80 percent.

External Cephalic Version

When is it the answer?

- Is first attempted in patients with transverse lie or breech presentation.
- The optimum time for external version is 37 weeks' gestation, and success rates are 60–70 percent.

Atony = *a tony,* or **without tone.**

Postpartum Hemorrhage

- **Uterine atony** is the *most common cause* of excessive postpartum bleeding. Consider in rapid or protracted labor, chorioamnionitis, medications ($MgSO_4$, halothane), and overdistended uterus. Manage with **uterine massage** and **uterotonic agents** (e.g., oxytocin, methylergonovine, or carboprost).

- **Carboprost** is a prostaglandin F2 alpha analog that causes myometrial contractions. Increasing contractions causes the blood vessels to get squeezed and decreases bleeding. Hypertension is a contraindication to its use.
- **Misoprostol** is a prostaglandin E1 analog that also induces contractions, and can be given in hypertension.
- **Methylergonovine** causes vasospasm, and is contraindicated in hypertension or scleroderma patients.

- **Lacerations:** Management involves **surgical repair.**
- **Retained placenta** is associated with accessory placental lobe or abnormal uterine invasion. Suspect this with any missing placental cotyledons. Manage through **manual removal** or **uterine curettage** under ultrasound guidance. **Placenta accreta/increta/percreta** is the diagnosis when the examination shows placental villi infiltration. Placental villi may be infiltrated to the deeper layers of the endometrium (accreta), myometrium (increta), or serosa (percreta). **Hysterectomy** may be needed to control the bleeding.
- **DIC** is most commonly related to abruptio placenta. It is also associated with severe preeclampsia, amniotic fluid embolism, or prolonged retention of a dead fetus. Suspect DIC when there is generalized oozing or bleeding from IV or laceration sites in the presence of a contracted uterus.
- **Uterine inversion:** Suspect this when there is a beefy-appearing bleeding mass in the vagina and failure to palpate the uterus. Management involves **uterine replacement,** followed by **IV oxytocin.**
- **Urinary retention** may occur with a hypotonic bladder. If residual volume is > 250 mL, give bethanechol (Urecholine). If this fails, urinary catheterize for no more than 2–3 days.

Atony = *a tony,* or **without tone.**

Postpartum Contraception

- **Breastfeeding:** Contraceptive use may be deferred for 3 months in women who are breastfeeding because of temporary anovulation.
- **Diaphragm and IUD placement:** Fitting and placement is deferred until the 6-week postpartum visit.
- **Combined estrogen-progestin formulations** (e.g., pills, patch, vaginal ring): These are not started until 3 weeks postpartum to prevent hypercoagulable state and risk of DVT. They are not used in breastfeeding women because of diminished lactation. Combined hormone contraception decreases secretion of FSH and LH by inhibiting midcycle secretion of gonadotropin (GnRH). FSH promotes follicular development; LH surge causes ovulation. Absence of these hormones suppresses ovulation.
- **Progestin contraception** (e.g., mini-pill, Depo-Provera, Implanon) can safely be used during breastfeeding. They can be begun immediately after delivery. Progestin is the only contraception that can be used while breastfeeding. It works by thickening cervical mucus and thinning endometria.

Postpartum Fever

PP Day	Diagnosis	Risk Factors	Clinical Findings	Management
0	Atelectasis	General anesthesia with incisional pain Cigarette smoking	Mild fever with mild rales Patient is unable to take deep breaths	Incentive spirometry and ambulation Chest x-rays are unnecessary
1	UTI	Multiple catheterizations and vaginal exams	High fever, CVA tenderness, (+) urinalysis, (+) urine culture	Single-agent intravenous antibiotics
2–3	Endometritis	C-section, prolonged rupture of membranes, multiple vaginal exams	Moderate-to-high fever, uterine tenderness, (–) peritoneal signs	Multiple-agent IV antibiotics (e.g., gentamycin and clindamycin)
4–5	Wound infection	Emergency c-section after PROM	Persistent spiking fever despite antibiotics Wound erythema, fluctuance, or drainage	IV antibiotics Wet-to-dry wound packing Closure by secondary intention
5–6	Septic thrombophlebitis	Prolonged labor	Persistent wide fever swings despite broad-spectrum antibiotics	IV heparin for 7–10 days
7–21	Infectious mastitis	Nipple trauma and cracking	Unilateral breast tenderness, erythema, and edema	PO nafcillin Breastfeeding should be continued

Contraindications to Breastfeeding

- Infections in the mother:
  - HIV
  - *Active* tuberculosis
  - HTLV-1
  - Herpes simplex *if* there is a lesion on the breast
- Use of drugs/medications
- Drugs of abuse (except cigarettes, alcohol)
- Cytotoxic medications (e.g., methotrexate, cyclosporine)
- Condition of the infant
  - Galactosemia

Section 7
Gynecology

contributing author Elizabeth August, MD

The Breast

Benign Breast Disease	Malignant Breast Disease (i.e., Breast Cancer)
1. Fibroadenoma	1. Ductal carcinoma in situ (DCIS)
2. Fibrocystic disease	2. Lobular carcinoma in situ (LCIS)
3. Intraductal papilloma	3. Invasive ductal carcinoma
4. Fat necrosis (think of this with trauma to the breast)	4. Invasive lobular carcinoma
5. Mastitis (inflamed, painful breast in women who are breastfeeding)	5. Inflammatory breast cancer
	6. Paget's disease of the breast/nipple

Nipple Discharge

If the history describes bilateral nipple discharge, think of prolactinoma. Order prolactin levels and TSH levels.

Most Common Cause

The most common cause of unilateral nonbloody nipple discharge is intraductal papilloma. It commonly presents with watery, serous or serosanguinous fluid discharge. The likelihood of cancer is greater if there is an associated palpable mass, involvement of more than one duct or bloody discharge.

- Nonbloody nipple discharge = most likely intraductal papilloma. May also be malignancy.
- Bloody nipple discharge = most likely malignancy.

Diagnostic Testing

- **Mammogram:** Look for underlying masses or calcifications.
- **Surgical duct excision:** Perform this for definitive diagnosis.
- Cytology is *not* helpful in the diagnosis and is never the answer for nipple discharge.

Surgical duct excision is *never* the answer for bilateral, milky nipple discharge. These patients should undergo workup for **prolactinoma.**

Breast Mass

Fibrocystic Disease

This classically presents in a woman age 20–50 with cyclical, **bilateral painful breast lump(s).** A clue to the diagnosis is that the **pain will vary with the menstrual cycle.** A simple cyst will have sharp margins and posterior acoustic enhancement on ultrasound. It will collapse on fine-needle aspiration FNA.

Treatment is **oral contraceptive pills/medications (OCP).** In patients with severe pain, danazol may be used.

Fibroadenoma

This classically presents as a **discrete, firm, nontender, and highly mobile breast nodule.** A clue to the diagnosis is a **mass that's highly mobile** on clinical exam. Fibroadenomas are made up of stromal and epithelial cells.

Diagnostic Testing

The steps in diagnosis of any patient (including pregnant women) with a breast mass are as follows:

1. Clinical **breast examination** (CBE)
2. Imaging: **Ultrasound or diagnostic mammography** (if patient > 40)
3. Fine-needle aspiration (FNA) **biopsy**

Treatment

No treatment is necessary. Surgical removal can be done if the mass is growing.

Never diagnose a simple cyst on clinical exam alone. The diagnosis must be confirmed with either ultrasound or FNA.

A 30-year-old woman complains of bilateral breast enlargement and tenderness, which fluctuates with her menstrual cycle. On physical examination, the breast feels lumpy, and there is a painful, discrete 1.5-cm nodule. A fine-needle aspiration is performed, and clear liquid is withdrawn. The cyst collapses with aspiration. Which of the following is the next step in management?

a. Clinical breast exam in 6 weeks
b. Core needle biopsy
c. Mammography
d. Repeat FNA in 6 weeks
e. Ultrasound in 6 weeks

Answer: **A.** Clinical breast exam in 6 weeks is appropriate follow-up for a cystic mass that disappears after FNA. If the mass recurs on the 6-week follow-up, FNA may be repeated, and a core biopsy can be performed.

When do you answer the following?

- **Ultrasound:**
  - First step in workup of **a palpable mass that feels cystic** on exam.
  - Imaging test for younger women with dense breasts.

- **Mammography (> 50 years old) and biopsy (or biopsy alone if < 40 years old):**
  - Cyst recurs > twice within 4 to 6 weeks.
  - There is bloody fluid on aspiration.
  - Mass does not disappear completely upon FNA.
  - There is bloody nipple discharge (excisional biopsy).
  - There are skin edema and erythema suggestive of inflammatory breast carcinoma (excisional biopsy).
- **Fine-needle aspiration or core biopsy** is needed for a **palpable mass.** May be done **after ultrasound or instead of ultrasound.**
- **Cytology:**
  - Any aspirate that is grossly bloody must be sent for cytology.
- **Observation with repeat exam in 6–8 weeks:**
  - Cyst disappears on aspiration, and the fluid is clear.
  - Needle biopsy and imaging studies are negative.

Mammogram should be done before biopsy. Biopsy distorts radiography.

Core biopsy is superior to FNA.

A 47-year-old woman completes her yearly mammogram and is told to return for evaluation. The mammogram reveals a "cluster" of microcalcifications in the left breast. What is the most appropriate next step in management?

a. Excision biopsy
b. Core needle biopsy
c. Repeat screening mammogram in 6 months
d. Repeat screening mammogram in 12 months
e. Ultrasound

Answer: **B.** A cluster of microcalcifications are mostly benign; however, approximately 15–20 percent represent early cancer. The next step in workup is core needle biopsy under mammographic guidance.

Breast Cancer

Preinvasive Diseases

Both **ductal carcinoma in situ (DCIS)** and **lobular carcinoma in situ (LCIS)** increase the risk of invasive disease. If biopsy reveals

- **DCIS,** then schedule **surgical resection with clear margins** (lumpectomy; i.e., breast conserving surgical resection) and **give radiation therapy (RT) and tamoxifen** for 5 years to prevent the development of invasive disease.
- **LCIS,** then **tamoxifen alone** given for 5 years to reduce risk of development of breast cancer. It is *not* necessary to perform surgery.

Note that LCIS is classically seen in premenopausal women.

Risks associated with **tamoxifen** use:
- Endometrial carcinoma
- Thromboembolism

Contraindications:
- Patient is active smoker
- Previous thromboembolism
- High risk for thromboembolism

Basic Science Correlate

Tamoxifen is an estrogen receptor antagonist in the breast tissue. It acts as an endometrial agonist.

- **Agonist** drugs bind to and activate a receptor. Agonists **cause an action.**
- **Antagonists** are drugs with high affinity (bind to receptors well) but no efficacy (do not make the receptors work). Antagonists **block an action.**

Invasive Breast Diseases

- **Invasive ductal carcinoma** is the most common form of breast cancer (85 percent of all cases). It is **unilateral.** It metastasizes to **bone, liver, and brain.**
- **Invasive lobular carcinoma** accounts for 10 percent of breast carcinomas. It tends to be **multifocal** (within the same breast), and 20 percent are bilateral.
- **Inflammatory breast cancer** is uncommon, grows rapidly, and metastasizes early. Look for a **red, swollen, and warm breast and pitted, edematous skin** (classic *peau d'orange* appearance).
- **Paget's disease of the breast/nipple** presents with a pruritic, erythematous, scaly nipple lesion. It's often confused with dermatosis-like eczema or psoriasis. Look for an **inverted nipple** or **discharge.**

Breast cancer screening guidelines per the U.S. Preventive Services Task Force (USPSTF):

- Mammogram every 1–2 years recommended for ages 50–74.
- Screening before age 50 is no longer routinely recommended. Women < 50 should only consider mammographic screening based on high individual risk for early onset breast cancer.
- Teaching breast-self exam is no longer encouraged.
- Clinical breast exams are no longer routinely advised.

Established **risk factors** for breast cancer:

- Age ≥ 50 years old
- Familial BRCA1/BRCA2 mutation carrier
- Exposure to ionizing radiation
- First childbirth after age 30 or nulliparity
- History of breast cancer
- History of breast cancer in a first-degree relative
- Hormone therapy
- Obesity (BMI ≥ 30 kg per m^2)

When are **BRCA1 and BRCA2 gene testing** indicated?

- Family history of early-onset (< 50 years of age) breast cancer or ovarian cancer
- Breast and/or ovarian cancer in the same patient
- Family history of male breast cancer
- Ashkenazi Jewish heritage

Treatment

- Primary treatment of invasive carcinoma when tumor size < 5 cm is **lumpectomy + radiotherapy ± adjuvant therapy ± chemotherapy.**
- **Sentinel node biopsy** is preferred over axillary node dissection.

- *Always* test for estrogen and progesterone receptors *and* HER2/neu receptor protein.
- Primary treatment of inflammatory, tumor size > 5 cm, and metastatic disease is **systemic therapy**.

A 68-year-old woman visits her primary care physician with a solid peanut-shaped hard mass in the upper outer quadrant of the left breast. A biopsy of the lesion reveals "infiltrating ductal breast cancer." What is the next step in management?

a. Lumpectomy plus radiotherapy
b. Modified radical mastectomy
c. Modified radical mastectomy plus radiotherapy
d. Neoadjuvant chemotherapy plus lumpectomy plus radiotherapy
e. Tamoxifen and radiotherapy

Answer: **A.** Breast-conserving surgical therapy (lumpectomy) plus radiotherapy is the standard of care for invasive disease. Modified radical mastectomy gives no survival benefit.

When is **breast-conserving therapy** *not* the answer?

- Pregnancy
- Prior irradiation to the breast
- Diffuse malignancy or ≥ 2 sites in separate quadrants
- Positive tumor margins
- Tumor > 5 cm

When is **adjuvant hormonal therapy** included in management?

- In *any* hormone receptor-positive (HR+) tumors, *regardless* of age and *regardless* of menopausal status, stage, or type of tumor

Benefit is greatest when both ER+ and PR+ receptors are present. Therapy is **nearly as good** when there are only ER+ estrogen receptors. Adjuvant hormonal therapy has the **least benefit** when only PR+ receptors are present.

- **Tamoxifen** competitively binds estrogen receptors.
  - Five-year treatment → 50 percent decrease in the recurrence, 25 percent decrease in mortality.
  - May be used in pre- or postmenopausal patients.
- **Aromatase inhibitors** (anastrozole, exemestane, letrozole) block peripheral production of estrogen.
  - This is the standard of care in HR+ postmenopausal women (more effective than tamoxifen).
  - Do *not* cause menopausal symptoms but *do* increase risk of osteoporosis.
- **LHRH analogs** (e.g., goserelin) or **ovarian ablation** (surgical oophorectomy or external beam RT) is an alternative or an addition to tamoxifen in premenopausal women.

Benefits of Tamoxifen	Adverse Effects of Tamoxifen
• ↓ incidence of contralateral breast cancer • ↑ bone density in postmenopausal women • ↓ fractures • ↓ serum cholesterol • ↓ cardiovascular mortality risk	• Exacerbates menopausal symptoms • ↑↑ risk of endometrial cancer (1% in postmenopausal women after 5 yrs therapy) • ↑↑ risk of thromboembolism TIP: All women with a history of tamoxifen use and vaginal bleeding need evaluation & endometrial biopsy.

When is **chemotherapy** included in management?

- Tumor size > 1 cm
- Lymph node-positive disease

When is **trastuzumab** included in management?

- It is indicated for metastatic breast cancer overexpressing HER2/neu.
- Trastuzumab is a monoclonal antibody directed against the extracellular domain of the HER2/neu receptor and is used to treat and control visceral metastatic sites.

If the case describes invasive breast cancer in an

- **HR-negative, pre- or postmenopausal woman**
  - Give chemotherapy ± RT alone.
- **HR-positive, *pre*menopausal woman**
  - Give chemotherapy ± RT + tamoxifen.
- **HR-positive, *post*menopausal woman**
  - Give chemotherapy ± RT + aromatase inhibitor.

Uterus

> Always make sure that the pregnancy (beta-HCG/urine pregnancy test) is *negative* before considering leiomyoma or adenomyosis.

Enlarged Uterus

An enlarged uterus may be caused by the following:

1. **Pregnancy** (discussed in Section 6: Obstetrics)
2. **Leiomyoma**
3. **Adenomyosis**

Leiomyoma

This is a **smooth muscle growth of the myometrium.** It is the most common benign uterine tumor. The case will describe an **African-American woman** (the disease is 5 times more common in African Americans) of childbearing age with an **enlarged, firm, asymmetric, nontender** uterus. **Beta-hCG is negative.**

> **Basic Science**
> Three layers form the uterus: **endometrium** (inner layer), **myometrium** (middle layer), and **perimetrium** (outer layer). The myometrium is made up of smooth muscle, composed mainly of the proteins myosin and actin.

Look for increased tumor growth and symptoms during pregnancy (growth corresponds to estrogen stimulation) and tumor shrinkage in menopause. Leiomyoma is most commonly asymptomatic (intramural location), but when symptomatic, it presents as one of the following:

- **Intermenstrual bleeding and menorrhagia** (submucosal location) with distortion of the uterine cavity seen on saline ultrasound (see image).
- **Bladder, rectum, or ureter compression symptoms** (subserosal location). This type may become "parasitic" (i.e., break away from the uterus and obtain its blood supply from momentum, intestinal mesentery).
- **Acute-onset pain in a pregnant woman** as tumor outgrows blood supply and degenerates.

> Asymmetric and nontender uterus = Leiomyoma

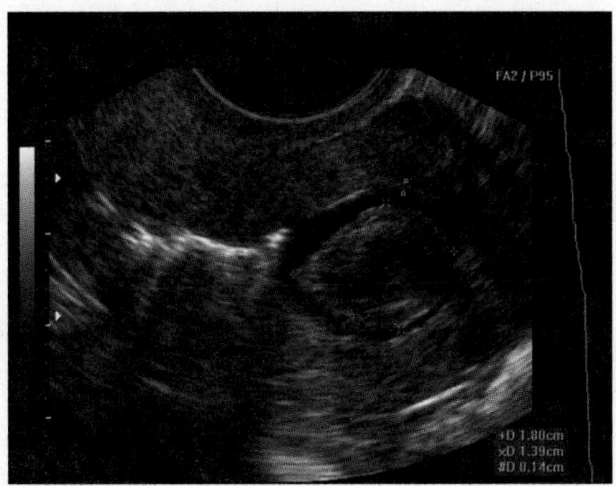

Intracavitary Leiomyoma

Adenomyosis

This is the **abnormal location of endometrial glands and stroma *within* the myometrium of the uterine wall.** When symptomatic, it causes **dysmenorrhea** and **menorrhagia.** The uterus feels **soft, globular, symmetrical, and tender.** Unlike leiomyoma, there is no change with high or low estrogen states.

> Symmetric and tender uterus = Adenomyosis

CCS Tip: The first test to order in a patient with an enlarged uterus is ß-hCG.

Diagnosis of Leiomyoma vs. Adenomyosis		
	Leiomyoma	**Adenomyosis**
Symptoms	Secondary dysmenorrhea and menorrhagia **± symptoms of bladder, ureter, or rectal compression**	Secondary dysmenorrhea and menorrhagia
1. Pelvic Exam	**Asymmetrically enlarged, firm, NONtender** uterus	**Symmetrically enlarged, soft, TENDER** uterus May be tender immediately before and during menses
2. Sonogram	Large intramural or subserosal myomas; saline infusion can show submucosal myomas	Diffusely enlarged uterus **with cystic areas** within the myometrial wall
3. Hysteroscopy	Direct visualize tumors	N/A
4. Histology	Definitive diagnosis	

Management of Leiomyoma vs. Adenomyosis		
	Leiomyoma	**Adenomyosis**
Observation/ Medical	Serial pelvic exams & observation for most patients	Levonorgestrel intrauterine system (IUS), may decrease heavy menstrual bleeding
Myomectomy	Preserves fertility Laparotomy, laparoscopy Must deliver next pregnancies by cesarean section because of increased risk of scar rupture in labor	N/A
Embolization of vessels	Preserves uterus Invasive radiology	N/A
Hysterectomy	Best choice when fertility is completed Definitive therapy: Transabdominal or transvaginal hysterectomy	

Postmenopausal Bleeding

A 65-year-old obese patient complains of vaginal bleeding for 3 months. Her last menstrual period was at age 52. She has no children. She has type 2 diabetes and chronic hypertension. Physical examination is normal with a normal-sized uterus and with no vulvar, vaginal, or cervical lesions. What is the next step in management?

a. Begin progestin therapy
b. Begin estrogen and progestin therapy
c. Perform an endometrial biopsy
d. Perform a Pap smear and endocervical sampling
e. Prescribe topical estrogen cream

Answer: **C.** The most common cause of postmenopausal bleeding is vaginal or endometrial atrophy, but the most important diagnosis to rule out is endometrial carcinoma (the most common gynecologic malignancy). Endometrial biopsy is the first step in management of any patient with postmenopausal bleeding.

Never give estrogen alone to a woman with a uterus. Always combine with progestins to prevent unopposed endometrial stimulation.

The most important risk factors for **endometrial carcinoma** are **unopposed estrogen states** (obesity, nulliparity, late menopause/early menarche, chronic anovulation) and a history of tamoxifen use.

All postmenopausal bleeding is suspected endometrial carcinoma until proven otherwise.

All reproductive age women with chronic anovulation (e.g., PCOS) are at high risk of endometrial carcinoma. Give **progestins** to prevent endometrial hyperplasia and cancer.

Diagnosis	Management
1. Pelvic Exam	If the endometrial biopsy reveals **atrophy and no cancer,** no further workup is needed
	If the endometrial biopsy reveals **adenocarcinoma → perform surgery staging:** (TAH and BSO, pelvic and para-aortic lymphadenectomy, and peritoneal washings) + ***Radiation therapy if:*** lymph node metastasis, > 50% myometrial invasion, positive surgical margins, or poorly differentiated + ***Chemotherapy if:*** metastasis
2. Hysteroscopy	Identifies endometrial or cervical polyps as source of bleeding
3. Ultrasonography	Measures thickness of endometrial lining In postmenopausal patients the endometrial lining stripe should < 5 mm thick

TAH: total abdominal hysterectomy; BSO: bilateral salpingo-oophorectomy; HRT: hormone replacement therapy

Ovaries: Ovarian Enlargement

Ovarian enlargement may be found incidentally on physical exam or may present with symptoms. The following conditions should be considered.

Simple Cyst: Physiologic Cysts (Luteal or Follicular Cysts)

This is the most common cyst that occurs during the reproductive years. It is **asymptomatic,** unless torsion has occurred (occurs with large cysts). The **β-hCG is negative;** ultrasound shows **fluid-filled simple cystic mass.**

Management

- **Transvaginal or transabdominal ultrasound** to assess initial visit. If it is asymptomatic, no further follow up is necessary.
- **Laparoscopic removal** if
  - cyst is > **7 cm diameter;** or
  - there has been **previous steroid contraception without resolution** of the cyst.

Fine needle aspiration of a complex ovarian cyst is **never the correct answer** on the test.

Complex Cyst: Benign Cystic Teratoma (Dermoid Cysts)

These are benign tumors. They can contain cellular tissue from all 3 germ layers. Rarely, squamous cell carcinoma can develop. The **β-hCG is negative;** ultrasound shows a complex mass.

Management

- **Laparoscopic/laparotomy removal,** either
  - **cystectomy** (to retain ovarian function); or
  - **oophorectomy** (if fertility is no longer desired).

The initial workup of an ovarian mass involves the following:
- ß-hCG
- Ultrasound
- Laparoscopy/laparotomy if complex or > 7 cm

A 31-year-old woman is taken to the emergency department complaining of severe, sudden lower abdominal pain that started 3 hours ago. On examination, the abdomen is tender, no rebound tenderness is present, and there is an adnexal mass in the cul-de-sac area. An ultrasound evaluation shows an 8-cm left adnexal mass. Beta-hCG is negative. What is the next step in management?

a. Appendectomy
b. Give high-dose estrogen and progestin
c. Laparoscopic evaluation of ovaries
d. Observation
e. Perform oophorectomy

Answer: **C.** Sudden onset of severe lower abdominal pain in the presence of an adnexal mass is presumed to be **ovarian torsion. Laparoscopy** and **detorsioning** of the ovaries is needed. If blood supply is not affected, **cystectomy** can be done. If there is necrosis, **oophorectomy** is needed. She should then receive a 4-week follow-up and yearly evaluation to ensure there is complete resolution.

Prepubertal or Postmenopausal Ovarian Mass

Any ovarian enlargement in prepubertal or postmenopausal women is always suspicious for an **ovarian neoplasm.**

Risk Factors	Protective Factors
• BRCA1 gene • Positive family history • High # of lifetime ovulations • Infertility	• Conditions that decrease # of ovulations - oral contraceptive pills (OCPs) - chronic anovulation - breastfeeding - short reproductive life

Diagnosis

Which cancer should you suspect in the following cases? What tumor markers will you order?

A 9-year-old girl presents with right adnexal pain and complex cystic mass on ultrasound.

Answer: **Germ cell tumor:** These are most common in **young women** and present in early-stage disease. The most common malignant epithelial cell type is **dysgerminoma.** Germ cells are the cells that give rise to the gametes. They undergo mitosis, meiosis, and cellular differentiation to develop into mature gametes (sperm or eggs).

Tumor markers: LDH, ß-hCG, a-FP

A 67-year-old woman presents with progressive weight loss, distended abdomen, and left adnexal mass.

Answer: **Epithelial tumor:** This is the most common ovarian cancer in postmenopausal women. The most common malignant subtype is serous.

Tumor markers: CA-125, CEA

A 58-year-old woman presents with postmenopausal bleeding. Endometrial biopsy shows endometrial hyperplasia. Pelvic ultrasound reveals a right ovarian mass.

Answer: **Granulosa-theca** (stromal tumor): This ovarian tumor **secretes estrogen** and can cause **endometrial hyperplasia.**

Tumor markers: Estrogen

A 48-year-old woman complains of increased facial hair and deepening of her voice. An adnexal mass is found on examination.

Answer: **Sertoli-Leydig cell** (stromal tumor): This ovarian tumor secretes **testosterone.** Patients present with **masculinization syndromes.**

Tumor markers: Testosterone

A 64-year-old woman with history of gastric ulcer and recent worsening dyspepsia presents with weight loss and abdominal pain. An adnexal mass is found.

Answer: **Metastatic gastric cancer** to the ovary **(Krukenberg tumor)**

Tumor markers: ***CEA****. This is a mucin-producing adenocarcinoma from the stomach that has metastasized to the ovary, most commonly to both ovaries.*

Management

- **Sonogram** (and CT scan for postmenopausal women)
- **Biopsy** via laparoscopy for simple cysts suggestive of malignancy (no septations or solid components) or postmenopausal without ascites
- **Tumor markers**
- **Cystectomy** for benign tissue
- Premenstrual women: **Salpingo-oophorectomy**
- Postmenopausal women: **Total abdominal hysterectomy** (TAH); bilateral salpingo-oopherectomy (BSO) and postoperative chemotherapy for malignant tissue

Cervix: Cervical Neoplasia

Basic Science Correlate

The most common HPV types associated with **cervical cancer** are HPV 16, 18, 31, 33, and 35.

HPV 6 and 11 are **benign condyloma acuminata.**

HPV is a non-enveloped DNA virus.

Pap smear classifications:

- Indeterminate smears:
  - **Atypical squamous cells of undetermined significance** (ASCUS)
- Abnormal smears:
  - **Low-grade squamous intraepithelial lesion** (LSIL): HPV, mild dysplasia, or CIN 1
  - **High-grade squamous intraepithelial lesion** (HSIL): Moderate dysplasia, severe dysplasia, CIS, CIN 2 or 3
  - **Cancer:** Invasive cancer

The following risk factors are associated with cervical neoplasia:

- Early age of intercourse
- Multiple sexual partners
- Cigarette smoking
- Immunosuppression

When is screening started?

- **Age 21,** regardless of the onset of sexual activity

What screening is used?

- **Conventional method:** 50 percent sensitivity
- **Liquid-based prep:** Sensitivity is increased to 75–80 percent
- **HPV DNA testing:** Useful in management of ASCUS

What is the frequency of screening?

- If < 30 years old and average risk, every 3 years with cytology only.
- If > 30 years old and average risk, every 3 years with cytology only or every 5 years with co-testing (cytology + HPV).
- If HPV tested concomitantly, can do Pap every 5 years.

Cervical cancer screening guidelines per the USPSTF:

- Pap screening not recommended for women > 65 with recent normal Pap smear.
- Pap smear not recommended for women with total hysterectomy for benign disease.
- HPV testing alone is not sufficient for screening.

A 35-year-old woman is referred because of a Pap smear reading of ASCUS. The patient states that her last Pap smear, done approximately 1 year ago, was negative. She has been sexually active, using combination oral contraception pills for the last 4 years. A repeat Pap smear after 3 months again reveals ASCUS. Which of the following is the next step in evaluation?

a. Endocervical curettage
b. Colposcopy and biopsy
c. HPV DNA typing
d. Repeat Pap smear in 6 months
e. Repeat Pap smear in 12 months

Answer: **B.** ASCUS is most commonly found in women with inflammation due to **early HPV infection.** Approximately 10–15 percent of patients with ASCUS have premalignant or malignant disease. Two Pap smears revealing ASCUS must be followed up with colposcopy and biopsy.

Management of abnormal Pap smears is a commonly tested exam topic.

Management

- If the case describes a patient with atypical squamus cells of undetermined significance (ASCUS) on the Pap smear and follow-up is *certain,* **repeat the Pap smear in 3–6 months** and **order HPV DNA typing.** If the result is negative, follow-up is routine. If the repeat Pap smear is again ASCUS, or HPV 16 and 18 are found, then order **colposcopy and biopsies.**
- If the case describes a patient with ASCUS on Pap smear and follow-up is *uncertain* (i.e., patient is not reliable to return for follow-up), order **colposcopy and biopsies.**

Workup of an Abnormal Pap		
Step in Workup	**When is this step the answer?**	**Next Step**
Repeat Pap	– First ASCUS Pap	Repeat Pap at 4- to 6-month intervals until there are 2 consecutive, negative Paps If a repeat Pap is again ASCUS, refer for colposcopy
HPV DNA testing	– First ASCUS Pap	If liquid-based cytology was used on the initial Pap, use specimen for DNA testing If conventional methods were used, a second Pap needs to be performed Colposcopy is then performed only if HPV 16 and 18 identified
Colposcopy and ectocervical biopsy	– An abnormal Pap smear – Two ASCUS Pap smears	Colposcopy is a magnification of the cervix (10–12 times) Abnormal lesions (e.g., mosaicism, inflammatory punctation, white lesions, abnormal vessels) are biopsied and sent for histology
Endocervical curettage (ECC)	– All NONpregnant patients with an abnormal Pap smear	All nonpregnant patients undergoing colposcopy for an abnormal Pap smear must undergo an ECC to rule out endocervical lesions
Cone biopsy	– Performed after colposcopy or ECC if Pap smear and biopsy findings are not consistent (suggests abnormal cells were not biopsied) – Abnormal ECC histology – An endocervical lesion – A biopsy showing microinvasive carcinoma of the cervix	NOTE: Deep cone biopsies can result in an *incompetent cervix* or *cervical stenosis.*

Management of Abnormal Histology		
Step in Management	**When is this step the answer?**	**Details**
Observation and follow-up	– **CIN 1** – **CIN 2 or 3 after ablation or excision**	– *Follow-up repeat Pap smears, colposcopy + Pap smear, or HPV DNA testing every 4 to 6 months for 2 years*
Ablative modalities	– **CIN 2 or 3**	– Cryotherapy – Laser vaporization – Electrofulguration
Excisional procedures	– **CIN 2 or 3**	– LEEP (loop electrosurgical excision procedure) – Cold-knife conization
Hysterectomy	– **Biopsy-confirmed** – **Recurrent CIN 2 or 3**	

Invasive Cervical Cancer

The average age of diagnosis is 45 years.

Diagnostic Testing

- **Cervical biopsy:** The most common diagnosis is squamous cell carcinoma.
- **Metastatic workup** is the next step in evaluation: Includes pelvic exam, CT scan (to look for metastatic disease), cystoscopy, and proctoscopy.

Treatment

- Management is simple hysterectomy or modified radical hysterectomy.
- Adjuvant therapy (radiation therapy and chemotherapy) is given when any of the following conditions is present:
  - Metastasis to lymph nodes
  - Tumor size > 4 cm
  - Poorly differentiated lesions
  - Positive margins
  - Local recurrence

Cervical Neoplasia in Pregnancy

A 25-year-old woman with a 15-week pregnancy by dates is found to have HGSIL (high-grade squamous intraepithelial lesion) on a recent Pap smear. On pelvic examination there is a gravid uterus consistent with 15 weeks' size, and the cervix is grossly normal to visual inspection. What is the next step in management?

a. Colposcopy and biopsy
b. Cone biopsy
c. Endocervical curettage
d. Hysterectomy
e. Repeat Pap after pregnancy

Answer: **A.** A pregnant woman with abnormal Pap smear is managed in the same way as a nonpregnant woman with the exception of endocervical curettage, which is not performed because of increased cervical vascularity. An abnormal Pap smear is evaluated with colposcopy and biopsy. Pregnancy does not predispose to abnormal cytology and does not accelerate precancerous lesion progression into invasive carcinoma.

Management of Abnormal Histology During Pregnancy	
Stage	**Management**
CIN/dysplasia	– Pap smear and colposcopy every 3 months during pregnancy – Repeat Pap and colposcopy 6–8 weeks postpartum. Any persistent lesions are then definitively treated postpartum
Microinvasive cervical cancer	– Cone biopsy to ensure no frank invasion – Deliver vaginally, reevaluate and treat 2 months postpartum
Invasive cancer	*Diagnosed before 24 weeks:* – Definitive treatment (radical hysterectomy or radiation therapy) *Diagnosed after 24 weeks:* – Conservative management up to 32–33 weeks – Cesarean delivery and begin definite treatment

Gardasil is also indicated for males age 9–26 for the prevention of genital warts caused by HPV.

Prevention of Cervical Dysplasia by Vaccination

- Give **quadrivalent HPV recombinant vaccine (Gardasil)** to all females 8–26 years of age.
- Protects against the **4 HPV types (6, 11, 16, 18)** that cause 70 percent of cervical cancer and 90 percent of genital warts.
- Testing for HPV before vaccination is *not* needed.
- Sexually active women can receive the vaccine.
- Women with previous abnormal cervical cytology or genital warts can receive the vaccine, but it may be less effective.
- It can be given to patients with previous CIN, but benefits are limited.
- The vaccine is *not recommended* for pregnant, lactating, or immunosuppressed women.
- Females who have been vaccinated for HPV must still follow Pap smear recommendations.

Pelvic Pain

The main differentials for a woman with pelvic pain are cervicitis, acute salpingo-oophoritis, chronic PID, and tuboovarian abscess.

The **initial workup** for pelvic pain:

1. Pelvic exam
2. Cervical culture
3. Laboratory: ESR (sedimentation rate), WBC (include blood culture if fever is present)
4. Sonogram

Cervicitis

This is the diagnosis when cervical discharge is found on routine exam, usually without other symptoms. Get cervical cultures (for chlamydia and gonorrhea). Manage positive results by giving a single dose of **oral azithromycin** and **IM ceftriaxone.**

> Always treat cervicitis to cover both chlamydia **and** gonorrhea.
> - Antibiotics that treat gonorrhea:
>   - Ceftriaxone IM
> - Antibiotics that treat chlamydia:
>   - Azithromycin PO
>   - Doxycycline PO

Acute Salpingo-oophoritis

This is suspected when there is **cervical motion tenderness** on exam and the patient complains of **lower pelvic pain after menstruation.**

Diagnostic Testing

- Cervical cultures will be positive.
- WBC and ESR are elevated.
- Rule out pelvic abscess with sonogram.

Treatment

- Outpatient: **One dose of IM ceftriaxone plus doxycycline**
- Inpatient: **IV cefotetan or cefoxitin plus doxycycline**

Chronic Pelvic Inflammatory Disease

This classically presents with **infertility** or **dyspareunia.** The patient may also have a history of ectopic pregnancy or abnormal vaginal bleeding.

Diagnostic Testing

Cervical cultures and laboratory tests will be **negative.** Sonogram will show **bilateral cystic pelvic masses** (hydrosalpinges).

Treatment

- Lysis of tubal adhesions, which may be helpful for infertility
- Severe, unremitting pelvic pain may require a pelvic clean-out (TAH, BSO)

Tuboovarian Abscess

This advanced form of pelvic inflammatory disease is diagnosed when the case describes an **ill-appearing woman** with **severe, lower abdominal/pelvic pain, back pain, and rectal pain,** with **systemic signs** and symptoms (nausea, vomiting, fever, tachycardia).

Diagnostic Testing

WBC and ESR are markedly elevated, there is **pus on culdocentesis,** and sonogram shows a **unilateral pelvic mass** that appears as a multilocular, cystic, complex adnexal mass. Blood cultures will grow **anaerobic organisms.**

Treatment

1. Admit to the hospital and give **cefoxitin** and **doxycycline.**
2. If no response within 72 hours or if there is abscess rupture, perform an **exploratory laparotomy ± TAH and BSO** or **percutaneous drainage.**

When are outpatient antibiotics the answer?

- All cases of **cervicitis**
- **Acute salpingo-oophoritis** when there is no systemic infection or pelvic abscess

When are inpatient antibiotics the answer?

- **Previous outpatient treatment failure, intrauterine device (IUD) in place, presence of fever, or pelvic abscess**
- All cases of **tubo-ovarian abscess**

Dysmenorrhea

Primary Dysmenorrhea

- Primary dysmenorrhea is the diagnosis when the case describes **recurrent, crampy lower abdominal pain** along with **nausea, vomiting, and diarrhea during menstruation.** Symptoms begin **2–5 years after onset of menstruation** (ovulatory cycles). There is no pelvic abnormality.
- Symptoms are related to **excessive endometrial prostaglandin F2,** which causes uterine contractions and acts on gastrointestinal smooth muscle.

Treatment

- **NSAIDs** are the first line of therapy.
- **Combination oral contraceptives** are the second line.

Secondary Dysmenorrhea

Secondary dysmenorrhea presents similar symptoms as primary dysmenorrhea but is due to another disorder. Most commonly, secondary dysmenorrhea occurs due to **endometriosis.** However, other pathology (such as **adenomyosis or leiomyomas)** can also be the underlying pathology.

Endometriosis

This involves endometrial glands outside the uterus. It classically presents in women over 30 with **dysmenorrhea, dyspareunia, dyschezia** (painful bowel movements), and **infertility.**

- The most common site is **the ovary,** causing adnexal enlargements (endometriomas), also known as a **chocolate cyst.**
- The second most common site is the **cul-de-sac**, causing **uterosacral ligament nodularity** and **tenderness on rectovaginal examination.** This location is associated with bowel adhesions and a fixed, retroverted uterus.
- Investigations: CA-125 may be elevated. Sonogram may show endometriomas. Definitive diagnosis is made with **laparoscopic visualization.**

Don't be fooled! Not all **elevations of CA-125** are due to ovarian cancer. It is also elevated in:
- Cirrhosis
- Endometriosis
- Peritonitis
- Pancreatitis

Treatment

- First-line therapy: **Continuous oral progesterone** or oral contraceptive pill (OCP). Progesterone inhibits endometrial growth.
- Second-line therapy: **Testosterone derivatives** (Danocrine or danazol) or **GnRH analogs** (Lupron or leuprolide)
- Laparoscopic lysis adhesions: Laser vaporization of lesions can improve fertility.
- TAH and BSO can be done for severe symptoms when fertility is not desired.

Vaginal Bleeding and Its Absence

Premenarchal Vaginal Bleeding

This is bleeding that occurs before menarche. The average age at menarche is 12. Causes are as follows:

- The most common cause is the **presence of a foreign body.**
- You must *rule out* **sarcoma botryoides** (cancer of vagina or cervix suggested by a grapelike mass arising from the vaginal lining or cervix), **tumor** of the pituitary adrenal gland or ovary, and sexual abuse.

Diagnostic Testing

- Perform **pelvic exam under sedation.**
- Order **CT or MRI of pituitary, abdomen, and pelvis** to look for estrogen-producing tumor.
- If workup is *negative,* the diagnosis is **idiopathic precocious puberty.**

Abnormal Vaginal Bleeding

A 31-year-old woman complains of 6 months of metromenorrhagia. The patient states that she started menstruating at age 13 and that she has had regular menses until the past 6 months. The pelvic examination, including a Pap smear, is normal. She has no other significant personal or family history. What is the next step in management?

a. Obtain ß-hCG
b. Obtain LH, FSH levels
c. Perform a pelvic ultrasound
d. Recommend oral contraceptive pill
e. Recommend progestin-only pill

Answer: **A.** Irregular bleeding in reproductive age should always be evaluated first for pregnancy. If pregnancy is ruled out, workup for anatomical causes of bleeding or anovulation can be started.

Primary Amenorrhea

Primary amenorrhea is diagnosed with **absence of menses at age 14 without secondary sexual development or at age 16 with secondary sexual development.**

Diagnostic Testing

- Physical exam and ultrasound:
  - Are **breasts** present or absent? Breasts indicate adequate estrogen production.
  - Is a **uterus** present or absent on ultrasound?
- Karyotype, testosterone, FSH

	Uterus Present	Uterus Absent
Breasts Present	**Workup as secondary amenorrhea** • Imperforate hymen • Vaginal septum • Anorexia nervosa • Excessive exercise • Pregnancy before the first menses	**Order testosterone levels and karyotype** • Müllerian agenesis – *XX karyotype, normal testosterone for female* • Complete androgen insensitivity (testicular feminization) – *XY karyotype, normal testosterone for male*
Breasts Absent	**Order FSH level and karyotype** • Gonadal dysgenesis (Turner's syndrome) – *X0 karyotype, FSH elevated* • Hypothalamic–pituitary failure – *XX karyotype, FSH low*	**RARE** • Not clinically relevant

A 17-year-old girl is brought to the clinic by her mother concerned because her daughter has never had a menstrual period. She reports that her daughter has good grades, studies hard but seems stressed out most of the time which is why she believed her period was delayed. On examination she seems to be well-nourished, with adult breast development and pubic hair present. Pelvic examination reveals a foreshortened vagina. No uterus is seen on ultrasound. What is the most appropriate advice?

a. CT scan of the brain is indicated to evaluate a pituitary tumor.

b. Estrogen and progesterone supplementation is indicated.

c. In vitro fertilization is an option for future fertility.

d. Surgical removal of intra-abdominal testes is recommended.

e. Vaginal reconstruction may be performed.

Answer: **E.** This patient has **Müllerian agenesis** resulting in an absence of uterus, cervix and upper vagina. Ovaries are intact and normal levels of estrogen are present. Vaginal reconstruction may be performed to elongate the vagina for satisfactory sexual intercourse.

Müllerian Agenesis

This is the diagnosis when karyotype reveals **normal female secondary sexual characteristics** and **normal estrogen and testosterone levels** (ovaries are intact). The only abnormality is **absence of all Müllerian duct derivatives** (fallopian tubes, uterus, cervix, and upper vagina).

Management involves the **surgical elongation of the vagina** for satisfactory sexual intercourse and counseling about infertility.

Androgen Insensitivity

This is the diagnosis when there is **no pubic or axillary hair,** a karyotype reveals **male genotype,** and ultrasound reveals **testes.** The testes produce *both* normal levels of estrogen for a female and normal levels of testosterone for a male.

Management involves the **removal of testes before age 20** because of increased risk of testicular cancer. Estrogen replacement will then be needed.

Gonadal Dysgenesis (Turner Syndrome, XO)

This is the diagnosis when karyotyping reveals **absence of one X chromosome (45, X), absence of secondary sexual characteristics,** and **elevated FSH.** Because the second X chromosome is essential to the development of normal ovarian follicles, streak gonads develop.

Management involves **estrogen and progesterone replacement** for development of secondary sexual characteristics.

Hypothalamic-Pituitary Failure

This is the diagnosis when there are **no sexual characteristics** but the **uterus is normal on ultrasound** and **FSH levels are low.** It may be due to stress, excessive exercise, or anorexia nervosa. **Kallmann syndrome** is the likely diagnosis when the case also describes **anosmia** (hypothalamus doesn't produce GnRH). CNS imaging (CT head) will rule out a brain tumor.

Management involves **estrogen and progesterone replacement** for development of secondary sexual characteristics.

Secondary Amenorrhea

This is diagnosed when one of the following conditions presents:

- Regular menses are replaced by an **absence of menses for 3 months.**
- Irregular menses are replaced by an **absence of menses for 6 months.**

Steps in the Workup of Secondary Amenorrhea

Steps in the Workup	Next Step in Management
1. Pregnancy Test (ß-hCG)	
2. Thyrotropin (TSH) (rule out hypothyroidism)	An elevated TRH in primary hypothyroidism → ↑ prolactin. Treat hypothyroidism with thyroid replacement for rapid restoration of menstruation
3. Prolactin (rule out elevation)	*If elevated:* 1) *Review medications:* Antipsychotics and antidepressants have antidopamine side effect → ↑ prolactin 2) *CT or MRI of head to rule out pituitary tumor* – Tumor < 1 cm: give bromocriptine (dopamine agonist) – Tumor > 1 cm: treat surgically 3) If the cause of elevated prolactin is idiopathic, treat with bromocriptine.
4. Progesterone Challenge Test (PCT)	• *Positive PCT:* Any withdrawal bleeding is *diagnostic of* ***anovulation.*** – *Treatment:* Cyclic progesterone to prevent endometrial hyperplasia. Clomiphene ovulation induction is done if pregnancy is desired. • *Negative PCT:* Inadequate estrogen or outflow tract obstruction
5. Estrogen–Progesterone Challenge Test (EPCT)	• 3 weeks of oral estrogen followed by 1 week of progesterone • *Positive EPCT:* Any withdrawal bleeding is *diagnostic of* ***inadequate estrogen. Next step is to get an FSH level.*** – ↑ *FSH is ovarian failure.* Y chromosome mosaicism may be the cause if patient is < 25 years. Order a **karyotype** for confirmation. – ↓ *FSH is hypothalamic–pituitary insufficiency.* Order a **brain CT/MRI** to rule out a tumor. Give estrogen-replacement therapy to prevent osteoporosis and cyclic progestins to prevent endometrial hyperplasia. • *Negative EPCT:* Diagnostic of an outflow tract obstruction or endometrial scarring (e.g., *Asherman syndrome*). Order a **hysterosalpingogram** to identify the lesion. Management: Adhesion lysis followed by estrogen stimulation of the endometrium. An inflatable stent prevents re-adhesion of the uterine walls.

Premenstrual Syndrome

Premenstrual Tension

This is defined as distressing physical, psychological, and behavioral symptoms recurring at the same phase of the menstrual cycle and disappearing during the remainder of the cycle.

Premenstrual Dysphoric Disorder (PMDD)

This is more severe, involving major disruptions to daily functioning and relationships.

Treatment

- **SSRIs** are the treatment of choice. SSRIs increase extracellular serotonin by blocking the presynaptic receptor. Blocking this receptor leaves more serotonin in the synaptic cleft for the postsynaptic cell to pick up.
- Low doses of **vitamin B6 (pyridoxine)** may improve symptoms.
- Diuretics have shown mixed results in the management of premenstrual fluid retention.

Endocrine Disorders

- **Hirsutism:** Excessive male-pattern hair growth in a woman.
- **Virilization:** Excessive male-pattern hair growth in a woman *plus* other masculinizing signs, such as clitoromegaly, baldness, lowering of voice, increasing muscle mass, and loss of female body contours.

Almost all cases of hirsutism are either **PCOS** or **idiopathic.** More serious causes of hirsutism (**androgen-secreting tumors**) need to be *excluded* in the workup.

Initial steps in workup:

- Testosterone
- DHEAS
- LH/FSH
- 17-hydroxyprogesterone

Polycystic Ovarian Syndrome (PCOS)

This is the diagnosis when there is **gradual-onset hirsutism, obesity, acne, irregular bleeding,** and **infertility.** There are chronic anovulatory cycles and **infertility.** Diagnosis is mostly clinical. However, an **elevated LH/FSH ratio** is used for confirmation. **Bilaterally enlarged ovaries** will be found on exam and ultrasound.

> **Anovulation** classically presents with a **history of amenorrhea** followed by **unpredictable bleeding** (prolonged unopposed estrogen stimulates the endometrium). Consider the following diagnoses:
> - Polycystic ovary syndrome (PCOS)
> - Hypothyroidism
> - Pituitary adenoma
> - Elevated prolactin
> - Medications (e.g., antipsychotics, antidepressants)

- **Anovulation** → no corpus luteum production of progesterone → unopposed estrogen → hyperplastic endometrium and irregular bleeding → **predisposition to endometrial cancer.**
- **Increased testosterone:** ↑LH levels → ↑theca cell production of androgens → hepatic production of SHBG is suppressed → **↑total testosterone and ↑free testosterone.**
- **Ovarian enlargement:** Ultrasound shows a necklacelike pattern of multiple peripheral cysts (20–100 cystic follicles in each ovary). ↑androgens → multiple follicles in various stages of development, stromal hyperplasia, and a thickened ovarian capsule → **bilaterally enlarged ovaries.**

Diagnostic Testing

- LH:FSH ratio = **3:1** (normal is 1.5:1).
- Testosterone level is **mildly elevated.**
- Pelvic ultrasound shows **bilaterally enlarged ovaries with multiple subcapsular small follicles and increased stromal echogenicity.**

Treatment

- **Oral contraceptive pill** treats irregular bleeding and hirsutism. The progestin component prevents endometrial hyperplasia.
- **Spironolactone** may also be used to suppress hair follicles.
- **Clomiphene citrate** or **human menopausal gonadotropin** (HMG) is the treatment of choice for infertility.
- **Metformin** enhances ovulation and manages insulin resistance.

Adrenal or Ovarian Tumor

This is the diagnosis when the question describes **rapid onset hirsutism** and **virilization** *without* a family history. **DHEAS is markedly elevated** in an adrenal tumor; **testosterone is markedly elevated** in an ovarian tumor. The next step is to order an **ultrasound** (adnexal mass) or CT (adrenal mass).

Management involves **surgical removal** of the tumor.

Congenital Adrenal Hyperplasia (21-Hydroxyolase Deficiency)

This is the diagnosis when the question describes **gradual-onset hirsutism** *without* virilization in the **second or third decade** that is associated with **menstrual irregularities** and **anovulation. Serum 17-hydroxyprogesterone** level is markedly elevated. Precocious puberty with short stature is common. Family history may be positive.

Management involves **corticosteroid replacement,** which will arrest the signs of androgenicity and restore ovulatory cycles.

Idiopathic Hirsutism

This is the diagnosis when there is **no virilization** and **all laboratory tests are normal.** It is the most common cause of hirsutism.

Treatment

- **Spironolactone** is the treatment of choice.
- **Eflornithine (Vaniqa)** is the first-line topical drug for the treatment of unwanted facial and chin hair.

Diagnosis	Testosterone	DHEAS	LH/FSH	17-OHP	Next Step in Management
	Produced by ovary & adrenal gland	*Produced by adrenal glands*	*Produced by the anterior pituitary gland*	*Precursor in cortisol synthesis & converted peripherally to androgens*	
Polycystic ovary syndrome	↑	NL /↑	↑LH ↓FSH	NL	**Ultrasound** to rule out other disorders/tumors Screen lipids and fasting blood glucose
Congenital adrenal hyperplasia	NL/↑	NL /↑	NL/NL	↑↑	**ACTH stimulation** confirms the diagnosis
Ovarian tumor	↑↑	NL	NL/NL	NL	**Ultrasound/CT** to image tumor
Adrenal tumor	↑	↑↑	NL/NL	NL	**Ultrasound/CT** to image tumor

Menopause Disorders

- *Menopause* is defined as **12 months of amenorrhea** with **elevation of FSH and LH.** The mean age is 51 years. Smokers experience menopause up to 2 years earlier.
- Diagnose with **serial levels of elevated gonadotropins** (FSH > 50 IU/mL).
- If menopause occurs between ages 40 and 50, it is **early menopause.** It is most often idiopathic but can also occur after radiation therapy or surgical oophorectomy.
- If menopause occurs before age 30, it is **premature ovarian failure** and may be associated with autoimmune disease or Y chromosome mosaicism.

The following menopausal symptoms are related to a **lack of estrogen:**

- **Amenorrhea:** Menses become anovulatory and decrease in the 3- to 5-year period known as perimenopause.
- **Hot flashes:** This is unpredictable, profuse sweating and heat that occurs in 75 percent of women. Obese women are less likely to undergo hot flashes (due to peripheral conversion of androgens to estrone).
- **Reproductive tract:** Decreased vaginal lubrication, increased vaginal pH, and increased vaginal infections can occur.
- **Urinary tract:** Increased urgency, frequency, nocturia, and urge incontinence can occur.
- **Psychic:** Depressed mood, emotional lability, and sleep disorders can occur.
- **Cardiovascular disease:** This is the most common cause of mortality (50 percent) in postmenopausal women.
- **Osteoporosis**

Osteoporosis

The most common site of symptomatic osteoporosis is in the **vertebral bodies,** leading **to crush fractures, kyphosis,** and **decreased height.** Hip and wrist fractures are the next most frequent sites.

The most common risk factor is **positive family history in a thin, white female.** Other risk factors are **steroid use, low calcium intake, sedentary lifestyle, smoking,** and **alcohol.**

Prevent with calcium and vitamin D, weight-bearing exercise, and elimination of cigarettes and alcohol.

DEXA scan results:
- T-score –1.5 to –2.5 = osteopenia
- T-score ≥ –2.5 = osteoporosis

Diagnostic Testing

- **Bone density** is assessed with a **DEXA scan** (dual-energy x-ray absorptiometry). The results are reported as a T-score: a T-score ≥ –2.5 indicates the presence of osteoporosis.
- **Calcium loss** is assessed with a **24-hour urine hydroxyproline** or **NTX** (N-telopeptide, a bone breakdown product).

Treatment

- First-line therapy is **bisphosphonates** and **SERMs.**
  - Bisphosphates (e.g., alendronate, risedronate) **inhibit osteoclastic activity.**
  - Selective estrogen receptor modulators (SERMs) **increase bone density.**
    - **SERMs** are protective against the heart and bones but are *not* effective for vasomotor symptoms of menopause.
    - **Tamoxifen (Nolvadex)** has endometrial and bone agonist effects but breast antagonist effects.
    - **Raloxifene (Evista)** has bone agonist effects but endometrial antagonist effects.

Denosumab is a RANKL inhibitor that inhibits osteoclast function.

- Calcitonin, denosumab, and teriparatide are second-line therapy.
- Teriparatide is a PTH analog that is used when biphosphates fail.
- Estrogen is *never* the primary treatment of osteoporosis because of associated risks of clots and endometrial cancer.

Hormone Replacement Therapy (HRT)

When is HRT the answer?	When is HRT NOT the answer?
Treatment of: • Menopausal vasomotor symptoms (hot flashes) • Genitourinary atrophy • Dyspareunia	*Treatment of:* • Osteoporosis *When the case describes a history of:* • Estrogen-sensitive cancer (breast or endometrial) • Liver disease • Active thrombosis • Unexplained vaginal bleeding

- Women *without* a uterus can be given **continuous estrogen.**
- All women *with* a uterus must also receive progestin therapy to prevent endometrial hyperplasia.

Benefits of HRT	Risks of HRT
↓Rate of osteoporotic fractures ↓Rate of colorectal cancer	↑Risk of DVT ↑Risk of heart attacks and breast cancer in combination therapy *Risk of breast cancer is only associated with therapy > 4 yrs*

Guidelines for Hormone Replacement Therapy

- *Only* start HRT for vasomotor symptoms.
- *Never* give HRT for the prevention of cardiovascular disease.
- Use the *lowest dose* of HRT to treat symptoms.
- Use the *shortest duration* of HRT to treat symptoms; reevaluate annually.
- Do not exceed 4 years of therapy (increased risk of breast cancer after 4 years of therapy).

Contraception

Low-dose contraceptive pills do *not* increase the risk of cancer, heart disease, or thromboembolic events in women with no associated risk factors (hypertension, diabetes, or smoking).

	Examples	Absolute Contraindication	Relative Contraindication	Benefits
Barrier Methods	Condoms Vaginal diaphragm ± spermicides	N/A	N/A	– Protective against STDs
Steroid Contraception	Combination (estrogen + progesterone) Progestin only (OCP called "mini-pill", injectable, implant, morning after pill)	– Pregnancy – Acute liver disease – Vascular disease (e.g., thromboembolism, DVT, CVA, SLE) – Hormone dependent cancer (e.g., breast CA) – Smoker > 35 – Uncontrolled hypertension – Migraines with aura – DM with vascular disease – Thrombophilia	– Migraines – Depression – DM – Chronic HTN – Hyperlipidemia	– ↓ovarian and endometrial CA – ↓dysmenorrhea – ↓dysfunctional uterine bleeding – ↓ectopic pregnancy
Intrauterine Device	– Levonorgestrel-impregnated – Copper-banded	– Pregnancy – Pelvic malignancy – Salpingitis	– Abnormal uterine size or shape – Immune suppression (including steroid therapy) – Nulligravidity – Abnormal Pap smears – History of ectopic pregnancy	Effective and avoids side effects of hormonal therapy

Infertility

A 35-year-old woman comes to the gynecologist's office complaining of infertility for 1 year. She and her husband have been trying to achieve pregnancy for > 1 year and have been unsuccessful. There is no previous history of pelvic inflammatory disease, and she had used oral contraception medication for 6 years. The pelvic examination is normal. Semen analysis is low volume and shows decreased sperm density and low motility. What is the next step in management?

a. Administer testosterone
b. Measure serum testosterone
c. Measure thyroid hormone
d. Repeat semen analysis
e. Refer for intrauterine insemination

Answer: **D.** Because semen samples are variable, an abnormal semen analysis is repeated in 4–6 weeks to confirm findings.

Infertility is defined as inability to achieve pregnancy after 12 months of unprotected and frequent intercourse.

Steps in workup for infertility:

1. The first step is **semen analysis.**
2. If semen analysis is normal, work up for **anovulation.**
3. If semen analysis is normal and ovulation is confirmed, work up for **fallopian tube abnormalities.**

Step	Diagnosis	Management
1. Semen Analysis	Normal values: • Volume > 2 mL; pH 7.2–7.8; sperm density > 20 million/mL; sperm motility > 50%; and sperm morphology > 50% normal.	• If values are abnormal, repeat the semen analysis in 4–6 weeks. • *Abnormal semen analysis:* Intrauterine insemination, intracytoplasmic sperm injection (ICSI), and in vitro fertilization (IVF) are fertility options. • *No viable sperm:* Artificial insemination by donor may be used.
2. Anovulation	• Basal body temperature (BBT) chart: NO midcycle temperature elevation • Progesterone: Low • Endometrial biopsy: Proliferative histology	• Hypothyroidism or hyperprolactinemia are causes of anovulation that can be treated. • *Ovulation induction:* – *Clomiphene citrate* is the agent of choice. – Human menopausal gonadotrophin (hMG) is used if clomiphene fails – *Most common side effect* = ovarian hyperstimulation. Ovarian size must be monitored during induction.
3. Tube Abnormalities: Hysterosalpingogram and Laparoscopy	• *Chlamydia Antibody:* A negative IgG antibody test for chlamydia rules out infection-induced tubal adhesions.	• *Hysterosalpingogram* (HSG): No further testing is performed if the HSG shows normal anatomy. • Laparoscopy: Performed with an abnormal HSG to visualize the oviducts and attempt reconstruction (tuboplasty). If tubal damage is severe, IVF should be planned.

Unexplained Infertility

The **semen analysis** is normal, **ovulation** is confirmed, and **patent oviducts** are noted. **No treatment** is indicated, and approximately 60 percent of patients with unexplained infertility will achieve a spontaneous pregnancy within the next 3 years.

In Vitro Fertilization

1. Eggs are aspirated from the ovarian follicles using an ultrasound-guided transvaginal approach.
2. They are fertilized with sperm in the laboratory, resulting in the formation of embryos.
3. Multiple embryos are transferred into the uterine cavity with a cumulative pregnancy rate of 55 percent after 4 IVF cycles.

Gestational Trophoblastic Disease (GTN)

This is an **abnormal proliferation of placental tissue** involving both the cyto-trophoblast and/or syncytiotrophoblast. It can be either benign or malignant.

- GTN is most common in **Taiwan** and the **Philippines.** Other risk factors are **maternal age extremes** (< 20 years old, > 35 years old) and **folate deficiency.**
- The most common symptom is **bleeding < 16 weeks gestation** and **passage of vesicles from the vagina.** Other symptoms of a molar pregnancy include hypertension, hyperthyroidism, and hyperemesis gravidarum and no fetal heart tones appreciated.
- The most common signs are **fundus larger than dates, absence of fetal heart tones, bilateral cystic enlargements of the ovary** (theca-lutein cysts).
- The most common site of distant metastasis is the **lungs.**

Benign: H. Mole	
Complete	**Incomplete**
Empty egg	Normal egg
46,XX (dizygotic ploidy)	69,XXY (*tri*ploidy)
Fetus absent	Fetus nonviable
20% → malignancy	10% → malignancy
No chemotherapy; serial ß-hCG titers until (–); f/up for 1 year on OCP	

A 32-year-old Filipino woman is 15 weeks' pregnant by dates. She presents with painless vaginal bleeding associated with severe nausea and vomiting. Her uterus extends to her umbilicus but no fetal heart tones can be heard. Her blood pressure is 162/98 mm Hg. A dipstick urine shows 2+ proteinuria. Which of the following is the most likely diagnosis?

a. Chronic hypertension
b. Chronic hypertension with superimposed preeclampsia
c. Eclampsia
d. Molar pregnancy
e. Preeclampsia

Answer: **D.** This patients presentation is typical for a molar pregnancy. Absence of fetal heart tones eliminates the other options.

Diagnostic Testing

- Sonogram reveals **homogenous intrauterine echoes without a gestational sac or fetal parts** ("snowstorm" ultrasound).

Management

- **Baseline quantitative β-hCG titer**
- **Chest x-ray** (rule out lung metastasis)
- **Suction dilation and curettage (D&C)** (to evacuate the uterine contents)
- Place the patient on **effective contraception** (oral contraceptive pills) to ensure no confusion between rising β-hCG titers from recurrent disease and normal pregnancy

Section 8
Radiology

Choosing an Imaging Study

When Is CT the Best Answer on the Test?

- **Noncontrast head CT:** This is the best initial test to **rule out hemorrhage** when the case describes trauma or acute neurological change.
- **Contrast head CT:** This is appropriate when you want to evaluate for **AV malformations** or **primary or metastatic tumors.**
- **Abdominal pelvic CT:** This is the best test to evaluate **retroperitoneal structures:** pancreatitis or pancreatic masses or nodal metastasis from colon, prostate, testicular, or renal malignancies.
- **High-resolution CT scan of chest:** This is the test of choice to evaluate **parenchymal lung disease** (interstitial fibrosis). It is also the best test to evaluate **bony structures.**

Keep the following in mind regarding CT scans:

- Do *not* order CT with contrast in patients with renal disease (creatinine ≥ 1.5).
- Do *not* give IV contrast in patients with multiple myeloma.
- *Always* discontinue metformin before doing a CT scan with IV contrast and only resume metformin 48 hours after the scan, when renal failure has been ruled out.
- Do *not* order MRI with contrast in patients with renal disease (creatinine ≥ 1.5) due to the risk of nephrogenic systemic fibrosis.

When Is MRI the Best Answer on the Test?

- MRI is the test of choice for evaluating **demyelinating diseases** (e.g., multiple sclerosis and some dementias).
- It is the best test to evaluate the **posterior fossa, base of the skull, and the orbit.**
- It is the best test to evaluate **acoustic neuromas, pituitary tumors, and small intraparenchymal brain tumors.**
- It is the test of choice for **bone tumors, bone and soft tissue infections** (e.g., osteomyelitis), **joint spaces, and aseptic necrosis of femoral head.**
- It is the test of choice for evaluating **disease of the spinal cord and spinal column** (e.g., herniated discs, degenerative disc disease, and spinal tumors).

When Are Nuclear Scans the Best Test?

- **HIDA (hepatobiliary) scan:** This is used for **evaluating biliary obstruction versus acute cholecystitis** and the **evaluation of biliary leaks postoperatively.** It is also the test of choice to evaluate **congenital abnormalities of the biliary tract,** including biliary atresia. It is *not* the test of choice for evaluating gallbladder stones.
- **Bone scan:** This is used for evaluating **metastatic bone lesions** (prostate, breast, kidney, thyroid, lung), **evaluating delayed fractures,** and **evaluating osteomyelitis and avascular necrosis of the femoral head.**
- **Adrenal scan:** This is the test of choice to **localize pheochromocytoma** when a MRI/CT scan is nondiagnostic.
- **V/Q scan:** This is the initial test of choice to evaluate for **pulmonary embolism** (PE). (A normal study rules out PE. An indeterminate scan requires further workup with CT angiogram. A perfusion defect with normal ventilation quite probably indicates PE.) Do *not* order a V/Q scan in a patient with COPD or extensive lung disease.
- **Gallium scan:** This is the test of choice for **localizing abscesses, staging lymphomas, and melanomas.**

Bone scan is not useful in purely lytic metastatic lesions. It is **never the correct answer** in a patient with multiple myeloma.

When Is Ultrasound the Best Test?

- It is the best initial test to **evaluate the gallbladder for stones** when a patient presents with right upper-quadrant pain.
- It is the best initial test for **assessing the uterus, adnexa, and ovaries** (with the *exception* of cervical carcinoma).
- It is the best initial test to **evaluate the prostate;** it also aids in **obtaining biopsy.**
- It is the best test to **evaluate for deep venous thrombosis (DVT).**

Images You Must Be Able to Recognize on the Exam

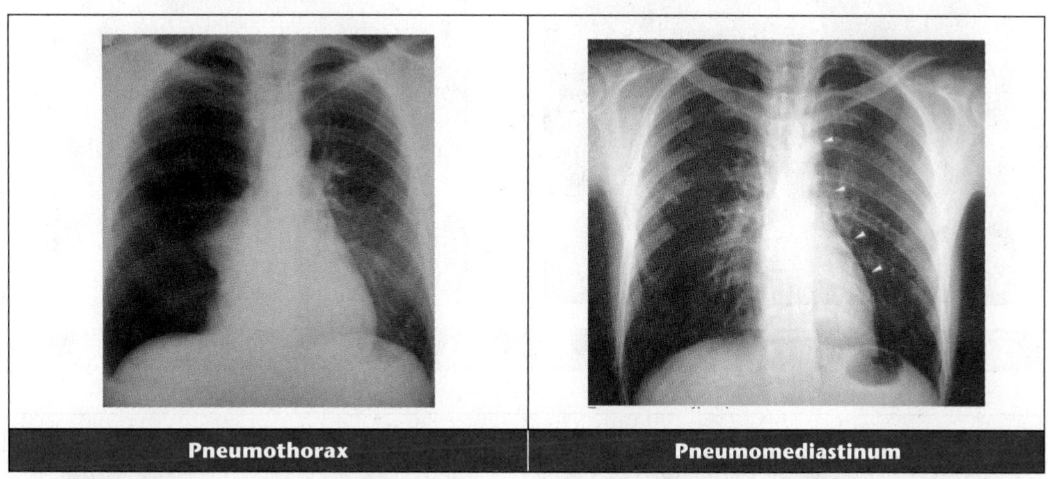

Pneumothorax | Pneumomediastinum

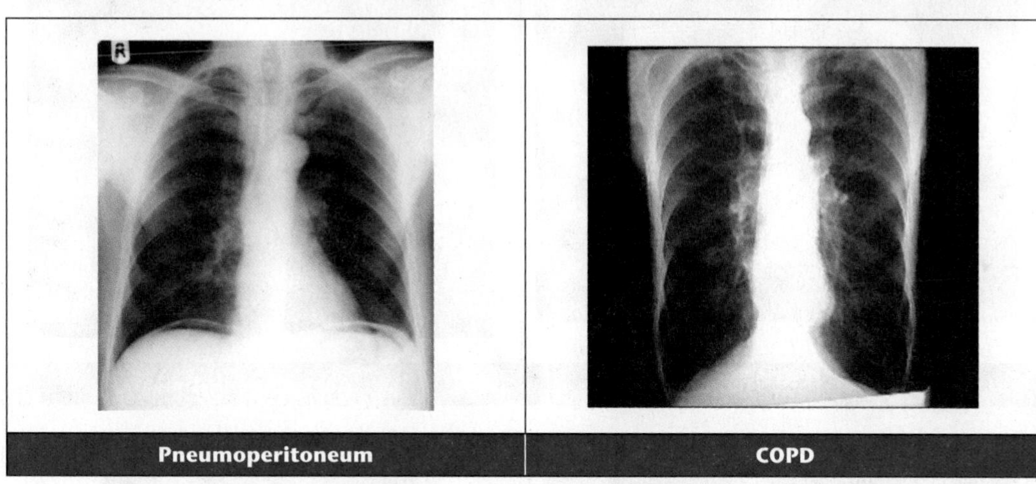

Pneumoperitoneum | COPD

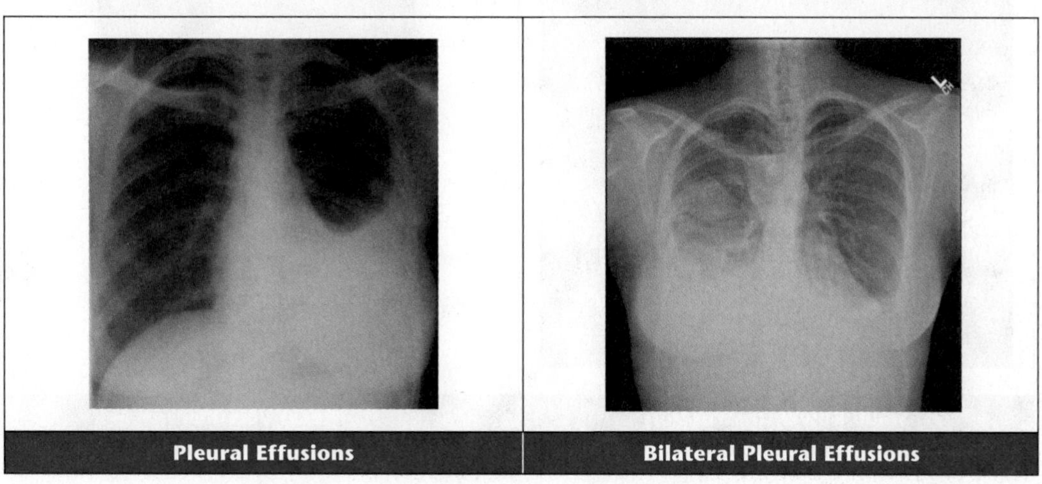

Pleural Effusions | Bilateral Pleural Effusions

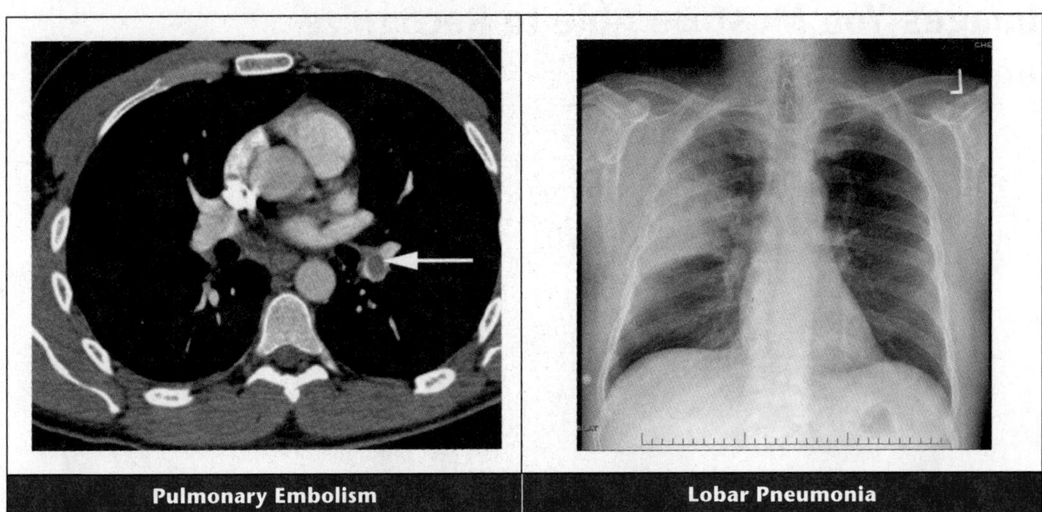

Pulmonary Embolism | Lobar Pneumonia

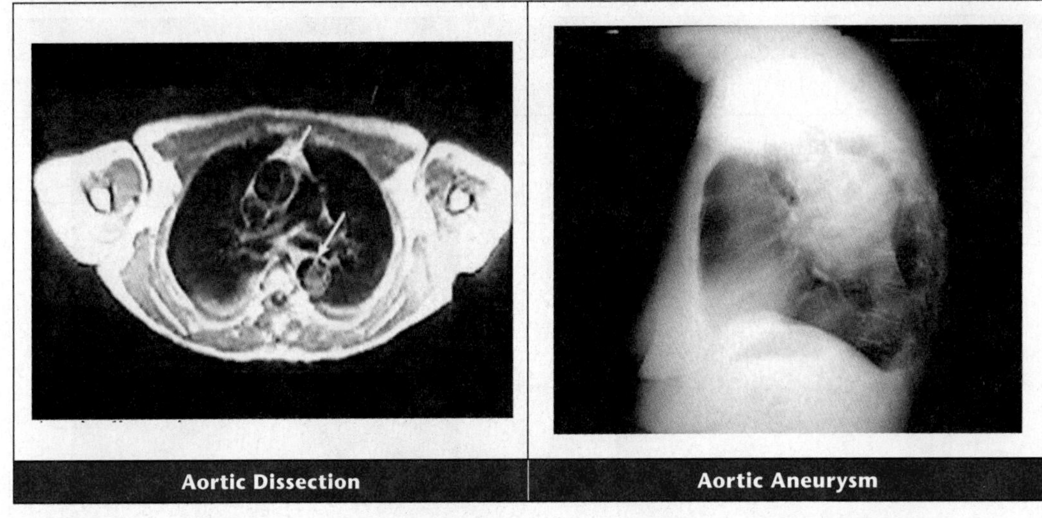

Aortic Dissection | Aortic Aneurysm

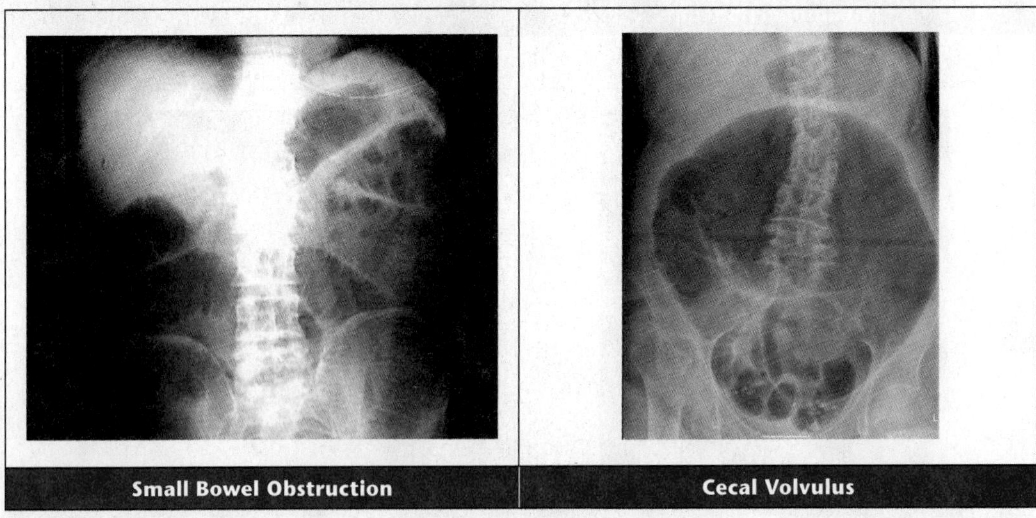

Small Bowel Obstruction | Cecal Volvulus

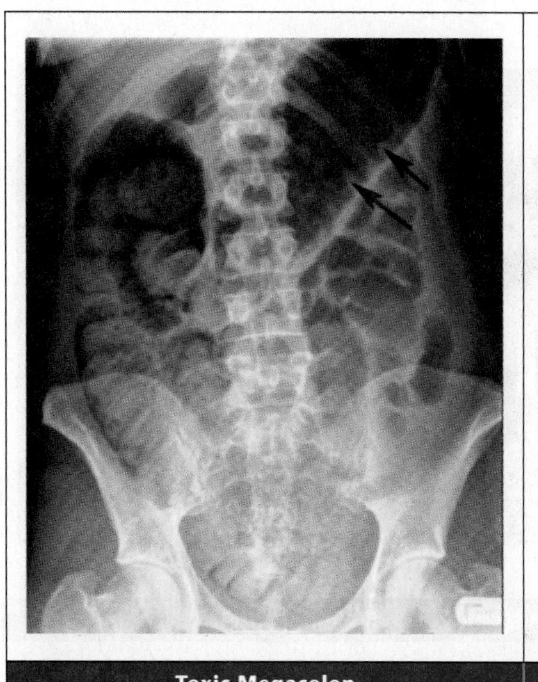

Toxic Megacolon

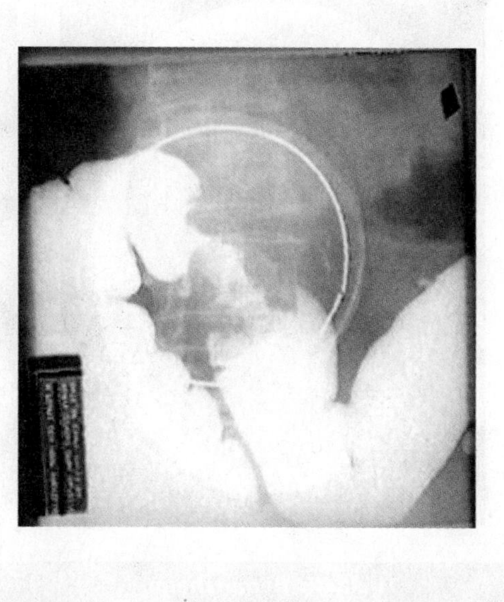

Carcinoma of the Colon

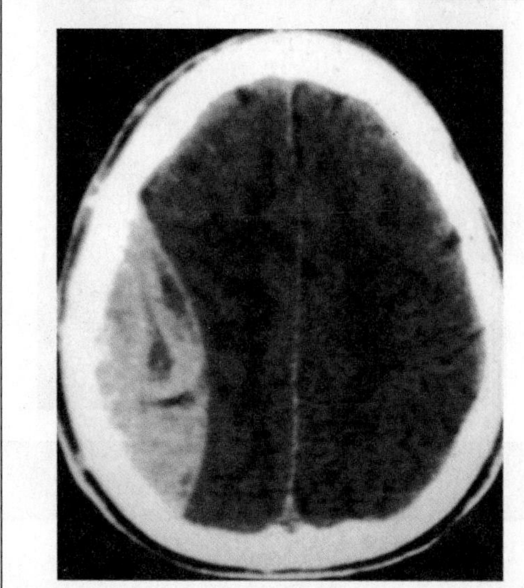

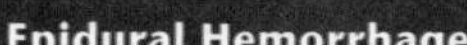

Epidural Hemorrhage

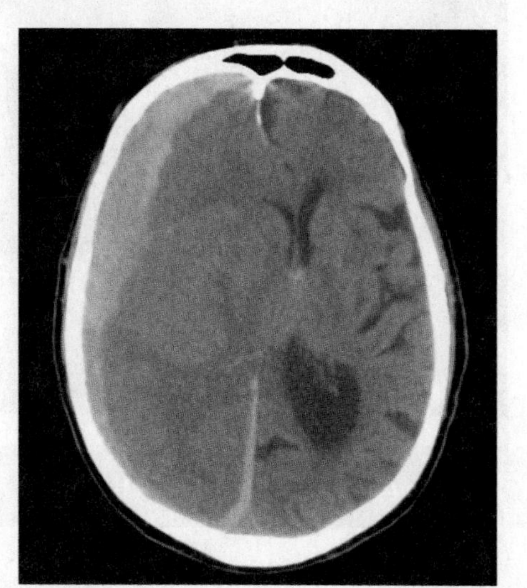

Subdural Hemorrhage

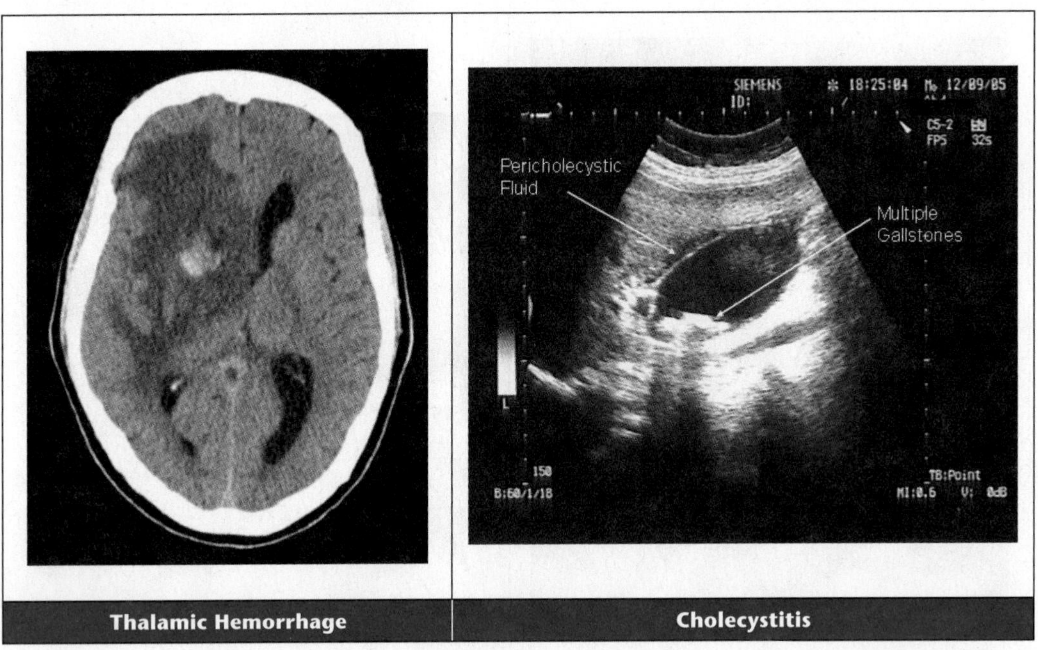

Thalamic Hemorrhage

Cholecystitis

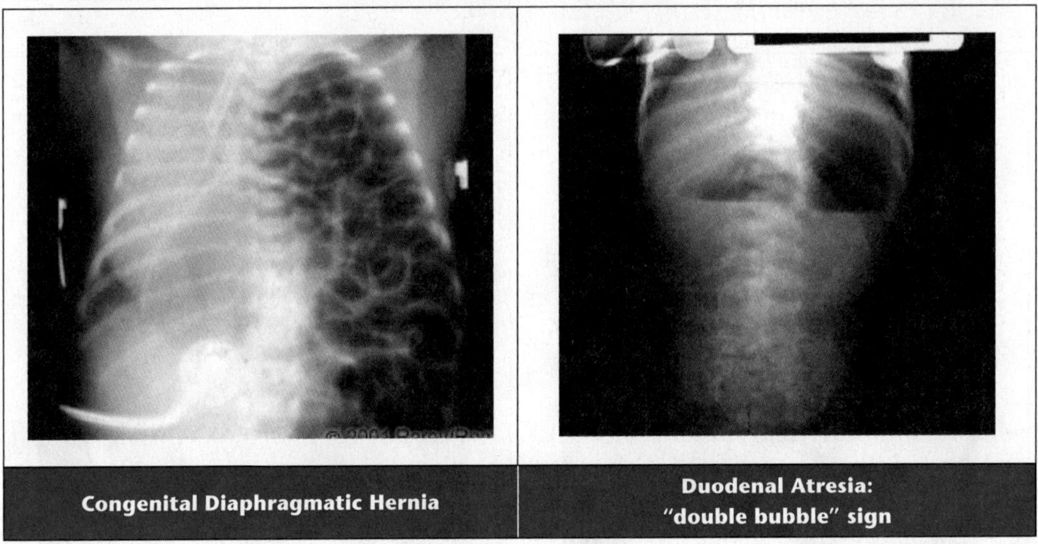

Congenital Diaphragmatic Hernia

Duodenal Atresia:
"double bubble" sign

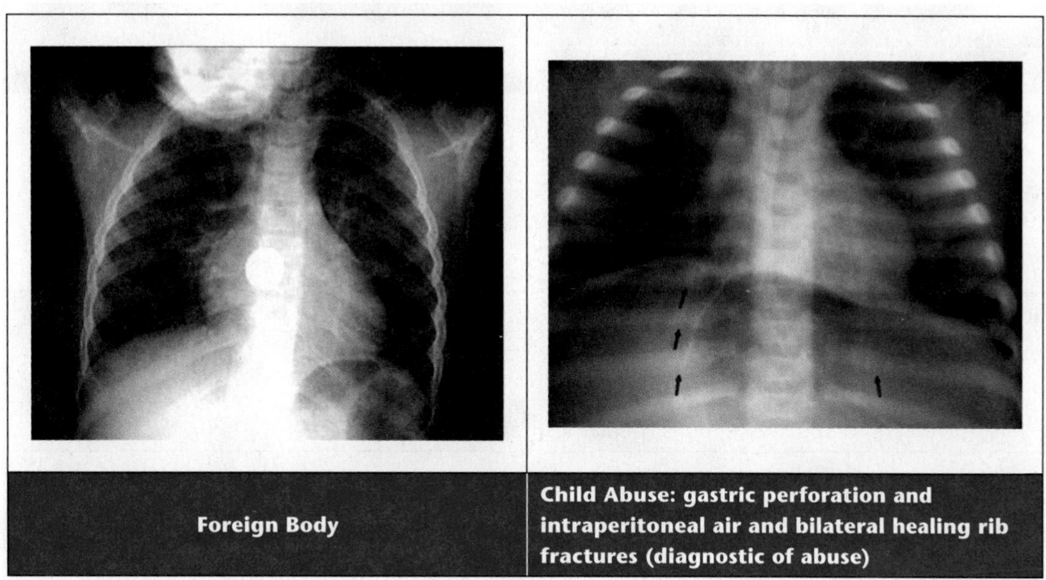

Foreign Body	Child Abuse: gastric perforation and intraperitoneal air and bilateral healing rib fractures (diagnostic of abuse)

Other Radiology Knowledge for the Exam

When you see...	Think of...
Bones	
Lytic bone lesions on x-ray films	Multiple myeloma Primary bone tumor Metastasis (most common: lung, renal or thyroid, breast)
Blastic bone lesions on x-ray films	Metastasis (most common: breast, prostate, lymphoma) Paget's disease Medulloblastoma in pediatrics
Chest	
Large mediastinum	Aortic aneurysm Lymphadenopathy
Lung infiltrated with an effusion	*Staphylococcus pneumoniae* *Streptococcus pneumoniae* Lung infarct Tuberculosis

When you see...	Think of...
Abdomen/Pelvis	
Small bowel obstruction	Adhesions Hernia Intussusception (pediatrics) Gallstone ileus Carcinoma
Large bowel obstruction	Carcinoma Hernia Diverticulitis Intussusceptions (pediatrics)
Gas in biliary system	Gallstone ileus Gas forming infection Instrumentation
Small kidney(s)	Renal artery disease Chronic hydronephrosis Chronic glomerulonephritis Chronic pyelonephritis
Large kidney(s)	Acute pyelonephritis Acute glomerulonephritis Renal vein thrombosis Carcinoma (unilateral) Wilms' tumor (pediatrics)
Brain/Neurology	
Ring-enhancing lesion in brain	Immunocompetent patients: • Metastatic tumors • Demyelinating disease • Pyogenic abscess Immunocompromised patients: • Toxoplasma encephalitis *(T. gondii)* • Primary CNS lymphoma (Epstein-Barr virus) • Tuberculosis (in endemic areas)
Hemorrhage into basal ganglia, cerebellum, or pons	Hypertensive brain hemorrhage
Hemorrhage into the cerebral hemispheres	Arteriovenous malformation Aneurysm Trauma Metastatic lesions Other causes: vasculitis, cocaine, coagulation abnormalities

Section 9
Psychiatry

contributing author Niket Sonpal, MD

Psychotic Disorders

Psychotic disorders present with a combination of positive and/or negative symptoms. The key differentiating feature is the **duration** of symptoms.

Diagnosis

Positive Symptoms	Negative Symptoms
Associated with dopamine receptors	**Associated with muscarinic receptors**
• Delusions (mostly bizarre) • Disorganized speech/behavior • Hallucinations	• Flattened affect • Social withdrawal • Anhedonia • Apathy • Poverty of thought *Tip:* Atypical antipsychotics are the most effective treatment for negative symptoms.

"Phrenia" > 6 months
"Phreniform" > 1 month but < 6 months

To merit a diagnosis of **schizophrenia**, symptoms must be present for a period of at least **1 month**, with a significant impact on social or occupational functioning for at least **6 months**. In addition to the negative symptoms, the individual must have at least one of these 3 symptoms: delusions, hallucinations, and disorganized speech. Schizophrenia presents at a younger age in males (15–24 years) than in females (25–34 years).

When symptoms are present for < **6 months but** > **1 month**, the diagnosis is **schizophreniform disorder.**

Catatonia is no longer so strongly associated with schizophrenia.

When symptoms are present for < **1 month** and the question states that there is a return to baseline, the diagnosis is **brief psychotic disorder** (look for a stressful life event that precipitates it).

Basic Science Correlate

L-Phenylalanine → L-Tyrosine → L-DOPA → Dopamine

Schizophrenia is not diagnosed if symptoms of pervasive developmental disorder are present, *unless accompanied by* prominent delusions or hallucinations.

When there is a history of symptoms for many years with **no impairment of baseline functioning,** think of:

- Delusional disorder (key is that **delusions are nonbizarre)**
- **Personality disorders**

These patients do not respond to antipsychotics. *Psychotherapy is the preferred therapy.*

Rule out medical illness and other forms of psychosis that aren't schizophrenia:

- Check **TSH** for hypo- or hyperthyroidism.
- Check basic electrolytes and calcium to rule out metabolic disorders.
- Test **serology** to rule out HIV.
- Test **VDRL** to rule out syphilis.
- Drug screen is the best initial test in a patient with psychosis.
- **Temporal lobe epilepsy** can present with hallucinations (auditory and olfactory distortions), feeling of *déjà vu,* or dissociation from surroundings.

The first step in management of any acute psychiatric condition is to determine if the patient needs hospitalization. Hospitalize if the patient is at risk of harm to self or to others. Hospitalize against the patient's will if the patient has suicidal or homicidal ideation.

Watch out for **suicidal ideation** in schizophrenia patients and schizophreniform patients. Fifty percent of schizophrenia patients attempt suicide in their lifetimes, and 10 percent of these attempts are successful. Schizophreniform patients are at greater risk of depression and suicide *after* the episode of psychosis resolves. The first step in management is *always* to hospitalize if there is any risk of suicide.

What is the greatest risk factor for progression to schizophrenia?

Answer: **Schizophreniform disorder.** Two thirds eventually progress to schizophrenia.

When the case describes any of the following features, the prognosis is poor:

- Early age of onset
- Negative symptoms
- Poor premorbid functioning
- Family history of schizophrenia
- Disorganized or deficit subtype

Prognosis

In general, **females** have a better prognosis and respond better to treatment than males.

Treatment

1. If the case describes bizarre or paranoid symptoms, **hospitalize the patient.**
2. Give **benzodiazepines** for agitation and start **antipsychotics.**
   - Antipsychotic medications are given for 6 months and are the *most effective* therapy to prevent further episodes.
   - Long-term antipsychotics are *only* given when there is a history of repeat episodes.
3. Initiate **long-term psychotherapy.**

Antipsychotics

Antipsychotics have an immediate **quieting effect** in acute psychotic attacks of any cause (e.g., schizophrenia, depression with psychotic features, mania in bipolar disorder). They also delay relapses.

There are 2 other indications for antipsychotics:

1. For **sedation** when benzodiazepines are contraindicated or as an adjunct during anesthesia
2. For **movement disorders: Huntington's disease** and **Tourette syndrome** (to suppress tics and vocalization)

Basic Science Correlate

Huntington's disease is a trinucleotide repeat disorder = CAG repeat = Glutamine.

Antipsychotics are chosen based on side effect profile, *not* efficacy:

- **Low-potency antipsychotics** have the highest risk of causing **orthostatic hypotension** (alpha blockade), **acute urinary retention, dry mouth, blurry vision, and delirium** (anticholinergic effect). Change to an atypical antipsychotic if these symptoms are present.
- **Thioridazine** is associated with **prolonged QT and arrhythmias.** *Always* get an EKG if the case describes **chest pain, shortness of breath,** or **palpitations** in a patient taking thioridazine. Thioridazine is also associated with **abnormal retinal pigmentation** after many years of use. Routine eye exam is needed for chronic therapy.
- **Impotence** and **inhibition of ejaculation** (α-blocker effect) are common reasons for noncompliance in males.
- **Weight gain** (due to hyperprolactinemia) is a common reason for noncompliance in females. Also ask about galactorrhea and amenorrhea.

Clozapine is associated with agranulocytosis (1 percent). **Always** check CBC with differential both before initiating therapy **and** weekly after starting therapy.

	Conventional Antipsychotics		Atypical Antipsychotics
	High Potency	**Low Potency**	
Examples	Fluphenazine, haloperidol	Thioridazine, chlorpromazine	Risperidone, olanzapine, quetiapine, clozapine
Advantages	Less sedating Fewer anticholinergic effects Less hypotension Useful as depot injections (e.g., haloperidol decanoate) for noncompliant patients Give IM route for acute psychosis when patient is unable or unwilling to take PO	Less likely to cause EPS	Drug of choice for initial therapy Greater effect on negative symptoms Little or no risk of EPS
Disadvantages	Greatest association with extrapyramidal systems (EPS)	Greater anticholinergic effects More sedation More postural hypotension	Clozapine is reserved for treatment-resistant patients because of risk of agranulocytosis.

Olanzapine has the greatest **weight gain** of any of the antipsychotics.

a. A newly diagnosed schizophrenic patient complains of insomnia. What is the most appropriate antipsychotic to initiate therapy?

b. A schizophrenic patient has been maintained on olanzapine for the past 6 months. He complains of daytime sedation, and he has lost 2 jobs in the past month because of impaired performance. What is the next step in management?

Answers:

a. Olanzapine, quetiapine, ziprasidone, and aripiprazole are first-choice medications when insomnia is a problem.

b. Prescribe risperidone, a first-choice medication for the treatment of schizophrenia when sedation is a problem.

Basic Science Correlate

Risperidone affects 6 receptors:
- 5HT
- D1
- D2
- $\alpha 1$
- $\alpha 2$
- H1

Movement Disorders

Extrapyramidal symptoms (EPS) are the most common reason for failure to comply with therapy. Be able to identify a patient with a medication-related movement disorder and know how to minimize the symptoms.

The following table shows common medication-related movement disorders and their management.

Acute Dystonia	Bradykinesia (Parkinsonism)	Akathisia	Tardive Dyskinesia	Neuroleptic Malignant Syndrome
Occurs in the first week	Within weeks	Weeks to chronic use	Months to years	Anytime
Muscle spasms (e.g., torticollis), difficulty swallowing *TIP: Young men are at higher risk*	Bradykinesia, tremors, rigidity, and other signs of parkinsonism *TIP: Elderly are at higher risk*	Motor restlessness Do not mistake for anxiety for agitation *TIP: Always review medication list*	Choreoathetosis and other involuntary movements after chronic use Often irreversible	Muscle rigidity, hyperthermia, volatile vital signs, altered LOC, ↑ WBC & CK
-Reduce the dose -Rx: Anticholinergics • benztropine • diphenhydramine • trihexyphenidyl	-Reduce the dose -Rx: Anticholinergics • benztropine • diphenhydramine • trihexyphenidyl	-Reduce the dose -Add benzodiazepines or beta-blockers -Switch to newer antipsychotics	-Stop older antipsychotics -Switch to newer antipsychotics (e.g., clozapine) *TIP: Symptoms commonly worsen after medication discontinuation*	-Stop antipsychotic *TIP: Transfer to ICU for monitoring, mortality rate is 20%*

Basic Science Correlate

High-potency D2 receptor antagonists produce a dystonic reaction by nigrostriatal dopamine D2 receptor blockade, which leads striatal cholinergic output. Thus, anticholinergics are the first-line treatment.

A 35-year-old male presents with poor adherence to chlorpromazine and haloperidol. He complains of tics and other uncontrolled movements. His wife reports that even when he takes his medications, they don't appear to help his paranoia. What is the next step in management?

a. Add risperidone
b. Add diphenhydramine
c. Change to clozapine
d. Increase the dose of chlorpromazine
e. Increase the dose of haloperidol

Answer: **C.** The case describes 2 main problems in management, poor response to therapy prescribed and movement disorder as a side effect from the regimen. Clozapine is the most effective antipsychotic for schizophrenia and also has no incidence of movement disorders. It is a second-line therapy because of the risk of seizures and agranulocytosis. Remember to monitor CBC to watch for bone marrow suppression.

Tardive dyskinesia can be treated with benztropine.

A 78-year-old male with a slow-growing stomach tumor in palliative care is brought in by the family, who have noticed increased sedation and difficulty eating. They are concerned because he continues to lose more weight. On examination, he has repetitive movements of his lips and tongue. He has limited facial expression. His medications include morphine, metoclopramide, and hydrochlorothiazide. Which of the following is the most appropriate management?

a. Decrease morphine
b. Discontinue metoclopramide
c. Start omeprazole
d. Start prochlorperazine
e. Place NG tube for supplemental feedings

Answer: **B.** Chronic use of dopamine antagonists, including antimetics (metoclopramide, prochlorperazine), can result in **tardive dyskinesia.** Management includes discontinuing the offending drug and, if indicated, beginning a newer antipsychotic.

Anxiety Disorders

Anxiety disorders are characterized by anxiety that interferes with daytime functioning and is not due to any other identifiable causes of symptoms. Other conditions that may present as an anxiety disorder include the following:

- **Medical causes:** Hyperthyroidism, pheochromocytoma, excess cortisol, heart failure, arrhythmias, asthma, and COPD
- **Drugs:** Corticosteroids, cocaine, amphetamines, and caffeine, as well as withdrawal from alcohol and sedatives

Adjustment Disorder

This is a normal psychological reaction (anxiety, depression, irritability) that occurs soon after profound changes in a person's life, such as divorce, migration, or birth of a handicapped child. Symptoms are not severe enough to be classified in another category. Adjustment disorder is *not* a true anxiety disorder.

> Do *not* treat adjustment disorder patients with medications; instead provide **counseling** to help with the patient adjust to the life stressor.

Panic Disorder

Panic disorder is the diagnosis when the case describes **brief attacks of intense anxiety with autonomic symptoms (e.g., tachycardia, hyperventilation, dizziness, and sweating).** Episodes occur **regularly,** with an obvious precipitant and in the absence of other psychiatric illness.

Treatment

Treatment is **cognitive-behavioral therapy** and/or **relaxation training and desensitization.** Relaxation and desensitization may be more useful when agoraphobic symptoms are present. Medications include SSRIs (e.g., fluoxetine), benzodiazepines (e.g., alprazolam, clonazepam), imipramine, and MAOIs (e.g., phenelzine).

Phobic Disorders

Phobic disorder is the diagnosis when the case describes a **persistent, unreasonable, intense fear of situations, circumstances, or objects.** It is differentiated from posttraumatic stress disorder (PTSD) and acute stress disorder (ASD), which has a **history of a traumatic event** (threat to life or limb). There are no known eliciting events in phobic disorders associated with the onset of symptoms.

Agoraphobia

Fear or avoidance of places due to anxiety about not being able to escape (public places, being outside alone, public transportation, or crowds). Agoraphobia is more common in women.

Social Anxiety Disorder

Most common phobia: Fear or avoidance of **objects or situations** other than those involved in agoraphobia. Commonly involves animals (e.g., carnivores, spiders), natural environments (e.g., storms), injury (e.g., injections, blood), and situations (e.g., heights, darkness).

Treatment

Exposure therapy (involves increasing exposure to stimulus in order to induce habituation and decreased anxiety). **Benzodiazepines** and **beta-blockers** are helpful when given prior to exposure.

Basic Science Correlate

Benzodiazepines work by increasing GABA through increased **frequency** of chloride ions across neuronal cell membranes, resulting in decreased excitability of neurons.

Barbiturates work by increasing GABA through increased **duration** of chloride ions across the neuronal cell membranes, resulting in decreased excitability of neurons.

A 19-year-old ballet dancer presents because of extreme anxiety on stage. She reports that she fell 3 months ago at a national ballet competition and since then suffers extreme anxiety, trembling, diaphoresis, and breathlessness when she has to go on stage. She denies any problems with ballet practice and has no other medical problems. Which of the following is the most likely diagnosis?

a. Acute stress disorder
b. Adjustment disorder with anxious mood
c. Panic disorder
d. Social phobia

Answer: **C.** Panic disorder presents with a clear precipitating event which subsequently results in anxiety in similar circumstances. Panic disorder is differentiated from social phobia, which has no clear precipitating cause.

Generalized Anxiety Disorder (GAD)

Excessive, poorly controlled **anxiety that occurs daily for more than 6 months. No single event or focus** is related to the anxiety. It often coexists with major depression, specific phobia, social phobia, and panic disorder.

Treatment

Treatment consists of **supportive psychotherapy,** including relaxation training and biofeedback. Medications include **SSRIs, venlafaxine, buspirone, and benzodiazepines.**

Distinguish GAD from panic attack or social phobia by what is causing the anxiety. If the question describes persistent worry of a panic attack or social encounter, then GAD is not the answer. In GAD, multiple life circumstances, not just one, are causing the anxiety.

Anxiolytic Medications

Anxiolytics Prescribed for Anxiety Disorders		
Anxiety Disorder	**Anxiolytic**	**Benefits**
Adjustment disorder with anxious mood	Benzodiazepines with brief psychotherapy	Rapid onset to therapy
Panic disorder	SSRIs, alprazolam, and clonazepam	Decrease frequency and intensity of panic attacks
Generalized anxiety disorder (GAD)	Venlafaxine, other SSRIS, and buspirone	Decrease overall anxiety
OCD	SSRIs and clomipramine	Decrease obsessional thinking
Social phobia	SSRIs and buspirone	Decrease fear associated with social situations

Benzodiazepines

- Do *not* change dosages abruptly.
- Use the lowest dose in the elderly.
- Advise against using machinery or driving.
- In order from shortest to longest half-life: Alprazolam (Xanax) < lorazepam (Ativan) < diazepam (Valium)

Buspirone

- Therapeutic effect can take up to 1 week
- Can be used safely with other sedative-hypnotics (no additive effect)
- Best option for people with occupations where driving or machinery is involved, as there is no sedation or cognitive impairment
- No withdrawal syndrome

Basic Science Correlate

Buspirone is a serotonin 5-HT1A receptor partial agonist.

Obsessive-Compulsive Disorder (OCD)

OCD is the diagnosis when the case describes **recurrent obsessions or compulsions.** The case must also describe that the **individual recognizes that the behavior is unreasonable and excessive** (i.e., there is insight). **Obsessions** are anxiety provoking; thoughts are intrusive and are commonly related to contamination, doubt, guilt, aggression, and sex. **Compulsions** are peculiar behaviors that reduce the anxiety and are most commonly habitual hand washing, organizing, checking, counting, and praying. Patients with Tourette syndrome often also have OCD. **Depression** and **substance abuse** are common in OCD.

Obsessive symptoms in psychotic disorders may be misdiagnosed as OCD. You can **differentiate psychosis from OCD** by looking for a lack insight and loss of contact with reality.

Treatment

Behavioral psychotherapy and pharmacotherapy (**SSRIs** and **clomipramine**).

Trauma- and Stress-Related Disorders

Acute Stress Disorder (ASD) and Posttraumatic Stress Disorder (PTSD)

These disorders involve severe anxiety symptoms that follow a life-threatening event. ASD is diagnosed when symptoms **last less than 1 month and occur within 1 month of stressor.** PTSD is diagnosed when symptoms **last longer than 1 month.**

Following are 3 key symptom groups:

1. **Re-experiencing of the traumatic event:** Dreams, flashbacks, or intrusive recollections
2. **Avoidance of stimuli** associated with the trauma or **numbing** of general responsiveness
3. **Increased arousal:** Anxiety, sleep disturbances, hypervigilance, emotional lability, or impulsiveness

Treatment

Give benzodiazepines acutely for anxiety symptoms. SSRIs and other antidepressants can be helpful for long-term therapy.

A school bus is involved in a major collision. Two children are killed, and 7 others are injured. What is the most important therapy to prevent PTSD?

a. Diazepam
b. Fluoxetine
c. Group counseling
d. Haloperidol
e. Individual psychotherapy

Answer: **C.** Group counseling is the most effective therapy to prevent PTSD following a traumatic event.

Mood Disorders

Major Depressive Disorder

This disorder is characterized by **depressed mood** or **anhedonia** and depressive symptoms lasting **at least 2 weeks.**

Look for other causes of depression where the first step in management is different, such as the following:

- **Hypothyroidism:**
  - Check TSH
  - First step in management is thyroxine
- **Parkinson's disease:**
  - Treat with anti-Parkinson medications
- **Medications:**
  - Corticosteroids, β-blockers, antipsychotics (especially in the elderly), and reserpine
  - Treat by discontinuing medication and switching to an alternative
- **Substance disorders:**
  - Alcohol (ask CAGE questionnaire), amphetamines
  - Treat with detoxification and antidepressants

SIGECAPS: Major depressive disorder = depressed mood +

S: changes in *sleep*
I: loss of *interests*/pleasure
G: thoughts of worthlessness or *guilt*
E: loss of *energy*
C: trouble *concentrating*
A: changes in *appetite* or weight
P: changes in *psychomotor activity*
S: thoughts about death or *suicide*

Treatment

- **Admit the patient** if there is suicidal/homicidal ideation or paranoia.
- Begin **antidepressant medications** (SSRI is first drug of choice).
- Give **benzodiazepines** if agitated.
- **Electroconvulsive therapy (ECT)** is the best choice if the patient is acutely suicidal (works quicker than antidepressants) or for patients worried about side effects from medications.

In patients with unipolar psychotic depression, the combination of an antidepressant and an antipsychotic is more effective than monotherapy with either drug.

Dysthymic Disorder

Dysthymic disorder is characterized by **low-level depression symptoms** that are **present on most days for at least 2 years.** However the question may describe superimposed acute major depression, which is common in these patients. Do *not* hospitalize these patients unless there's suicidal ideation.

Treatment

Long-term individual, insight-oriented psychotherapy is the best treatment. If this fails, a trial of SSRIs is the next step in management.

Seasonal Affective Disorder

The diagnosis is seasonal affective disorder when the case describes **depressive symptoms in the winter months** (shorter daylight hours) and absence of depressive symptoms during summer months (longer daylight hours). Treatment is **phototherapy** or **sleep deprivation.**

Bipolar Disorder

Bipolar disorder is the diagnosis when the case describes episodes of **depression, mania, or mixed symptoms for at least 1 week** that cause distress or impaired functioning.

Bipolar disorder is the *most commonly missed* diagnosis in the USMLE, because it can easily be mistaken for depression or mania alone. The questions will describe a history of both manic symptoms and depressive symptoms, as well as periods of normal mood. **Rapid cycling bipolar** is indicated by > 4 episodes of mania per year.

Mania symptoms include grandiosity, less need for sleep, excessive talking or pressured speech, racing thoughts or flight of ideas, distractibility, goal-focused activity at home or at work, or sexual promiscuity. **Major depressive symptoms** include depressed mood or loss of pleasure or interest.

CCS Tip: If the history suggests drug use, first get a drug screen to rule out **amphetamine use** as a cause of mania. If the history gives elevated blood pressure or low TSH, consider medical conditions, such as **pheochromocytoma** and **hyperthyroidism.**

Steps in Management of Acute Mania

1) **Hospitalize**
2) **Mood stabilizers** to induce remission. Lithium is the drug of choice (takes 1 week for effect).
3) **Antipsychotics** to control acute mania. Drug of choice is risperidone.
4) Give **IM depot phenothiazine** in noncompliant, severely manic patients.
5) Give antidepressants *only* in patients with recurrent episodes of depression and *only* with mood stabilizers (to prevent inducing manic episode).

a. What is the most common cause of progression to rapid cycling bipolar?
b. How should you manage rapid cycling bipolar?
c. What other medical conditions predispose a patient to rapid cycling bipolar?
d. What drug has been shown to prevent suicidal ideation in bipolar disorder?
e. A 32-year-old known bipolar patient who is undergoing maintenance therapy with lithium presents with a positive pregnancy test. How will you manage this patient's bipolar disorder?

Answers:

a. **Use of antidepressants:** Do not give antidepressants prophylactically unless the question describes previous severe depressive episodes. In that case, antidepressants are only given for a few weeks.
b. **Gradually stop** all antidepressants, stimulants, caffeine, benzodiazepines, and alcohol.
c. **Hypothyroidism:** Check TSH in any patient with rapid cycling bipolar and replace thyroid hormones if needed.
d. **Lithium**
e. **Discontinue lithium** (to avoid heart abnormalities): Choose **ECT therapy** for first-trimester patients with manic episodes. Use **lamotrigine** in 2nd or 3rd trimester.

Treatment

- First-line treatment: monotherapy with lithium, lamotrigine, or risperidone
- Second-line treatment: **aripiprazole**, divalproex, **quetiapine**, and **olanzapine**
- Patients with multiple recurrences require combination therapy.
- Always plan for psychotherapy and cognitive behavioral therapy.
- Avoid teratogenic drugs such as lithium, valproate, and carbamazepine in female patients.

> Lithium can lead to Ebstein's anomaly and diabetes insipidus.

Cyclothymia

When the patient presents with a history of **recurrent episodes of depressed mood and hypomanic mood for at least 2 years,** the diagnosis is cyclothymia. It resembles a milder form of bipolar affective disorder.

Treatment

Psychotherapy is the first step in management. Many people function without medications and learn to manage their hypomanic dispositions (especially artists). Start **divalproex** when functioning is impaired. Divalproex is more effective in cyclothymia than lithium.

Grief and Depression

Grief	Depression
Sadness, tearfulness, decreased sleep, decreased appetite, decreased interest in the world	
Symptoms wax and wane	Symptoms are pervasive and unremitting
Shame and guilt are less common	Shame and guilt are common
Suicidal ideation is less common	Suicidal ideation is more common
Symptoms can last up to 1–2 years	Symptoms continue for more than 1 year
Patient usually returns to baseline level of functioning within 2 months	Patient does not return to baseline functioning
Treatment includes **supportive therapy**	Treatment includes **antidepressant medications**

A 32-year-old woman who gave birth 4 months ago is brought in by her husband because of depressed mood. The husband reports that she has been depressed since the birth of her child, refuses to eat, has trouble sleeping, and is unable to concentrate. The woman reports that she has lost interest in everything and sometimes can't even get out of bed. She reports that she's recently had visions of seeing her deceased mother talking to her and criticizing her skills as a new mother. She also admits that she hears her voice talk to her constantly too. She denies homicidal or suicidal ideation. Which of the following is the best initial treatment?

a. Psychotherapy
b. Behavioral therapy
c. Sertraline
d. Risperidone
e. Phenelzine

Answer: **D.** Patients with both mood and psychotic symptoms respond to both antidepressants and antipsychotic medication. However, you must **treat the worst symptom first.** In this case, the antipsychotic would be most indicated to reduce her psychotic symptoms.

A 45-year-old woman presents 2 months after the sudden loss of her son in a car accident. She reports "not being able to cope well." She is constantly teary, has lost her appetite, and has decreased 2 dress sizes. She finds herself laying out a dinner plate every night for him. Recently, she believes she has heard his voice and every night she has nightmares about the car accident. She denies suicidal ideation. Which of the following is the most appropriate next step in management?

a. Group therapy
b. Amitriptyline
c. Fluoxetine
d. Zolpidem
e. Supportive therapy

Answer: **E.** This patient is undergoing normal grief reaction. Auditory hallucinations without other psychotic symptoms are normal in grief reaction.

Postpartum Depression

	Postpartum Blues or "Baby Blues"	Postpartum Depression	Postpartum Psychosis
Onset	After any birth	Usually after 2nd birth	Usually after 1st birth
Mother's emotions toward baby	Cares about baby	Many have thoughts about hurting the baby	Many have thoughts about hurting the baby
Symptoms	Mild depressive	Severe depressive	Look for psychotic symptoms along with severe depressive symptoms
Treatment	Self-limited; no treatment necessary	Antidepressants	Mood stabilizers or antipsychotics and antidepressants *TIP:* Avoid medications if patient is breastfeeding; instead choose electroconvulsive therapy (ECT).

Suicide and Suicidal Ideation

Management of the Suicidal Patient	
Ask about risk factors:	**Emergency Assessment**
• **History of suicide threats and attempts is the most important predictor of suicide** • Family history of suicide • Perceived hopelessness (demoralization) • Schizophrenia/borderline or antisocial PD • Drug use, especially alcohol • Males/age > 65 • Socially isolated/recently divorced or widowed • Chronic physical illness • Low job satisfaction or unemployment	• Take all suicide threats seriously • Detain and hospitalize (usually a couple of weeks) • Never transport patient to emergency department without medically trained personnel accompanying patient • Do not identify with the patient • Do not leave patient unsupervised • Treatment of choice = psychotherapy + antidepressant medications (SSRIs are first choice) • For acute, severe risk of self-harm, treatment of choice is electroconvulsive therapy (ECT)

Indications for Electroconvulsive Therapy (ECT)

- Major depressive episodes that are unresponsive to medications
- High risk for immediate suicide
- Contraindications to using antidepressant medications
- Good response to ECT in the past

ECT is safe in pregnancy.

Caution: The biggest complication of ECT is **transient memory loss,** which worsens with prolonged therapy and resolves after several weeks. Use of ECT is *cautioned* in patients with space-occupying intracranial lesions (e.g., brain metastasis), as ECT induces transient intracranial pressure.

Antidepressants and Mood Stabilizers

Guidelines for Use of Antidepressants

- SSRIs are first-line therapy.

Basic Science Correlate

SSRIs inhibit the reuptake of serotonin in the synaptic cleft, resulting in more signaling across the synapses.

In TCA overdose, the most urgent next step is to check an EKG for life-threatening arrhythmias.

SSRIs are first-line therapy for many conditions because of their therapeutic effect and low side effect profile. Always think of SSRIs first in patients with the following disorders:

- Major depressive disorder
- Bipolar disorder
- Anxiety disorders: Panic disorder, OCD, social phobia, generalized anxiety disorder
- Bulimia nervosa

- TCAs are avoided because of risk of toxicity (think: **T**CA may be **T**oxic).
- MAOIs are more helpful in atypical depressive disorders.
- Choose an antidepressant based on side effect profile.
- Switch to another antidepressant if patient does not respond after 8 weeks or if the patient does not tolerate the side effects.
- Treat patients for 6 months and attempt to discontinue after tapering. Consider long-term therapy for multiple episodes of depression.
- When the question describes a patient concerned about weight gain or sexual side effects, give **bupropion** (causes modest weight loss). Note: Bupropion is associated with **seizures.**
- When the question describes a patient who has poor appetite, loss of weight, or insomnia, give **mirtazapine.** Mirtazapine is associated with weight gain.
- **Amitriptyline** is used to treat chronic pain (especially effective in neuropathic pain).
- **Imipramine** is useful in enuresis.
- **Trazodone** is strongly sedating and is often used to treat depressed patients who have severe insomnia.
- SSRIs and TCAs are **safe in pregnancy** *except* for paroxetine (Paxil).

A young male recently started on antidepressants develops prolonged erection. What is the antidepressant he was most likely taking?

Answer: **Trazodone**

An elderly patient presents with depression and agitation. What is the most appropriate medication?

Answer: Give an **antidepressant with sedative effects** (e.g., doxepin, trazodone). Amitriptyline is also sedating but has anticholinergic effects, which may be problematic in elderly.

A 25-year-old male with history of seizures is diagnosed with depression. Which medications should be avoided?

Answer: Seizures are common with **TCAs and bupropion**, and these medications should be avoided in patients with seizure disorders. The best first-line therapy in patients with seizures is SSRIs.

A middle-aged woman is brought into the ER with confusion and disorientation. An overdose of prescription medications is suspected. Blood pressure is 90/53 mm Hg, HR 111/min. Pupils are dilated, mucous membranes are dry, and she has facial flushing.

1. **What is the most likely cause of acute intoxication?**
2. **What is the most important test to determine severity and prognosis in this patient?**
   a. EKG
   b. EEG
   c. Serum sodium
   d. Serum tricyclic levels
   e. Urinalysis
3. **EKG is performed and shows PR and QRS prolongation and sinus tachycardia. What is the most appropriate next step in management?**
   a. Calcium carbonate
   b. Diazepam
   c. Gastric lavage
   d. Insulin and glucose
   e. Sodium bicarbonate

Answers:

1. **Tricyclic antidepressants (TCAs):** TCAs have anticholinergic effects and are an alpha blocker, causing peripheral vasodilatation and hypotension and also affecting sodium channels in cardiac tissue.
2. **A.** EKG is the single most important test to guide therapy and prognosis. Watch out for prolonged QRS, QT, and PR intervals. Most serious complication is ventricular tachycardia and fibrillation.
3. **E.** Sodium bicarbonate attenuates TCA cardiotoxicity by alkalinization of blood, which uncouples TCA from myocardial sodium channels and increases extracellular sodium concentration, thereby improving the gradient across the channel.

A 42-year-old woman with a history of hypertension, diabetes, and depression presents to the clinic with dry eyes and dry mouth. Her medications include hydrochlorothiazide, metformin, and amitriptyline. Which of the following is the next step in management?

a. Discontinue amitriptyline and change to sertraline
b. Order antinuclear antibodies
c. Order SS-Ro and SS-La
d. Prescribe eye drops
e. Refer to ophthalmologist

Answer: **A.** Discontinue amitriptyline and switch to another antidepressant medication with little/no anticholinergic effects. Anticholinergic effects are most severe with amitriptyline, but there are almost none with most SSRIs.

Lithium

Lithium is the first-line medication for **bipolar and schizoaffective disorders** and treatment and prophylaxis of mood episodes. Side effects are a major reason for noncompliance. These include the following:

- **Acne and weight gain** are the most common problems.
- **Dose-related tremors, GI distress, and headaches** (decrease the dose)
- **Hypothyroidism** (5 percent)
- **Polyuria** secondary to medication-induced diabetes insipidus
- Do *not* use in first trimester of pregnancy. Lithium causes **cardiac defects.**

Divalproex

Divalproex is the first-line choice for **rapid-cycling bipolar disorder** or when lithium is ineffective, impractical, or contraindicated.

Carbamazepine

Carbamazepine is the **second-line therapy for bipolar disorder** when lithium and divalproex are ineffective or contraindicated. It is not commonly used because of serious **agranulocytosis** and significant **sedation.**

Basic Science Correlate

Carbamazepine affects the inactivated state of voltage-gated Na^+ channels, making fewer channels available to open. Carbamazepine is a CYP450 inducer, and it increases the clearance of warfarin, phenytoin, theophylline, and valproic acid.

Medication Overdoses

> **High yield topic:**
> Know the different features of lithium toxicity, MAOI-induced hypertension, serotonin syndrome, and neuroleptic malignant syndrome.

Lithium Toxicity

Suspect lithium toxicity when the question describes an **elderly** patient who takes **lithium** with **renal failure** or **hyponatremia** (may be caused by diuretics, vomiting, dehydration). The question will describe nausea, vomiting, acute disorientation, tremors, increased DTRs, and even seizures. The treatment of choice is **dialysis.**

> **Basic Science Correlate**
>
> Lithium can also result in nephrogenic diabetes insipidus. Lithium accumulates in the collecting duct through epithelial sodium channels. This leads to resistance to ADH by increasing urinary prostaglandin E2, which induces lysosomal degradation of aquaporin 2 water channels.

Neuroleptic Malignant Syndrome (NMS)

The question will describe a patient who **recently started taking antipsychotics** (particularly haloperidol) or a Parkinson's patient who has **recently stopped levodopa.** Look for **high fever, tachycardia, muscle rigidity, altered consciousness, elevated CPK, and autonomic dysfunction.** This syndrome is unrelated to dosage or previous drug exposure. There is a 20 percent mortality rate.

> **Basic Science Correlate**
>
> Antipsychotics cause NMS through D2 receptor blockade in the hypothalamus, nigrostriatal pathways, and spinal cord. This leads to muscle rigidity, tremor via extrapyramidal, and elevated temperature in the hypothalamus. In the periphery, antipsychotics lead to increased calcium release from the sarcoplasmic reticulum, which leads to rigidity and muscle cell breakdown.

Treatment

- **Transfer to the ICU**
- **Discontinue antipsychotic**
- Give **bromocriptine** to overcome dopamine receptor blockade. Bromocriptine is a potent dopamine D2 receptor agonist.
- Give muscle relaxants **dantrolene** or **diazepam** to reduce muscle rigidity

Serotonin Syndrome

Serotonin syndrome is the diagnosis when the case describes a **history of SSRI use** and the **use of migraine medication** (triptans) **or a MAOI.** The patient will present with **agitation, hyperreflexia, hyperthermia, and muscle rigidity with volume contraction** secondary to sweating and insensible fluid loss.

Treatment

- IV fluids
- Cyproheptadine to decrease serotonin production. Cyproheptadine is a histamine-1 receptor antagonist with nonspecific 5-HT1A and 5-HT2A antagonistic properties.
- Benzodiazepine to reduce muscle rigidity

MAOI-Induced Hypertensive Crisis

Consider this diagnosis if the history describes a patient with **acute hypertension and a history of MAOI use** and either **antihistamines, nasal decongestants, or consumption of tyramine-rich foods** (cheeses, pickled foods). May also be seen in patients who take a MAOI and a TCA concurrently.

Basic Science Correlate

MAOIs inhibit the breakdown of dietary amines. This raises levels of tyramine, which in turn displaces norepinephrine from the storage vesicles, leading to hypertensive crisis.

Treatment

Treat as hypertensive crisis. There is no specific antihypertensive indicated.

What is the first assessment prior to prescribing antidepressants?

a. Complete blood count
b. Family history of depression
c. Previous use of antidepressants
d. Suicidal ideation
e. Thyroid function tests

Answer: **D.** Always assess for suicidal ideation prior to starting antidepressants, as there is an increased risk in suicidal ideation in some patients within the first 2 weeks. Know how to manage acute suicidal ideation. If the patient is acutely suicidal, you must hospitalize and consider electroconvulsive therapy, which can help mood in an acute setting.

Somatic Symptom and Related Disorders

A somatic symptom disorder is the correct diagnosis when the case describes **physical symptoms without medical explanation.** The symptoms are severe enough to **interfere with the patient's ability to function** in social or occupational activities.

A 47-year-old woman presents to the clinic with shortness of breath, chest pain, abdominal pain, back pain, double vision, and difficulty walking due to weakness in her legs. She remembers being sick all of the time for the past 10 years. According to her husband, she constantly takes medications for all of her ailments. She has visited numerous physicians and none has been able to diagnose her condition correctly. What is the next step in management?

a. Order ANA
b. Order CT of the abdomen
c. Order CT of the head
d. Hospitalize
e. Schedule regular monthly visits

Answer: **E.** Scheduling regular monthly visits to establish a single physician as the primary caregiver is the most important first step in management.

Management

1. Maintain a **single physician** as the primary caretaker.
2. Schedule **brief monthly visits.**
3. *Avoid* diagnostic testing or therapies.
4. Schedule **individual psychotherapy.**
5. Do *not* hospitalize the patient.

Conversion Disorder

Conversion disorder is the diagnosis when there are **one or more neurologic symptoms** that **cannot be explained by any medical or neurologic disorder.** Most common symptoms are mutism, blindness, paralysis, and anesthesia/paresthesias. Look for psychologic factors associated with the onset or exacerbation of symptoms. A clue to diagnosis is that patients often **are unconcerned about their impairment** (*la belle indifference*). You must first rule out other medical conditions.

Management

- Supportive physician-patient relationship
- Psychotherapy

Factitious and Malingering Disorders

In both factitious disorder and malingering, the case will suggest that a patient has **intentionally feigned symptoms.**

- The diagnosis is **factitious disorder** when the case describes a patient that has **seen many doctors** and **visited many hospitals,** has **large amount of medical knowledge** (e.g., health care worker), and **demands treatment.** They are typically agitated and threaten litigation if tests return negative.
- The diagnosis is **factitious disorder by proxy** if the signs and symptoms are **faked by another person,** as in a mother making up symptoms in her child. The motivation is to assume the caretaker role.
- **Malingering** is the diagnosis when obvious gain (shelter, medications, disability insurance) results from feigned symptoms. Malingering patients are more **preoccupied with rewards or gain** than with alleviation of presenting symptoms.

A 23-year-old nursing student presents to the emergency department with fever and chills at home. She has had multiple admissions in other hospitals because of pneumonia and chronic pain problems. She was found to be tampering with the blood culture bottles and dipping her temperature thermometer in hot water. Which of the following is the most likely diagnosis?

a. Conversion disorder
b. Factitious disorder
c. Factitious disorder by proxy
d. Malingering
e. Obsessive-compulsive disorder

Answer: **B.**

A 46-year-old homeless man presents to the hospital reporting that he had a seizure this morning. He is adamant that he be admitted, however, he refuses all blood work and imaging studies. He cannot answer questions about the seizure and cannot describe his symptoms at the time of the seizure. Instead he demands to be admitted and is wondering why you're taking so long. When you ask about his social history, he admits that he is homeless at the moment as he was "kicked out of the shelter" because of drug-taking and alcohol abuse. Which of the following is the most likely diagnosis?

a. Conversion disorder
b. Factitious disorder
c. Factitious disorder by proxy
d. Malingering
e. Borderline personality disorder

Answer: **D.**

Treatment

- **Supportive psychotherapy** is the treatment of choice.
- Do *not* confront or accuse the patient (the patient will become angry, more guarded, and suspicious).
- Only **provide the minimum amount of treatment and workup** needed. Aggressive management of the patient's symptoms only reinforces the behavior.

Eating Disorders and Other Impulse Control Disorders

Eating Disorders

Following are the 3 main eating disorders that you need to distinguish on the exam:

1. **Anorexia nervosa**
2. **Bulimia nervosa**
3. **Body dysmorphic disorder**

Anorexia Nervosa

The diagnosis is anorexia nervosa when the case describes a **young female** who is **underweight** because of **food restriction and excessive exercise.** The question may also include a **history of purging** (50 percent of anorexia nervosa patients also purge), but the diagnosis will still be anorexia nervosa.

Bulimia Nervosa

The diagnosis is bulimia nervosa when the case describes a **young female** in **normal weight range** with episodes of **binge eating followed by guilt, anxiety, and self-induced vomiting, laxative, diuretics, or enema use.** These episodes must occur at least once a week. Food restriction is *not* a feature of bulimia nervosa. Look for painless parotid gland enlargement and dental enamel erosions. Electrolyte disturbances are common (metabolic alkalosis, hypochloremia, and hypokalemia caused by emesis; metabolic acidosis caused by laxative abuse). There is a risk of cardiomyopathy with excessive syrup of ipecac use.

Treatment

Treat anorexia nervosa and bulimia nervosa as follows:

- **Hospitalize for IV hydration** if electrolyte disturbances are present
- **Olanzapine** in anorexia nervosa helps with weight gain
- **SSRI antidepressants** (especially fluoxetine) prevent relapses
- Prescribe **behavioral psychotherapy**

Body Dysmorphic Disorder

The diagnosis is body dysmorphic disorder when the case describes a **young woman** who is preoccupied with an **imagined or slight defect in appearance,** causing distress and **impaired ability to function in a social or occupational setting.** The distress is most commonly related to facial features, although any body part may be the focus of anxiety. The patients are often isolated and housebound.

Treatment

- **High doses of SSRIs** are first-line therapy.
- If the only concern is body shape and weight, anorexia nervosa is the more accurate diagnosis.
- If the only concern is sex characteristics, gender identity disorder is the more accurate diagnosis.

Disruptive, Impulse Control, and Conduct Disorders

These occur in people who are unable to resist impulses. The question will describe anxiety prior to the impulse that is relieved after the patient acts on the impulse.

> Check urine toxicology for cocaine in patients with intermittent explosive disorder.

- **Intermittent explosive disorder:** This is the diagnosis when the case describes episodes of **aggression out of proportion to the stressor.** There may be a history of head trauma. If there is a history of drug intake, intermittent explosive disorder is *not* the diagnosis. It must be found in someone age > 6 and occur, on average, twice weekly for 3 months or involve more destructive episodes (assault) 3 times within a 12-month period. Treatment of choice is **SSRIs** and **mood stabilizers.**
- **Kleptomania:** This is the diagnosis when the case describes an individual who **repeatedly steals items to relieve anxiety.** The person does *not* steal because she needs the object, and the individual often secretly replaces the object after stealing it.
- **Pyromania:** This is the diagnosis when the case describes an individual who **repeatedly lights fires.** Pyromania is *not* the diagnosis if the motive is personal gain (i.e., insurance money) or to show anger, which differentiates this from conduct disorder.
- **Pathologic gambling:** This is the diagnosis when the case describes **obsession with gambling despite the consequences.** Treatment of choice is group psychotherapy (e.g., gambling anonymous).

Individuals with impulse control disorders do not believe their actions are excessive or out of proportion (i.e., they lack insight), unlike in OCD.

Psychosocial Problems

Types of Abuse

Class	Child Abuse	Adult Maltreatment/ Elder Abuse	Spousal Abuse
Definition of abuse	• **Physical is the most common** (look for bruises, burns, lacerations, broken bones, shaken baby syndrome—do eye exam) • Neglect • Sexual exploitation (STDs) • Mental cruelty	• **Neglect is the most common** (50% of all reported cases) • Physical • Psychological • Financial	• **Physical is the most common—it is the** number one cause of injury to American women • Psychological • Financial
Physician's role in care	1. Mandatory reporting up to age 18. You must report *all* suspected cases. 2. Protect the child (separate from parents) and consider admission to hospital.	1. You must report *all* suspected cases. 2. Protect patient from abuser and consider admission to hospital.	1. Reporting is not indicated. 2. Provide information about local shelters and counseling.
Those at risk	• Younger than 1 year • Stepchildren • Premature children • Very active children • "Defective" children	• Caretaker is the most likely source of abuse; spouses are often caretakers	• More frequent in families with drug abuse, especially alcoholism • Victim often grew up in a violent home (about 50%) • Married at a young age • Dependent personalities • Pregnant, last trimester (highest risk)
Exam points	• Be careful not to mistake benign cultural practices, such as "coining" or "moxibustion," for child abuse. • Treat female circumcision as abuse.	• Mandatory reporting to Adult Protective Services	

Personality Disorders (PD)

When the case describes **self-aggression** or **self-mutilation,** the diagnosis is often **passive-aggressive personality disorder** (example of acting out).

Personality disorders are pervasive, inflexible, and maladaptive thoughts or behaviors. More males have antisocial and narcissistic PDs; more females have borderline and histrionic PDs.

Treatment

- Psychotherapy
- Use of mood stabilizers and antidepressants is sometimes useful for Cluster B PDs.

FEATURES	EXAMPLES
Cluster A: **Peculiar thought processes, inappropriate affect**	
Paranoid PD: • **Distrust and suspiciousness** - Individuals are mistrustful and suspicious of the motivations and actions of others and are often secretive and isolated. - They are emotionally cold and odd. - They often take legal action against other people. • **Often confused with paranoid schizophrenia.** • **Main defense mechanism is projection.**	A 62-year-old man lives in an apartment and constantly accuses his neighbors of stealing his mail and prying into his apartment. He believes that all his neighbors are conspiring to have him removed from the building.
Schizoid PD: • **Detachment and restricted emotionality** - Individuals are emotionally distant and fear intimacy with others. - They are absorbed in their own thoughts and feelings and disinterested. • **Main defense mechanism is projection**	A 68-year-old man lives in the country-side manning a lighthouse near a remote village. He is seen in town 2–3 times a year to purchase supplies. He has no known friends or family.
Schizotypal PD: • **Discomfort with social relationships, thought distortion, eccentricity** - Like schizoid PD except they also have magical thinking, clairvoyance, ideas of reference, or paranoid ideation. • **Symptoms aren't severe enough for classification of schizophrenia**	A 28-year-old man lives in a small coastal town attempting to start his own internet herbal business. He believes that the herbs have magical powers and he sells their magical properties of healing for a living. He believes that spirits are guiding him to wealth.
Cluster B: **Mood lability, dissociative symptoms, preoccupation with rejection**	
• **Histrionic PD:** - Colorful, exaggerated behavior and excitable, shallow expression of emotions - Use of physical appearance to draw attention to self - Sexually seductive - Discomfort in situations where not the center of attention.	A 30-year-old woman presents to the doctor's office dressed in a sexually seductive manner and insists that the doctor comment on her appearance. When the doctor refuses to do so, she becomes upset.

FEATURES	EXAMPLES
Borderline PD: • Unstable affect, mood swings, marked impulsivity, unstable relationships, recurrent suicidal behaviors, chronic feelings of emptiness, identity disturbance, and inappropriate anger. Become intensely angered if they feel abandoned. • **Main defense mechanism is splitting.**	A 30-year-old woman presents to the clinic. She reports that she has been to many doctors, she said they were all wonderful until they started ignoring her or cutting her visits short, then she realized what terrible doctors they were. She starts the visit saying that the assistant at the front desk is the "worst she's ever seen" because she didn't smile at her. The other assistant was just wonderful according to her.
Antisocial PD: • Usually characterized by continuous antisocial or criminal acts, inability to conform to social rules, impulsivity, disregard for the rights of others, aggressiveness, lack of remorse, and deceitfulness.	A 26-year-old man is caught lighting forest fires during a recent spate. He has a history of legal problems since childhood. He reports that his mother is to blame. He denies feeling regret. He has no friends and is found to be hostile to everyone at the police station.
Narcissistic PD: • Usually characterized by a sense of self-importance, grandiosity, and preoccupation with fantasies of success. This person believes he is special, requires excessive admiration, reacts with rage when criticized, lacks empathy, is envious of others, and is interpersonally exploitative.	A patient is in the hospital for chest pain and becomes very agitated because he feels he is not getting enough attention. He reports that he is an important CEO and demands a special VIP room and more consideration and a dedicated nurse to attend his needs.
Cluster C: **Anxiety, preoccupation with criticism or rigidity**	
Avoidant PD: • Individuals have social inhibition, feelings of inadequacy, and hypersensitivity to criticism. They shy away from starting anything new or attending social gatherings for fear of failure or rejection. They desire affection and acceptance and are open about their isolation and inability to interact with others.	A 45-year-old single man fears an upcoming social party being hosted by his parents. He dreads having to meet other people and doesn't feel comfortable speaking with others. He is planning on staying at home to avoid speaking to others.
Dependent PD: • **Submissive and clinging behavior related to a need to be taken care of.** Individuals are consumed with the need to be taken care of. They are clingy and worry about abandonment. They feel inadequate and helpless and avoid disagreements with others. They usually focus dependency on a family member or spouse.	A 28-year-old woman seeks counseling because of a recent relationship breakup. They were dating for 6 months. She continues to call her ex 15–20 times a day even though he does not pick up. She says she can't understand why they broke up because she never disagreed with him. She never left the house without him, and she always asked for his opinion, even for little decisions. She cannot imagine a life without him.
Obsessive-Compulsive PD: • Individuals are preoccupied with orderliness, perfectionism, and control. They are often consumed by the details of everything and lose their sense of overall goals. They are strict and perfectionistic, overconscientious, and inflexible. Associated with difficult interpersonal relationships. • **Differentiated from obsessive-compulsive disorder.**	A 38-year-old man presents with his wife for marital counseling. The wife reports that he is inflexible and has unrealistic demands of orderliness and an inflexible schedule. Both partners agree that his demands are causing marital problems.

Substance Use Disorders

Step 3 will test your ability to **recognize substance abuse** and **know the best management** for acute substance use and acute withdrawal.

Alcohol Dependence (Alcoholism)

Alcohol dependence is the frequent use of alcohol resulting in **tolerance and physical and psychological dependence. Alcohol abuse** is when episodes of alcohol use result in **failure to fulfill obligations, craving or strong urge to use a substance, or exposure to physically dangerous situations.** Tolerance is *not* included in the diagnosis of alcohol abuse.

Basic Science Correlate

Ethanol is converted to acetaldehyde by alcohol dehydrogenase.

Basic Science Correlate

Alcohol follows zero-order elimination kinetics, in which a constant quantity per time unit of the drug is eliminated.

Diagnosis

The most accurate diagnosis is made with the **CAGE questionnaire.** Laboratory tests are *never* included in the diagnosis of alcohol abuse.

CAGE: An answer of yes to any 2 of the following questions is suggestive of alcohol abuse:

- Have you ever felt that you should Cut down your drinking?
- Have you ever felt Annoyed by others who have criticized your drinking?
- Have you ever felt Guilty about your drinking?
- Have you ever had an Eye-opener to steady your nerves or alleviate a hang-over?

When the question describes a patient with alcohol abuse, do the following:

- **Order toxicology** to look for use of other drugs: breath, blood, and urine drug screens.

- Look for **secondary effects** of alcohol use (but *not* for diagnosis): elevated GGTP, AST, ALT, and LDH.
- If there's suggestion of IV drug use (e.g., track marks), order HIV, hepatitis B, hepatitis C, and PPD (for tuberculosis).

Management

If the question asks for the most effective management of alcohol abuse or prevention of relapse, the correct answer is Alcoholics Anonymous (AA).

Basic Science Correlate

Disulfiram inhibits the enzyme acetaldehyde dehydrogenase, leading to a rise in acetaldehyde. Acetaldehyde is responsible for the vomiting, headache, tachycardia, and sweating.

Acute Outpatient Management of Alcohol Dependence	Acute Inpatient Management Pearls	Chronic Maintenance Management
1) Prevent further ETOH intake 2) Prevent individual from driving a car, operating machinery 3) Sedate patient if he or she becomes agitated 4) Transfer to inpatient	1) Look for withdrawal symptoms 2) Prevent Wernicke-Korsakoff (ataxia, nystagmus, ophthalmoplegia, amnesia): Give IV or IM thiamine and magnesium ASAP; also give B12 and folate 3) Benzodiazepine of choice is **chlordiazepoxide** or **diazepam** 4) Choose short-acting benzodiazepam *only* if the question describes patient with severe liver disease (prevent toxic metabolites)—**lorazepam** or **oxazepam** 5) Do *not* give seizure prophylaxis; repeated seizures should be treated with diazepam 6) Haldol is *never* the answer (reduces seizure threshold)	1) Refer to inpatient rehabilitation or outpatient group therapy (e.g., AA) 2) Never give drug therapy without group psychotherapy 3) Naloxone and acamprosate decrease relapse rate *only* when given with psychotherapy 4) Disulfiram has poor compliance and hasn't been shown to be effective

Withdrawal Syndrome	Minor Withdrawal Symptoms	Alcoholic Hallucinosis	Withdrawal Seizure	Delirium Tremens
Onset After Last Drink	6 hours	12–24 hours	48 hours	48–96 hours
Symptoms	Insomnia, tremulousness, mild anxiety, headache, diaphoresis, palpitations	Visual hallucinations There may also be auditory and tactile hallucinations.	Tonic-clonic seizures	Hallucinations, disorientation, tachycardia, hypertension, low-grade fever, agitation, and diaphoresis
Exam Tips	Give thiamine, folate, multivitamin, and glucose	If there are hallucinations with disorientation, altered mental status, alcoholic hallucinosis is *not* the answer.	Get CT scan if repeated seizures to rule out structural or infectious cause.	Time of onset is important. This is the diagnosis if the case describes symptoms 2 days after last drink.

A 38-year-old man presents to the emergency department with acute-onset, right lower quadrant abdominal pain. He undergoes an appendectomy. Two days after surgery, he is found in his room disorientated and agitated, and he is claiming to see snakes in his room. Physical exam reveals tachycardia and temperature of 101.2°F. Which of the following is the most likely diagnosis?

a. Alcoholic hallucinosis
b. Delirium tremens
c. Korsakoff's psychosis
d. Fentanyl withdrawal
e. Pulmonary embolism

Answer: **B.** Delirium tremens should always be suspected. The clue is that symptoms occur more than 2 days after the last drink. The question doesn't need to give you a history of alcohol use.

Substance	Signs and Symptoms of Intoxication	Treatment of Intoxication	Signs and Symptoms of Withdrawal	Treatment of Withdrawal
Alcohol	Talkative, sullen gregarious, moody	Mechanical ventilation if severe	Tremors, hallucinations, seizures, delirium	Long-acting benzo's No seizure prophylaxis Disulfiram or naloxone for adjunct to supervised therapy after acute withdrawal
Amphetamines, cocaine	Euphoria, hypervigilance, autonomic hyperactivity, weight loss, pupil dilatation, disturbed perception, stroke, myocardial infarction	Short-term use of antipsychotics, benzodiazepines, inderal, vitamin C to promote excretion	Anxiety, tremors, headache, increased appetite, depression, risk of suicide	Antidepressants
Cannabis	Impaired motor coordination, impaired time perception, social withdrawal, increased appetite, dry mouth, tachycardia, conjunctival redness	None	None	None

(continued next page)

Basic Science Correlate

Cocaine blocks the reuptake of norepinephrine serotonin and dopamine, while amphetamines induce the release of dopamine.

Substance	Signs and Symptoms of Intoxication	Treatment of Intoxication	Signs and Symptoms of Withdrawal	Treatment of Withdrawal
Hallucinogens (e.g., LSD)	Ideas of reference, hallucinations, impaired judgment, dissociative symptoms, pupil dilatation, panic, tremors, incoordination	Supportive counseling (talking down), antipsychotics, benzodiazepines	None	None
Inhalants	Belligerence, apathy, assaultiveness, impaired judgment, blurred vision, stupor, coma	Antipsychotics if delirious or agitated	None	None
Opiates	Apathy, dysphoria, constricted pupils, drowsiness, slurred speech, impaired memory, coma, death	Naloxone	Fever, chills, lacrimation, runny node, abdominal cramps, muscle spasms, insomnia, yawning	Clonidine, methadone
PCP	Panic reactions, assaultiveness, agitation, nystagmus, HTN, seizures, coma, hyperacusis	Talking down, benzodiazepines, antipsychotics, support respiratory function	None	None
Barbiturates and Benzodiazepines	Inappropriate sexual or aggressive behavior, impaired memory or concentration	Flumazenil	Autonomic hyperactivity, tremors, insomnia, seizures, anxiety	Substitute short- with long-acting barbiturates (chlordiazepoxide or phenobarbitol)

Basic Science Correlate

Opiates bind to mu, kappa, and/or delta receptors.

Treatment

- Naltrexone implant has been shown to be effective in long-term treatment of opioid dependence, alcohol dependence, and (most recently) poly-drug dependence.
- Acamprosate and disulferam have been used in alcohol dependence.
- Antidepressants are the wrong answer for patients with alcohol dependence without a comorbid mental disorder.

Human Sexuality

Homosexuality

Homosexuality is *not* a mental illness but instead is classified as a variant of human sexuality.

Gender Identity Disorder and Transsexualism

This is the answer when the case describes an individual who **insists that he/she is the opposite gender** and experiences **intense discomfort about his or her sex.** It is *not* the diagnosis when the question describes an individual **who desires to be another gender because of the perceived advantages of the other sex** (e.g., a boy who says he wants to be a girl so that he will receive the same special treatment as his younger sister).

Pharmacological Agents That Cause Sexual Dysfunction

Drug	Effect
α1-blockers	Impaired ejaculation
SSRIs	Inhibited orgasm
β-blockers	Erectile dysfunction
Trazodone	Priapism
Dopamine agonists	↑ erection and libido
Neuroleptics	Erectile dysfunction

Paraphilic Disorder

Paraphilias involves **recurrent, sexually arousing preoccupations,** which are usually focused on humiliation and/or suffering and the use of nonliving objects and nonconsenting partners. Occurs for **more than 6 months** and causes **impairment in patient's level of functioning.** Treatment of choice: **Individual psychotherapy and aversive conditioning.** If severe impairment, give antiandrogens or SSRIs to help reduce patient's sexual drive.

Types of Paraphilias

- **Voyeurism:** Recurrent urges to observe an unsuspecting person who is engaging in sexual activity or disrobing. This is the earliest paraphilia to develop.
- **Pedophilia:** Recurrent urges or arousal toward prepubescent children. Most common paraphilia.
- **Exhibitionism:** Recurrent urge to expose oneself to strangers
- **Fetishism:** Involves the use of nonliving objects usually associated with the human body.
- **Frotteurism:** Recurrent urge or behavior involving touching or rubbing against a nonconsenting partner
- **Masochism:** Recurrent urge or behavior involving the act of humiliation
- **Sadism:** Recurrent urge or behavior involving acts in which physical or psychological suffering of a victim is exciting to the patient.

Section 10
Emergency Medicine/ Toxicology

General Management of Overdose Patient

A 46-year-old woman is brought to the emergency department by her husband after a suicide attempt. She is confused, lethargic, and disoriented. Her respiratory rate is 8 per minute, and her blood pressure is 120/80 mm Hg. What is the most important step?

a. Oxygen
b. Bolus of normal saline
c. Naloxone, thiamine, dextrose
d. Endotracheal intubation
e. Gastric emptying
f. Urine toxicology screen

Answer: **C.** The most important step for an acute change in mental status of unclear etiology is to administer antidotes such as naloxone, dextrose, and thiamine. Oxygen does not make a specific difference. Gastric emptying is not as useful as a specific antidote and should only be used if it is very clear that the overdose occurred during the last hour. When you have an acute change in mental status, **hypoglycemia** is a very common cause, as is an **opiate overdose.** On a CCS case, give naloxone, thiamine, and dextrose and give oxygen and saline while checking the toxicology screen—all at the same time.

When do I answer "gastric emptying"?

This response is almost *always* wrong. Gastric emptying is *only* useful in the first hour after an overdose.

- 1 hour: 50 percent of pills can be removed
- 1–2 hours: 15 percent of pills can be removed
- 2 hours: It is useless

You can *never* perform gastric emptying when caustics (acids and alkalis) have been ingested.

Ipecac can *never* be used in a patient with altered mental status because the patient will aspirate (and you will fail). Ipecac is *always* wrong in children.

Intubation and lavage can *rarely* be performed *if* the patient has ingested the substance within the last 1–2 hours and there is *no* response to naloxone, dextrose, and thiamine.

When do I answer "naloxone, thiamine, and dextrose"?

These medications are used for an acute mental status change of unclear etiology.

When do I answer "charcoal"?

Charcoal will *not* harm anyone. In other words, give it. Charcoal can help in most overdose cases. If you have a toxicology case and do not know what to do—give charcoal.

CCS Tip: In overdose cases, do multiple things simultaneously. If there is a change in mental status from an overdose, give naloxone, thiamine, and dextrose at the same time as checking a toxicology screen, giving oxygen, and checking routine labs.

Following is the overdose case "menu":

- **Specific antidote** if the etiology is clear
- **Toxicology screen**
- **Charcoal**
- **CBC, chemistry, urinalysis**
- **Psychiatry consultation** if the overdose is the result of a suicide attempt
- **Oxygen** for carbon monoxide poisoning or any dyspneic patient

The following table lists specific antidotes for various kinds of poisoning.

Substance	Antidote
Acetaminophen	N-acetyl cysteine
Aspirin	Bicarbonate to alkalinize the urine
Benzodiazepines	Do *not* give flumazenil; it may precipitate a seizure
Carbon monoxide	100 percent oxygen, hyperbaric in some cases

(continued next page)

Substance	Antidote
Digoxin	Digoxin-binding antibodies
Ethylene glycol	Fomepizole or ethanol
Methanol	Fomepizole or ethanol
Methemoglobinemia	Methylene blue
Neuroleptic malignant syndrome	Bromocriptine, dantrolene
Opiates	Naloxone
Organophosphates	Atropine, pralidoxime
Tricyclic antidepressants	Bicarbonate protects the heart

Acetaminophen

Clinical Course

- **First 24 hours:** Nausea and vomiting, which resolve
- 48–72 hours later: Hepatic failure

Treatment

It is safe to give **charcoal and N-acetyl cysteine (NAC).** Know the following about treating an acetaminophen overdose:

- Give **N-acetyl cysteine (NAC)** to *any* patient with a possible overdose of a toxic amount.
- NAC is benign.
- NAC is useful to prevent liver toxicity for up to 24 hours after the ingestion. After 24 hours, there is *no* specific therapy to prevent or reverse the liver toxicity of acetaminophen.
- Vomiting patients can get NAC through the IV route.

If the amount of ingestion is equivocal, then **get an acetaminophen level** to determine if there will be toxicity but do *not* wait for the results to give NAC if the overdose is large.

- 10 g → toxic
- 15 g → fatal

The amounts needed for toxicity and fatality are lower if there is **underlying liver disease** or **alcohol abuse.**

Extra NAC never hurt anyone. Untreated acetaminophen overdose will kill the patient.

A man is brought to the emergency department a few hours after ingesting a bottle of extra-strength acetaminophen tablets. What is the next best step in management?

a. Urine toxicology screen
b. N-acetyl cysteine
c. Acetaminophen level
d. Transfer to the ICU
e. Liver function tests
f. Gastric emptying

Answer: **B.** The specific antidote is more important than waiting for a level with acetaminophen overdose. On a CCS case, do both. Do not transfer patients to the ICU without doing something for them first.

Aspirin/Salicylate Overdose

Aspirin acts as a direct **stimulant to the brainstem,** causing hyperventilation. A patient with an aspirin overdose will *always* be hyperventilating. In addition, aspirin is a **toxin to the lungs,** causing **acute respiratory distress syndrome (ARDS).**

The easiest way to identify the aspirin overdose patient is **tinnitus.**

Other findings in cases of aspirin overdose are the following:

- **Metabolic acidosis:** This is from the loss of Krebs cycle in mitochondria. You end up with lactic acidosis from hypoxic metabolism. The anion gap is elevated.
- **Respiratory alkalosis:** This always precedes the metabolic acidosis.
- **Renal insufficiency:** Salicylates, like other NSAIDs, are directly toxic to the kidney tubule.
- **Elevated prothrombin time:** Aspirin interferes with the production of vitamin K-dependent clotting factors.
- **CNS:** Confusion can occur from aspirin overdose. Severe cases can lead to seizures and coma.
- **Fever**

Diagnostic Testing

On CCS, you should order the following:

- **CBC**
- **Chemistry panel**
- **ABG**
- **PT/INR/PTT**
- **Salicylate (ASA) level**

Treatment

Treatment is as follows:

- **Alkalinize the urine** to increase excretion.
- Use **charcoal** to block absorption.
- **Dialysis** is used in severe cases.

CCS Tip: Alkalinize the urine with D5W with 3 amps of bicarbonate. Alkalinization of the urine facilitates excretion of the following:

- Salicylates (ASA)
- Tricyclic antidepressants (This will show up on the urine tox you ordered.)
- Phenobarbital
- Chlorpropamide

On CCS, remember to order an aspirin, acetaminophen, *and* alcohol (ETOH) level on *all* overdose patients. There is a very high frequency of co-ingestion.

Benzodiazepines

Benzodiazepine overdose (by itself) is *not* fatal. Let the patient sleep! Move the clock forward on CCS, and the overdose will pass.

Do *not* administer flumazenil for benzodiazepine overdoses to patients in the emergency department. You do not know who has chronic dependency, and flumazenil can induce benzodiazepine withdrawal and seizures.

Carbon Monoxide

The **most common cause of death in fires** is carbon monoxide (CO) poisoning; 60 percent of deaths in the first 24 hours after a fire are due to carbon monoxide poisoning.

Carboxyhemoglobin (COHg) does not release oxygen to tissues. Hence, CO poisoning is the same as anemia and asphyxiation. CO poisoning presents with the following:

- **Shortness of breath**
- **Lightheadedness and headaches**
- **Disorientation**
- Severe disease causes **metabolic acidosis** from tissue hypoxia.

CO poisoning also commonly presents in families that are "snowed in" and can't leave their house with a wood-burning stove. Everyone is **fatigued and has a headache.** Look for the phrase "He feels better when he is shoveling snow."

Treatment

If CO poisoning is suspected, **call an ambulance.** Give **100 percent oxygen** to all survivors from a fire until you have their CO levels.

Digoxin

The most common presentation of digoxin overdose is **GI disturbance** (nausea, vomiting, diarrhea, pain). This condition also presents with the following:

- Patient sees yellow "halos" around objects and has blurred vision.
- Arrhythmia: Anything is possible. You may see PR prolongation; there may also be "paroxysmal atrial tachycardia with block."
- Encephalopathy

*Hypo*kalemia may lead to digoxin toxicity, but digoxin toxicity leads to *hyper*kalemia from poisoning of the sodium/potassium ATPase.

Treatment

Administer **digoxin-binding antibodies** (Digibind) for severe disease. Severe means **central nervous system and cardiac abnormalities.**

Ethylene Glycol and Methanol

Overdoses from both of these substances present with the following:

- **Intoxication**
- **Metabolic acidosis with increased anion gap**

Ethylene glycol presents with the following:

- **Renal insufficiency** from direct toxicity
- **Hypocalcemia** from precipitation of the oxalic acid with the calcium
- **Kidney stones**

Methanol presents with the following:

- **Visual disturbance**
- **Retinal hyperemia** from the toxicity of the formic acid

Treatment

Overdoses from both substances are treated with the following:

- **Ethanol** or **fomepizole**
- **Dialysis** to remove them from the body before they are metabolized into the toxic metabolite

Methemoglobinemia

This condition involves hemoglobin locked in an oxidized state that will not allow it to pick up oxygen. The patient will present with the following:

- **Cyanosis**
- **Shortness of breath**
- **Dizziness**
- **Headache**
- **Confusion**
- **Seizures**

Look for a **history of use of nitrate, anesthetics, dapsone,** or **other oxidants,** as well as any of the drugs ending in *-caine.* (e.g., lidocaine, benzocaine, bupivacaine). Methemoglobinemia can be from as little as the anesthetic spray put into the throat of a patient who will be intubated. Nitroglycerin can also cause methemoglobinemia.

Diagnostic Testing

- **Normal pO_2 on ABG with chocolate-brownish blood** (oxidized blood)
- **Methemoglobin level**

> Cyanotic + Normal pO_2 → Should make you think of methemoglobinemia.

Treatment

- Administer 100 percent oxygen.
- Methylene blue restores the hemoglobin to its normal state.

Neuroleptic Malignant Syndrome/Malignant Hyperthermia

All heat disorders present with **rhabdomyolysis** and possibly **confusion** or **seizures** when the disorder is severe. Also, a potentially **life-threatening rhythm disturbance** can occur from the hyperkalemia.

Neuroleptic Malignant Syndrome (NMS)

Look for the ingestion of **neuroleptic medication,** such as **phenothiazines.** NMS has *no* specific diagnostic test. **CPK and potassium levels** can be elevated. **Muscle rigidity** is common.

Treat with the dopamine agonists **cabergoline** or **bromocriptine. Dantrolene** is also effective.

Malignant Hyperthermia

Look for a history of **anesthetic use.** There is *no* clinical distinction between NMS and malignant hyperthermia, just different risks of medications. Treat with **dantrolene.**

Heat Stroke

This is a heat disorder from **exertion and high outside temperatures.** You can *only* get heat stroke when the outside temperature is high and you are dehydrated or exerting yourself. Although these patients can get the same **confusion, seizures, hyperkalemia, and arrhythmias** that NMS and malignant hyperthermia get, the treatment is entirely different.

Treatment

Treat heat stroke with the **physical removal of heat** from the body by spraying the patient with water and fanning the patient in an air-conditioned room or using ice baths/packs. Do *not* infuse iced saline into the body, since this can stop the heart.

The following table compares heat stroke and heat exhaustion.

	Heat Exhaustion	Heat Stroke
Presenting Symptoms	Excessive sweating Nausea/vomiting	Dry skin Altered mental status
Body Temperature	Elevated	Elevated
Treatment	Normal saline IV (room temp) and removal of patient from hot to cool environment	Spraying patient with water and applying ice baths/packs

The following table compares heat stroke, neuroleptic malignant syndrome, and malignant hyperthermia.

	NMS	Malignant Hyperthermia	Heat Stroke
Risk	Antipsychotic medications	Anesthetics	Exertion on hot days
Presentation	High temperature Confusion Arrhythmia Hyperkalemia	Same	Same
Lab testing	CPK and potassium elevated	Same	Same
Treatment	Bromocriptine Dantrolene	Dantrolene	Hydration and external cooling (ice baths/packs, spraying with water and evaporation)

Opiate Intoxication

Opiate toxicity leads to **death from respiratory depression.** One *cannot* die from opiate withdrawal.

Treat **acute overdoses** with **naloxone.**

Organophosphates

Organophosphates **inhibit acetylcholinesterase,** blocking the metabolism of acetylcholine and, therefore, enormously increasing the effect of acetylcholine.

Look for either of these in the presentation:

- **Crop duster** exposed to insecticides
- **Nerve-gas attack**

Make *sure* not to spread the contaminant. When caring for victims of a nerve-gas attack, be certain to be protected. The toxin is absorbed through the skin.

Organophosphate overdose presents with the following symptoms:

- **Salivation**
- **Lacrimation**
- **Urination**
- **Diarrhea**
- **Wheezing from bronchospasm**

Treatment

- Best initial therapy: **Atropine**
- Most effective therapy: **Pralidoxime**
- **Remove the clothes and wash the rest off the patient.**

Tricyclic Antidepressants

Death over overdose on tricyclic antidepressants occurs from the following:

- **Seizures**
- **Arrhythmia**

A patient with a history of depression comes in with an overdose resulting from a suicide attempt. There was a bottle of amitriptyline nearby. What is the most urgent step?

a. Charcoal
b. Gastric lavage
c. Transfer to ICU
d. EKG
e. EEG
f. Head CT
g. Administer bicarbonate

Answer: **D.** In tricyclic overdose, the most urgent step is to perform an EKG to see if there is **widening of the QRS.** Those with a wide QRS are most likely to develop **ventricular tachycardia** or **torsade de pointes.** If there is a wide QRS or an arrhythmia, **give bicarbonate and transfer to the ICU.** Gastric lavage is not as important as protecting the heart. Alkalinizing the patient with bicarbonate carries its own risks. Therefore, finding out for sure if the patient really needs the bicarbonate is more important.

Other effects of tricyclics are related to their anticholinergic effects:

- **Dilated pupils**
- **Dry mouth**
- **Constipation**
- **Urinary retention**

Spider Bites

Black Widow

The bite of a black widow spider presents with **abdominal pain, rigidity, and hypocalcemia.** The patient presents as though there is a perforated abdominal organ, but there is pain *without* tenderness.

Treat with **antivenin.**

Brown Recluse Spider

The bite of this spider presents with local necrosis, bullae, and dark lesions.

Treat by **debriding the wound.** Occasionally, steroids and dapsone are of benefit.

Burns

The most important step when a patient has been in a fire is to give **100 percent oxygen.** The most common cause of death in fires is carbon monoxide poisoning. After that, the most important thing is to **determine who needs to be intubated and who can be managed just with fluids.**

After giving oxygen, **intubate** the patient if any of the following is present:

- **Hoarseness**
- **Wheezing**
- **Stridor**
- **Burns inside the nose or the mouth**

If evidence of respiratory injury is *not* present, then the most important step in management is to **give fluids** as follows:

- 4 mL of lactated Ringers or normal saline *for*
  - each percentage with a second- or third-degree burn *for*
  - each kilogram.

The most common cause of death late is **infection.**

Hypothermia

Look for an **alcoholic falling asleep outside in winter.** Hypothermia kills with **rhythm disturbance.**

The most urgent step is to perform an **EKG: "J-waves of Osborn,"** which look like ST segment elevation, are the most specific finding.

Ophthalmology

Glaucoma

Acute angle closure glaucoma is an **ophthalmologic emergency** that presents with a **red eye and a fixed midpoint pupil.**

Treatment

The best initial therapy is **pilocarpine drops** to constrict the pupil. **Mannitol** can be used as an osmotic diuretic to help open the angle. Following are other therapies that are used:

- **Acetazolamide:** Decreases production of aqueous humor
- **Prostaglandin analogs:** Latanoprost, travoprost
- **Beta blockers topically:** Timolol
- **Alpha agonists:** Apraclonidine

Retinal Detachment

This presents with a sudden loss of vision like **"a curtain coming down." Consult ophthalmology** and perform a **dilated retinal examination.**

Treatment

Treat by doing the following:

1. Tilt the head back.
2. **Reattach the retina** with surgery, cryotherapy, or by injecting an expansile gas into the eye.
3. If these fail, place a band around the eye to get the retina close to the sclera.

Red Eye

Diagnosing and treating "red eye" requires knowing the basic ophthalmology expected on Step 3. The following table summarizes the various causes of red eye.

	Glaucoma	Conjunctivitis	Uveitis	Abrasion
Presentation	Midpoint fixed pupil Rock-hard, painful eye Corneal haziness	Viral: Bilateral watery discharge, itchy eyes Bacterial: Unilateral purulent discharge, eyelids stuck together	Photophobia	History of trauma, most commonly from contact lenses
Diagnosis	Tonometry	Clinical presentation	Slit lamp examination	Fluorescein stain picks up on the damaged cornea
Treatment	Pilocarpine drops Acetazolamide Mannitol Topical beta blockers	Bacterial form is treated with topical antibiotics	Steroids	*No* specific therapy Do *not* patch abrasions caused by contact lenses

Section 11
Ethics

Autonomy

Autonomy is the most frequently tested subject on Step 3. The following is the most fundamental ethical concept:

- **An adult with the capacity to understand his or her medical problems can refuse any therapy or test.**

It does not matter if the treatment or test is simple, safe, and risk-free. It does not matter if the person will die without the treatment or test. The patient can refuse the treatment or test.

Respecting autonomy is *more important* than trying to do the right thing for a patient. Trying to do the right thing for a patient is called **beneficence.**

A 35-year-old mentally intact patient is refusing radiation for a stage I lymphoma. The treatment has a 95 percent chance of cure and virtually no adverse effects. What do you do?

a. Try to discuss it with him.

b. Honor his wishes.

c. Order a psychiatric consultation.

d. Arrange an ethics committee consultation.

e. Get a court order.

Answer: **A.** Even though an adult patient with capacity can refuse anything, USMLE wants you to discuss things first. Even though you may eventually honor his wishes, if an answer says "meet," "confer," or "discuss," then do that first.

Capacity

Capacity is determined by physicians. *Competence* is a legal term and is determined by courts and judges. An adult who is alert and not mentally handicapped is deemed to have *capacity* to understand her own medical procedures and treatments.

Psychiatry Consultation

"Psychiatry consultation" is the answer when **a patient's capacity to understand is not clear.** A psychiatry consultation is *not* necessary in the following situations:

- The patient is clearly competent.
- The patient is in a coma and clearly does not have the capacity to understand.

Minors

Minors, by definition, **are not determined to have the capacity** to understand their medical problems until the age of 18.

However, Step 3 does like to test your understanding of the **emancipated minor.** Emancipation means that although the patient is under 18, he can make his own decisions. Emancipated minors are **living independently** and **self-supporting, married,** or **in the military.**

Partial emancipation is considered to be present for the following issues:

- **Sex**
- **Reproductive health**
- **Substance abuse**

If the patient is a minor and seeks treatment for contraception, sexually transmitted diseases, HIV, or prenatal care, she is partially emancipated. In other words, she can make these decisions on her own, and her privacy is to be respected like that of an adult. **An exception is abortion:** 36 states have parental notification laws for abortion.

How does USMLE get around issues that are not universal across the United States? For such questions, the answer is a safe, universally correct answer, such as "Recommend that the patient inform the parents."

Limitations on the Ability of Parents to Refuse Treatment for a Minor

Parents cannot refuse lifesaving therapy for minors. For example, if a blood transfusion would be lifesaving, the parents cannot refuse. Doing so would be considered child abuse. Jehovah's Witnesses may refuse therapy for themselves but not for a child.

Informed Consent

Informed consent is based on **autonomy.** Only a fully informed patient with the capacity to understand the issues can grant "informed consent." For the consent to be informed, the patient must be informed as follows:

- The patient is informed of the **benefits** of the procedure (how will it help).
- The patient is informed of the **risks** of the procedure.
- **Alternatives** to the procedure are given.
- The information is in a **language the patient can understand.**
- The informed consent **must be given for each procedure (specificity).**

Emergency Procedures

Consent is implied in an emergency when there is not sufficient time to determine capacity or prior wishes. If prior wishes are fully known, then this information takes precedence. Consent obtained via telephone is considered valid. If the patient's proxy is not present at the time of the procedure, consent obtained via the telephone counts.

Pregnant Women

Pregnant women can refuse therapy, even if the life of the fetus is at risk. Until the fetus comes out of the body, it is considered part of the woman's body. For example, a woman can refuse a blood transfusion while pregnant. She can also refuse antiretroviral therapy during pregnancy, even if the life of the fetus is at risk. Once the baby comes out, however, she cannot refuse treatment for the baby.

Confidentiality

The patient has an absolute right to privacy concerning his own medical information. The following persons do *not* have a right to any of the medical information of the patient:

- Relatives, employers, friends, and spouses
- Other physicians: If a physician seeks medical information about a patient, you cannot release it without the express consent of the patient.

- Members of law enforcement: You cannot release medical information to courts or police without a court order or subpoena.

Hence, *only* a patient can obtain or ask for his or her medical information to be released. A current physician cannot obtain a patient's previous medical records without her direct consent.

Breaking Confidentiality to Prevent Harm to Others

An *exception* to the privacy rule is in the circumstance of **protecting other people.**

- If a patient has a **transmissible disease,** such as tuberculosis or HIV, the physician can violate the patient's confidentiality to protect innocent third parties. If you have tuberculosis, for example, your doctor can contact your close associates without your consent if they are at risk. If you have syphilis, HIV, or gonorrhea, your doctor can safely inform others without your consent that they may be at risk.
- The classic example is of a patient with a **psychiatric illness who may be planning to harm others.** They physician has the right to break your confidentiality to alert the person at risk to prevent harm.

This issue comes down entirely to whether another person may be harmed by the patient's illness or actions. If you have a dangerous disease and your doctor does *not* inform the innocent third party at risk, then that physician is liable for harm that befalls the innocent person.

End-of-Life Issues

Autonomy as applied to end-of-life issues is the most important subject for the test and for patient autonomy.

Withholding and Withdrawing of Care

Withholding of care and withdrawing of care are considered **indistinguishable** from the point of view of the test and of proper ethical behavior. **An adult with capacity can withhold or withdraw any form of therapy.** If the patient begins therapy, he or she has the right to withdraw that care. The reasons for the withdrawal or withholding of care are *not* important.

Advance Directives

An advance directive is a set of instructions from **an adult patient with capacity directing the care of himself or herself prior to losing capacity.**

Health Care Proxy

The strongest advance directive is a **health care proxy.** The proxy is both a document describing the care the person desires as well as the **appointment of an agent** to be the decision maker. The agent as a decision maker does not take hold until the patient loses the capacity to make a decision. If I appoint a proxy but I am still here, alert, and communicative, you *cannot* ask the agent for consent for my procedures.

Living Will

A living will is a written document **outlining the care** desired by the patient. If a patient does not have a health care proxy, the living will can be very useful to outline the care she wants. If the patient writes out, "I never want to be intubated," this is valid. If she writes, "No heroic measures," this is not valid. To be useful, a living will must be **clear and precise.**

Do Not Resuscitate (DNR) Orders

The DNR order means the **refusal of endotracheal intubation and cardiopulmonary resuscitation** in the event of the loss of the ability to breathe or the heart stopping. A DNR order does *not* mean the elimination of testing or medical therapy.

Patient with No Capacity and No Advance Directive (Proxy or Living Will)

This is the most complex and the most common circumstance. In this case, the care is based on the best understanding of the patient's wishes for herself. Family and friends attempt to outline what they heard the patient say she wanted. This is *not* the same as saying "This is what is best for the patient." Decisions are based on the best possible understanding of clearly expressed wishes. If there is no clear expression of wishes, then the weakest basis on which to act is the "best interests of the patient."

Ethics Committee

The ethics committee is used for cases in which the following are true:

- **The patient is not an adult with capacity.**
- **There are no clearly stated wishes on the part of the patient.**

Also, the ethics committee is the answer if

- **the caregivers, such as the family, are split or in disagreement about the nature of the care.** If some family members say, "He never wanted to be on a ventilator, ever," and some family members say, "He might have wanted a ventilator sometime," then this is a case for an ethics committee.

Court Order

This option comes into play only when **all the other options have not given clarity.** If there is disagreement after all the other steps, including an ethics committee, which cannot reach a clear determination of care, then a court order is the answer. You do *not* need a court order if the proxy clearly states wishes or the family is in agreement.

Fluid and Nutrition Issues

An adult patient with capacity may refuse all forms of nutrition. There is *no* ethical basis for forcing fluids or nutrition upon a patient. If the patient is not an adult with the capacity to understand, the proxy or living will can direct the removal of fluid and nutrition, provided the patient's clearly expressed wishes while competent stated that no artificial nutrition be started. In the absence of clearly stated wishes on the issue of fluids and nutrition, they should be given.

Physician-Assisted Suicide and Euthanasia

- **Physician-assisted suicide** means providing the patient with the means to end her own life. **This is always wrong.**
- **Euthanasia** means the physician directly administers the means of ending the patient's life. **This is always wrong.**

These are *not* the same as providing pain medications that may end the patient's life. It is ethical to give pain medication, even if the only way to relieve pain may result in the inadvertent shortening of life. The primary difference is **intent:**

- In physician-assisted suicide, the primary intent is to end life.
- With a life shortened by pain medication, the primary intent is to relieve suffering.

Futile Care

There is *no* obligation on the part of the physician to provide care that will not work. There is no obligation to provide treatments without possible benefit.

A patient with widely metastatic cervical cancer develops renal failure. The family insists that dialysis be started. What do you tell them?

Answer: You do not have to provide dialysis to a person who will certainly die and not benefit from the treatment.

Brain Death

You are *not* obliged to provide care for a brain-dead patient. Brain death = dead.

Reproductive Issues

Abortion

A woman's right to an abortion varies by trimester of pregnancy:

- **First trimester:** A woman has an **unrestricted** right to an abortion.
- **Second trimester:** A woman has access, but her rights are **less clear.**
- **Third trimester:** There is **no clear access** to abortion in the third trimester. In the third trimester, the fetus is potentially viable.

You do not need the consent of the father for the abortion.

Donation of Gametes

Patients have an **unrestricted right** to donate sperm and eggs. There is *no* ethical problem with being a **paid donor** for sperm and eggs. Note that one cannot be a paid donor for organs, such as the kidney or corneas.

HIV Issues

A **patient has a right to confidentiality** of his HIV status. However, this confidentiality can be broken to protect the uninfected, such as sexual and needle-sharing partners.

There is **no obligation for HIV-positive health care workers to disclose their HIV status.** This includes surgeons. A surgeon does *not* have to disclose her HIV status to patient.

Physicians have the legal right to refuse to treat any patient. It is *not* illegal to refuse to take care of HIV-positive persons—it is **unethical** to refuse care to HIV-positive patients simply because they are HIV-positive, but it is **legal** to do so.

Doctor-Patient Relationship

Accepting a Patient

A physician does not have an obligation to accept a patient. The need of a person does not compel the physician to accept that person as a patient. For example, if there is only 1 neurosurgeon at a hospital and a patient needs neurosurgery, this situation does not compel the physician to accept the patient.

Once having accepted a patient, however, **the physician cannot simply abandon the patient.** The physician has an obligation to inform the patient that he must find another physician, and the physician must render care until a substitute caregiver can be identified.

Gifts

- **Ethically acceptable:** Gifts from patients that are **small** and **not tied to specific treatments and tests**
- **Ethically unacceptable:** Gifts given with the intention of getting **a specific prescription**

Sexual Contact

- **Psychiatrists:** Sexual contact between a patient and a psychiatrist is *never* acceptable.
- **Other physicians:** They must end the doctor-patient relationship first.

Elder Abuse

Elder abuse can be reported even against the will of the patient. Elder abuse does not imply a specific age; it has to do with the **fragility** of the patient. If the patient is frail and vulnerable, the abuse can be reported even against the patient's will.

Impaired Drivers

Impaired drivers, such as patients suffering from a seizure disorder, cannot have their license taken away by a physician. Only the department of motor vehicles can remove or restrict a license. These laws are not clear from state to state.

Torture

Physician participation in torture, on any level, is always wrong. You cannot even agree to certify the patient dead.

Impaired Physicians

Impaired physicians must be reported to an authority figure:

- For **physicians in training,** the reporting should be to the program director or department chair.
- For **faculty,** reporting is to the department chair or the dean of the medical school.
- For **those in practice,** reporting is to the state medical board of the office of profession medical conduct.

The impairment must involve **potential danger to medical care.** If you see a physician stealing a car, his behavior is *not* reportable to the department chair. If you see a physician at a bar dancing naked on the table top, but her medical performance is not impaired, this is *not* reportable.

Index

A

C

D

E

F

G

H

I

N

O

P

Q

R

S

W

X

Z